Hemostasis and Th

MW01268204

Hemostasis and Thrombosis

Practical Guidelines in Clinical Management

EDITED BY

Hussain I. Saba MD, PhD

Professor of Medicine
Director of Hematology/Hemophilia/Hemostasis & Thrombosis Center
USF College of Medicine;
Professor Emeritus
Department of Malignant Hematology
Moffitt Cancer Center and Research Institute
Tampa, FL, USA

Harold R. Roberts MD

Emeritus Professor of Medicine and Pathology
Division of Hematology/Oncology
University of North Carolina
Chapel Hill, NC, USA

WILEY Blackwell

Library of Congress Cataloging-in-Publication Data

Hemostasis and thrombosis (Saba)
 Hemostasis and thrombosis : practical guidelines in clinical management / edited by Hussain I. Saba, Harold R. Roberts.
   p. ; cm.
 Includes bibliographical references and index.
 ISBN 978-0-470-67050-7 (pbk.)
 I. Saba, Hussain I., editor of compilation. II. Roberts, H. R. (Harold Ross), editor of compilation. III. Title.
 [DNLM: 1. Blood Coagulation Disorders–therapy. 2. Hemostatic Disorders–therapy. 3. Thrombosis–therapy. WH 322]
 RC647.C55
 616.1'57–dc23

                        2013042714

A catalogue record for this book is available from the British Library.

Contents

Color plate section can be found facing page 212

Contributors

Louis Aledort MD, MACP
The Mary Weinfeld Professor of Clinical
Research in Hemophilia
Division of Hematology and Medical Oncology
The Tisch Cancer Institute
Mount Sinai School of Medicine
New York, NY, USA

Noman Ashraf MD
Assistant Professor
Department of Hematology/Oncology
University of South Florida/James A. Haley VA
Hospital
Tampa, FL, USA

Lodovico Balducci MD
Professor of Oncologic Sciences
H. Lee Moffit Cancer Center & Research
Institute
Tampa, FL, USA

Charles E. Bane Jr. DVM
Department of Pathology, Microbiology, and
Immunology
Vanderbilt University
Nashville, TN, USA

Margareta Blombäck MD, PhD
Professor Emeritus
Department of Molecular Medicine and
Surgery
Division of Clinical Chemistry and Blood
Coagulation
Karolinska Institutet
Stockholm, Sweden

Giancarlo Castaman MD
Consultant Hematologist
Department of Cell Therapy and Hematology
Hemophilia and Thrombosis Center
San Bortolo Hospital
Vicenza, Italy

Meera Chitlur MD
Associate Professor of Pediatrics and Director of
Hemophilia/Hemostasis Clinic
Wayne State University
Children's Hospital of Michigan
Detroit, MI, USA

Samir Dalia MD
Fellow in Hematology and Oncology
H. Lee Moffitt Cancer & Research Center
University of South Florida
Tampa, FL, USA

Stephanie J. Davis, MD
Resident
Department of Internal Medicine
University of North Carolina Hospitals
Chapel Hill, NC, USA

Benjamin Djulbegovic MD, PhD
Distinguished Professor
University of South Florida & H. Lee Moffit
Cancer Center & Research Institute
Tampa, FL, USA

Nils Egberg MD, PhD
Associate Professor
Department of Molecular Medicine and
Surgery
Division of Clinical Chemistry and Blood
Coagulation
Karolinska Institutet
Stockholm, Sweden

Jawed Fareed PhD
Professor of Pathology & Pharmacology
Hemostasis & Thrombosis Research
Laboratories
Loyola University Chicago
Maywood, IL, USA

Massimo Franchini, MD
Director
Department of Transfusion Medicine and
Hematology
C. Poma Hospital
Mantova, Italy

David Gailani MD
Professor of Pathology, Microbiology and
Immunology
Division of Hematology/Oncology
Vanderbilt University
Nashville, TN, USA

Jean-Philippe Galanaud MD
Assistant Professor of Vascular Medicine
Clinical Investigation Centre and Department
of Internal Medicine
Montpellier University Hospital
Montpellier, France

David Green MD, PhD
Professor Emeritus of Medicine
Feinberg School of Medicine
Northwestern University
Chicago, IL, USA

Maureane Hoffman MD, PhD
Professor of Pathology
Duke University Medical Center
Durham, NC, USA

Debra Hoppensteadt PhD
Professor of Pathology and Pharmacology
Loyola University Medical Center
Maywood, IL, USA

Walter P. Jeske PhD
Professor of Thoracic and Cadiovascular
Surgery
Loyola University Medical Center
Maywood, IL, USA

Susan R. Kahn MD, MSc, FRCPC
Professor of Medicine
Division of Internal Medicine
Lady Davis Institute, Jewish General Hospital
Department of Medicine
McGill University
Montreal, QC, Canada

Raj S. Kasthuri MD
Associate Professor
Department of Medicine
Division of Hematology/Oncology
University of North Carolina at Chapel Hill
Chapel Hill, NC, USA

Craig M. Kessler MD, MACP
Professor of Medicine and Pathology
Director, Division of Coagulation
Division of Hematology and Oncology
Lombardi Comprehensive Cancer Center
Georgetown University Medical Center
Washington, DC, USA

Asma Latif MD
Clinical Fellow
Division of Hematology and Medical Oncology
The Tisch Cancer Institute
Mount Sinai School of Medicine
New York, NY, USA

Agnes Y. Y. Lee MD, MSc, FRCPC
Medical Director, Thrombosis Program
Associate Professor of Medicine
Division of Hematology
University of British Columbia
British Columbia Cancer Agency
Vancouver, BC, Canada

Ton Lisman PhD
Associate Professor
Section of Hepatobiliary Surgery and
Liver Transplantation
Department of Surgery
University Medical Center Groningen
University of Groningen
Groningen, The Netherlands

Rustem I. Litvinov MD, PhD, DrSci
Senior Research Investigator
Department of Cell and Developmental Biology
University of Pennsylvania
Perelman School of Medicine
Philadelphia, PA, USA

Jeanne M. Lusher MD
Distinguished Professor of Pediatrics and
Marion I Barnhart Chair in Hemostasis
Research
Wayne State University
Children's Hospital of Michigan
Detroit, MI, USA

Pier Mannuccio Mannucci MD
Scientific Director
IRCCS Cà Granda Foundation
Maggiore Policlinico Hospital
Milan, Italy

Paul E. Monahan MD
Associate Professor
Department of Pediatrics
Division of Hematology/Oncology
University of North Carolina at Chapel Hill
Chapel Hill, NC, USA

Dougald M. Monroe, PhD
Professor
University of North Carolina at Chapel Hill
School of Medicine
Division of Hematology/Oncology
Chapel Hill, NC, USA

James H. Morrissey PhD
Professor
Department of Biochemistry
University of Illinois at Urbana-Champaign
Urbana, IL, USA

Anne T. Neff MD
Associate Professor
Department of Medicine Division of
Hematology/Oncology
Vanderbilt University
Nashville, TN, USA

Erica A. Peterson MD, MSc
Fellow, Thrombosis Program
Division of Hematology
University of British Columbia and
Vancouver Coastal Health
Vancouver, BC, Canada

Robert J. Porte MD, PhD
Professor of Surgery
Section of Hepatobiliairy Surgery and Liver
Transplantation
Department of Surgery
University Medical Center Groningen
University of Groningen
Groningen, The Netherlands

Francesco Rodeghiero MD
Director
Department of Cell Therapy and Hematology
San Bortolo Hospital
Vicenza, Italy

Sabiha R. Saba MD
Associate Professor
Department of Pathology and Cell Biology
USF College of Medicine
Tampa, FL, USA

Alvin H. Schmaier MD
Robert W Kellemeyer Professor of
Hematology/Oncology
Division of Hematology and Oncology
Department of Medicine
Case Western Reserve University
Cleveland, OH, USA

Anjali A. Sharathkumar MD, MS
Assistant Professor
Director, Hemophilia and Thrombophilia
Program
Northwestern University Feinberg School of
Medicine
Chicago, IL, USA

Evi X. Stavrou MD
Assistant Professor
Division of Hematology and Oncology
Department of Medicine
Case Western Reserve University
Cleveland, OH, USA

Alberto Tosetto MD
Consultant Hematologist
Department of Cell Therapy and Hematology
Hemophilia and Thrombosis Center
San Bortolo Hospital
Vicenza, Italy

John W. Weisel PhD
Professor
Department of Cell & Developmental Biology
University of Pennsylvania Perelman
School of Medicine
Philadelphia, PA, USA

Preface

Since the discovery and early concept of hemostasis and thrombosis, there has been a progressive and remarkable change in the ongoing availability of knowledge in this area. The available knowledge has become extensive and dynamic. The information has led to the understanding of the formation of the steps involved in blood clotting reactions. Advances and understanding in the management of bleeding diseases has led to safe management of diseases such as hemophilia, von Willebrand Disease (VWD) and other hemophoid disorders; appropriate management of inhibitors has been achieved. Alterations in hemostasis and thrombosis have been investigated in the pathogenesis of liver disease as well as cancer. The important influence of platelet polyphosphates on hemostasis and thrombosis has also been explored. Significant advances have been made in the proper use of anticoagulation agents. Critical knowledge also led to advances in the area of disseminated intravascular coagulation (DIC) as well. This book presented here, *Hemostasis and Thrombosis: Practical Guidelines in Clinical Management*, represents the current understanding of important European and American academics on the subject.

Hussain I. Saba
Tampa, Florida, USA

Acknowledgments

First of all, I thank Almighty God who gave me the strength and wisdom to complete this book.

I wish to acknowledge my gratitude and sincere appreciation to Dr. Harold R. Roberts at UNC Chapel Hill, NC, my friend, advisor, and colleague, for his support in the completion of this book. Our long-term academic association has offered me the opportunity to learn not only some of the principles of scientific research but also, simultaneously, the value of critical thinking. I am also in debt to him for many conversations pertaining not only to science but also to the broad aspect of human life and the human condition. From these discussions it has become apparent, to me at least, that science cannot encompass the real world and part of reality lies also in the realm of metaphysics. The realization has, perhaps, influenced both of us more than we know. I would like to acknowledge Sabiha R. Saba, Hasan I. Zeya and John C. Herrion for their support of my pursuit of knowledge in the area of hematology and hematological research.

My sincere thanks to Genevieve Morelli for her kind support on this project. Her organizational skills and efforts in contacting, proofing, and coordinating the work of the authors, editors, and publisher of this work have been remarkable and appreciated.

I would also like to thank Rukhsana Azam and Monique Johnson for the help and support I received in the development and publication of this book.

Hussain I. Saba
Tampa, Florida, USA

CHAPTER 1

Theories of Blood Coagulation: Basic Concepts and Recent Updates

Dougald M. Monroe[1] and Maureane Hoffman[2]
[1] University of North Carolina at Chapel Hill, School of Medicine, Division of Hematology/Oncology, Chapel Hill, NC, USA
[2] Duke University, Department of Pathology, Durham VA Medical Center, Durham, NC, USA

Historical background

Any mechanistic description of blood coagulation should account for a number of simple observations about the blood coagulation process. Blood that is circulating inside the body tends not to clot. However, blood that escapes from the vasculature does clot. This suggests that there is a material outside blood that is necessary for the clotting process. This point was emphasized by the study of Foà and Pellacani who showed that "tissue juice" (filtered saline extract of brain), when injected into the circulation of a rabbit, could cause intravascular thrombus formation [1]. This result was further clarified by Macfarlane and Biggs who showed that blood had all the factors needed to clot (intrinsic factors) but that this process was slow and that clotting was accelerated by the addition of tissue extracts (extrinsic factors) [2].

A clotted mass of blood was called a thrombus. When this thrombus was washed, a material, thrombin, could be eluted that would immediately clot fresh blood. It was further shown that there existed in blood an inactive agent, prothrombin, which could be converted to active thrombin. The agent responsible for this conversion was called thromboplastin (or thrombokinase). Attempts to discover the nature of thromboplastin led to much of our current mechanistic understanding of coagulation.

In 1875, Zahn made the important observation that bleeding from a blood vessel was blocked by a white (not red) thrombus [3]. Bizzozero and Hayem, working separately, studied a colorless corpuscle in blood called a thrombocyte or platelet [4,5]. This cell could be shown to be

Hemostasis and Thrombosis: Practical Guidelines in Clinical Management, First Edition.
Hussain I. Saba and Harold R. Roberts.
© 2014 John Wiley & Sons, Ltd. Published 2014 by John Wiley & Sons, Ltd.

associated with fibrin and was postulated to be a major component of the
white thrombus [4]. It was therefore suggested that there was a platelet
thromboplastin that was critical for clotting (in modern usage, platelet
procoagulant function is described as such and the term thromboplastin
is used to mean the protein tissue factor [TF] which is the coagulation
initiator in tissues).

It is known that in some families there is an inherited bleeding tendency
(hemophilia). Eagle studied individuals with this disorder and showed that
the platelet function in those patients was normal but that there was still
a deficiency in prothrombin conversion [6]. This established that there
was a plasma component required for clotting in addition to a requirement
for platelets. Further studies in patients with different bleeding tendencies
established that there are a number of elements that make up the plasma
clotting component. Because these factors were discovered by multiple
investigators in different parts of the world (and given a different name
by each group), a systematic nomenclature was established using Roman
numerals [7] (Table 1.1).

While studies on deficient plasmas had established what the important
components were, the mechanisms of action and the interactions between
these components were not immediately clear. Early coagulation schemes
started from the model of prothrombin being converted to thrombin and
visualized all of the circulating coagulation proteins as zymogens that were
converted during coagulation into active enzymes [8,9]. Once the proteins
involved in coagulation were isolated and their structure and functions
were studied, it became clear that coagulation function was organized

Table 1.1 Systematic nomenclature of clotting factors.

Factor*	Comments
I	Fibrinogen
II	Prothrombin
III	Lipid, platelet surface, or Thromboplastin (not used)
IV	Calcium (not used)
V	
VI	Activated factor V (not used)
VII	
VIII	Hemophilia A factor
IX	Hemophilia B factor
X	
XI	Hemophilia C factor
XII	

*Activated forms of the factor are indicated by appending the
letter "a" to the name.

Table 1.2 Composition and physiologic location of coagulation complexes.

Cofactor	Enzyme	Substrate	Cell surface
Tissue factor	Factor VIIa	Factor X / Factor IX	Many cells (but generally not circulating cells)
Factor VIIIa	Factor IXa	Factor X	Platelets
Factor Va	Factor Xa	Prothrombin	Platelets release factor Va on activation; many other cells
Thrombomodulin	Thrombin	Protein C	Endothelial cells
Protein S	Activated protein C	Factor Va / Factor VIIIa	Endothelial cells

around a mechanism of an active enzyme being paired with a cofactor [10]. In the absence of the cofactor, the enzyme has limited activity; typically a cofactor will accelerate the activity of a coagulation enzyme as much as 1000-fold [11]. Thus, each step in coagulation is regulated at two levels: 1) activation of the zymogen to an active enzyme and 2) the presence of (and sometimes activation of) the requisite cofactor. Since some cofactors, such as thromboplastin (tissue factor) and thrombomodulin, are integral membrane proteins, the functions of these complexes can be limited to cells and tissues that express the protein (Table 1.2).

The coagulation factors show only weak activity in solution, and binding to an appropriate cell surface accelerates their activity up to 1000-fold. This surface binding is dependent on calcium and, therefore, blood can be anticoagulated by the addition of chelating agents such as citrate or EDTA that bind calcium [12]. This chelation does not alter protein properties and can be readily reversed by reintroduction of calcium in excess of the chelating agents. Clinical assays use plasma prepared from blood chelated with citrate to analyze clotting factor function by addition of an appropriate activator and calcium and measuring the time to clot formation.

Localization of the coagulation reactions to a desired surface represents a powerful mechanism for limiting coagulation to surfaces at the site of injury. One component of coagulation factor binding to cells is the phospholipid composition of the outer leaflet of the cell membrane. Phospholipids with acidic head groups, phosphatidic acid (PA) and phosphatidylserine (PS), promote binding of coagulation factors [13]. In addition, phosphatidylserine acts as an allosteric regulator of function and accounts for the ability of PS-containing membranes to enhance coagulation factor activity [14]. While generic phospholipid surfaces can support coagulation reactions (and are used in clinical assays), it is clear that cells, in addition to having appropriate lipid surfaces, have regulatory elements that control the coagulation reactions [15,16].

Functional platelets are required as a surface for hemostasis, and patients with low platelet counts (thrombocytopenia) or platelet function defects (thrombocytopathia) such as Bernard–Soulier syndrome or Glanzmann's thrombasthenia have a bleeding tendency. Circulating platelets, like essentially all cells in blood as well as endothelial cells, have outer membranes with low levels of acidic phospholipids. When platelets adhere at a site of injury the composition of their membrane changes such that acidic phospholipids, including phosphatidylserine, are now expressed on the outer surface of the membranes [17]. This change in surface lipid composition, along with changes in platelet surface proteins and release of procoagulant factors from platelet granules, provides a surface that supports robust coagulation.

Cell-based model of coagulation

In a mild injury, the coagulation process starts with hemostatic platelet aggregates which can be found at the ends of transected blood vessels [18]. Early in the process, these aggregates consist of activated (degranulated) platelets packed together. In time, small amounts of fibrin are deposited between the platelets. At longer times more fibrin becomes associated with the platelet masses. This fibrin extends into the tissues and provides stability to the area of injury [18,19].

In hemophilia A or B, the process is somewhat different [20]. Early in the process, the platelets are loosely associated but are not activated. Even at longer times platelets are only poorly activated and fibrin is not seen between the platelets. The result is that the platelet mass is not stabilized. Whereas normal individuals show extensive fibrin extending into the tissues, in hemophilia a thin layer of fibrin can be seen only at the margins of the wound area and does not extend significantly into the tissues [19,20].

These observations of hemostasis suggest that coagulation can be conceived of as a series of overlapping steps: initiation; amplification; and propagation.

Initiation

Blood coagulation is initiated by an injury to a blood vessel; this injury could be a denudement of some of the endothelium or a break in the vessel. In either case, two processes begin immediately. One process is that platelets quickly adhere to the site of injury. This adherence requires von Willebrand factor which binds to both collagen in the exposed subendothelium and the abundant platelet protein glycoprotein Ib. This adherence brings platelets into contact with collagen which, through the platelet collagen receptor glycoprotein VI, activates platelets [21]. This activation causes changes in platelet surface receptors and leads the platelets to degranulate. Degranulation releases a number of stored proteins including a partially activated form of factor V [22].

The second process that begins with a break in the vasculature is that plasma concentrations of coagulation proteins are brought into the area of injury and presented to extravascular cells. Cells surrounding the vasculature tend to be rich in the protein called tissue factor (thromboplastin); the high concentration of tissue factor around blood vessels has been described as contributing to a hemostatic envelope [23]. At least some of the tissue factor already has factor VII bound [24] and factor VII binds tightly to any free tissue factor. On cells this tissue factor-bound factor VII is rapidly converted to factor VIIa. This conversion can be via cellular proteases, by autoactivation by other factor VIIa molecules, or by factor Xa generated by factor VIIa–tissue factor complexes [25,26].

These factor VIIa–tissue factor complexes catalyze two reactions: activation of factor X and activation of factor IX [27]. The factor Xa that is formed can complex with the partially active factor V released from platelets; this factor Xa–Va complex converts at least some prothrombin to thrombin. Formation of factor Xa also starts the process of regulating coagulation. The inhibitor TFPI (tissue factor pathway inhibitor) can bind to factor Xa and factor VIIa to turn off the factor VIIa–tissue factor complex [28,29]. This inhibition requires factor Xa so that the factor VIIa–tissue factor complex is not turned off until some factor Xa has been formed. Factor Xa in a complex with factor Va is protected from the abundant plasma inhibitor antithrombin, but once released from the complex, factor Xa inhibition by antithrombin is rapid with an expected half-life of about 4 minutes.

Amplification

The initial thrombin formed during the initiation phase is probably not sufficient to provide for robust fibrin formation and hemostasis. However, the thrombin formed on the initiating cell can transfer to platelets where the initial hemostatic signal is amplified by activating platelets and cofactors. On the platelet surface, thrombin is relatively protected from inhibition by antithrombin (in plasma, thrombin has a half-life of just over 1 minute). Thrombin can bind to at least two receptors on the platelet surface: glycoprotein Ib and protease-activated receptor (PAR)-1 [30,31]. Thrombin binding to and cleavage of PAR-1 transmits signals that lead to platelet activation (outside-in signals) [32]. This activation results in changes in the surface lipid content with increased exposure on the outer leaflet of acid phospholipids [17]. Activation also leads to inside-out signals that alter the conformation and function of some surface proteins including the fibrin binding protein complex of glycoproteins IIb and IIIa [33].

Activation also results in release of internal stores of a number of components from alpha granules and dense granules. The released components include partially active factor V, fibrinogen, ADP which acts as signal for further platelet activation, and polyphosphates [34,35].

Thrombin bound to glycoprotein Ib can cleave PAR-1 and PAR-4 [36]. This thrombin can also cleave factor VIII, releasing factor VIIIa onto the platelet surface. Factor VIII circulates in a complex with von Willebrand factor [37]; since both thrombin and von Willebrand factor are bound to glycoprotein Ib, it suggests that factor VIII may be presented to thrombin in such a way as to allow for rapid activation. Thrombin on the platelet surface can also fully activate platelet surface factor V, a reaction that is enhanced by platelet-released polyphosphates [35]. Either the partially active factor V released from platelets or plasma-derived factor V can be activated by thrombin. Thrombin activation of platelets is augmented in platelets bound directly to collagen (as opposed to platelets aggregated onto other platelets or onto fibrin) [38]. These platelets, sometimes called COAT platelets, have higher levels of acidic phospholipids as well as significantly increased binding of factors X, IX, VIII, and V [17,39].

The amplification process leads to platelets which are primed to varying degrees for thrombin generation. These platelets have an appropriate lipid surface with activated receptors and activated cofactors bound to the surface.

Propagation

Factor IXa formed during the Initiation phase binds to the platelet surface. Factor IXa is available even in the presence of plasma levels of anti-thrombin since the half-life of activated factor IXa is about an hour in plasma. Factor IXa can bind either to platelet surface factor VIIIa [40] formed in the amplification phase or to a platelet receptor and be transferred to factor VIIIa [41]. The factor IXa/VIIIa complex activates factor X on the platelet surface. Factor Xa can then move quickly into a complex with factor Va. The resulting factor Xa/Va complex provides the rapid burst of thrombin critical to giving good fibrin structure and providing for a stable clot.

Formation of factor Xa on the platelet surface plays a critical role in regulating the clotting process [42]. The rate of factor X activation determines the rate and amount of thrombin generation. Deficiencies in platelet surface factor Xa generation caused by a lack of or reduction in factor VIII or IX levels (hemophilia A or B, respectively) result in reduced or absent factor Xa and thrombin generation. Therapies to treat hemophilia involve restoring a robust rate of platelet surface factor Xa generation [43]. Factor Xa generation appears to be regulated in part by release of TFPI from platelets, and agents that block TFPI are under consideration as possible therapeutic agents in hemophilia [44].

Thrombin generation on platelets initiates a positive feedback loop through factor XI. Factor XI can be activated on platelets by thrombin [45,46]. This thrombin activation is enhanced by polyphosphates released from platelets [35]. The platelet surface factor XIa can activate factor IX, leading to enhanced factor Xa and thrombin generation. The amount of enhancement from factor XI shows wide variations on platelets from different individuals and may account for some of the variable bleeding associated with factor XI deficiency (hemophilia C) [45].

In some cases, particularly in cases of intravascular injury where there is substantial blood flow across the injured surface, there may be a contribution to the propagation phase from circulating tissue factor [47]. While healthy individuals have little or no circulating tissue factor [48], in some pathologic conditions, such as pancreatic cancer, there are measurable levels of circulating tissue factor in the form of microparticles [49]. If the microparticles also have surface molecules that can associate with platelets or other cells at the site of injury, then tissue factor on these microparticles may contribute to factor X activation and thrombin generation at a site of injury [50].

Very small amounts of thrombin (less than 1 nM or 0.1 U/mL) are required to promote fibrin formation, and much of the thrombin generation occurs after a clot has formed [51]. The thrombin formed binds to fibrin where it can remain active for many hours; the binding of thrombin to fibrin resulted in fibrin being described as antithrombin I [52]. Furthermore, platelet factor Xa/Va complexes appear to be active long after clot formation (hours) and can rapidly generate thrombin when presented with fresh plasma as a substrate [51]. It is likely that the persistence of fibrin-bound thrombin and the prolonged ability to generate thrombin are protective mechanisms to stabilize clots. Disruption of a clot would mean that thrombin is immediately available to cleave fibrinogen and refresh the fibrin clot. Also, new prothrombin present in plasma could be activated to further replenish thrombin stores and provide for clot stability.

Control and localization

Multiple mechanisms exist to prevent a clot from spreading into healthy vasculature. Flow is an important control mechanism and reduced flow is associated with venous thrombosis. Flow removes procoagulant proteins from the area of active thrombin generation, reducing their concentrations below the threshold required to maintain coagulation. Once thrombin, factor Xa, and other procoagulant proteases are removed from the relatively protected area of the clot, they are subject to inhibition by antithrombin, TFPI, and other plasma inhibitors. This inhibition is enhanced by the carbohydrate components of proteoglycans found on endothelial cells [53]. Also, endothelial cells have surface-associated TFPI that promotes rapid inactivation of factor Xa [54].

Platelet activation also represents a control mechanism. Thrombin cleavage of PARs is important for platelet activation, but the final activated state is dependent on signaling through other platelet receptors [55]. Platelets bound to collagen (and that thus signal through glycoprotein IV) have very high levels of procoagulant factors and are associated with enhanced thrombin generation and fibrin formation. Other platelets appear to have less procoagulant activity and have a more structural role in stabilizing the fibrin clot [56]. It appears that growth of a clot may in part be constrained by structural platelets that do not strongly support thrombin generation and, therefore, do not strongly support the positive feedback loop that generates the burst of thrombin.

Platelets support a thrombin-driven positive feedback loop that activates additional platelets, promotes thrombin generation, and leads to fibrin formation. In contrast, thrombin on healthy endothelial cells leads to a negative feedback loop that shuts off further thrombin generation. Endothelial cells express the thrombin-binding protein, thrombomodulin [57]. Thrombin bound to thrombomodulin can no longer cleave fibrinogen; however, thrombin bound to thrombomodulin gains the ability to activate protein C [58]. Activation of protein C is enhanced by another endothelial cell protein called EPCR (endothelial cell protein C receptor) [59].

Activated protein C cleaves and inactivates both factor VIIIa and factor Va in a reaction that is enhanced somewhat by protein S [60]. This inactivation is more efficient on the endothelial cell surface than on platelets and suggests that the protein C pathway localizes thrombin generation rather than strictly shutting it down [61]. One of the sites on factor V that is cleaved by activated protein C is altered by the common factor V Leiden mutation [62]; this mutation is associated with venous thrombosis, suggesting that the negative feedback loop on healthy endothelium is a critical component of maintaining vascular patency.

Clinical assays

Coagulation function is generally measured in clinical assays that incorporate the elements of either the Initiation phase (prothrombin time or PT) or the propagation phase (activated partial thromboplastin time or aPTT). These assays are done on platelet-poor plasma so that the platelet contributions to clotting are not studied. The normal controls of these assays tend to be very reproducible, and the cell-free plasma can be frozen and stored. Other assays integrate the initiation and propagation phases and may include platelet function, such as thrombin generation (thrombogram or calibrated automated thrombography (CAT) [63] or whole blood clotting (thromboelastogram) [64].

The PT assay is done by adding very high levels of thromboplastin (TF) to plasma. Factor VII binds to this TF and is activated. The factor VIIa/TF complex activates factor X and the factor Xa/Va complex generates thrombin which clots the plasma. The endpoint of the assay is the time required for clot formation. Because thromboplastin is generally external to the blood, the assay is sometimes referred to as assaying the extrinsic pathway.

The aPTT assay is done by adding, in the absence of calcium, a negatively charged activator to plasma. The negative charge assembles a complex of high-molecular-weight kininogen and factor XII that converts all of the factor XI in the sample to factor XIa [65]. When recalcified, the factor XIa activates factor IXa which forms a complex with factor VIIIa. This factor IXa/VIIIa complex activates factor Xa which, in complex with factor Va, cleaves prothrombin to thrombin and clots the plasma. The endpoint of the assay is the time required for clot formation. Since all of the protein components are found in plasma, this assay is sometimes referred to as assaying the intrinsic pathway.

Since thrombin generation in the aPTT requires factors IX and VIII, it is used to monitor factor levels during therapy in hemophilia. The assay is very sensitive to the levels of the contact factors, factors XI and XII. However, patients with factor XI deficiency have a variable bleeding diathesis that is not strictly correlated with plasma levels [66]. This may be a function of how factor XI interacts with platelets and would not be assayed by the aPTT. Factor XII deficiency is not associated with any bleeding, nor is the deficiency protective of thrombosis in humans [67]. Bacterial polyphosphates are able to promote factor XII activation and may play a role in coagulation associated with the innate immune response; platelet polyphosphates are shorter than bacterial polyphosphates and do not promote activation of factor XII [35].

Summary

This overview provides a conceptual model of hemostasis as being initiated by injury leading to exposure of collagen and thromboplastin. Platelets adhere and are activated. Coagulation factors are activated, assemble on the platelet surface, and give robust thrombin generation leading to stable clot formation and clot retraction. Subsequent chapters will detail mechanisms of the processes involved in promoting hemostasis. Many of the same players (thromboplastin, platelets, coagulation factors), albeit with slightly different roles, are also involved in pathological coagulation leading to thrombosis or bleeding. Dysregulation resulting in thrombosis and other coagulation abnormalities will also be discussed in subsequent chapters.

References

1. Foà P, Pellacani P. Sul fermento übrinogeno e sullc azioni tossiclie esercitate da aleuni organi freschi. *Arch per le sc med* 1883;VII:113–65.
2. Macfarlane RG, Biggs R. A thrombin generation test; the application in haemophilia and thrombocytopenia. *J Clin Pathol* 1953;6:3–8.
3. Zahn F. Untersuchungen über Thrombose: Bildung der Thromben. *Virchows Arch Pathol Anat Physiol Klin Med* 1875;62:81–124.
4. Bizzozero J. Ueber einen neuen formbestandtheil des blutes und dessen rolle bei der thrombose und der blutgerinnung. *Virchows Arch Pathol Anat Physiol Klin Med* 1882;90:261–332.
5. Hayem G. Sur le mécanisme de l'arrêt des hémorrhagies. *C R Acad Sci* 1882;95:18–21.
6. Eagle H. Studies on blood coagulation, IV: the nature of the clotting deficiency in hemophilia. *J Gen Physiol* 1935;18:813–19.
7. Jackson CM. Recommended nomenclature for blood clotting-zymogens and zymogen activation products of the international committee on thrombosis and hemostasis. *Thromb Haemost* 1977;38:567–77.
8. Davie E, Ratnoff O. Waterfall sequence for intrinsic blood clotting. *Science* 1964;145:1310–12.
9. Macfarlane R. An enzyme cascade in the blood coagulation mechanism, and its function as a biochemical amplifier. *Nature* 1964;202:498–9.
10. Jobin F, Esnouf MP. Studies on the formation of the prothrombin-converting complex. *Biochem J* 1967;102:666–74.
11. Rosing J, Tans G, Govers-Riemslag JW, et al. The role of phospholipids and factor Va in the prothrombinase complex. *J Biol Chem* 1980;255:274–83.
12. Pekelharing C. *Untersuchen über des Fibrinferment.* Amsterdam: J. Müller, 1892.
13. Bull RK, Jevons S, Barton PG. Complexes of prothrombin with calcium ions and phospholipids. *J Biol Chem* 1972;247:2747–54.
14. Majumder R, Weinreb G, Lentz BR. Efficient thrombin generation requires molecular phosphatidylserine, not a membrane surface. *Biochemistry* 2005;44:16998–7006.
15. Wood JP, Silveira JR, Maille NM, et al. Prothrombin activation on the activated platelet surface optimizes expression of procoagulant activity. *Blood* 2011;117:1710–18.
16. Haynes LM, Bouchard BA, Tracy PB, Mann KG. Prothrombin activation by platelet-associated prothrombinase proceeds through the prethrombin-2 pathway via a concerted mechanism. *J Biol Chem* 2012;287:38647–55.
17. Bevers EM, Comfurius P, Zwaal RF. The nature of the binding for prothrombinase at the platelet surface as revealed by lipolytic enzymes. *Eur J Biochem* 1982;122:81–5.
18. Wester J, Sixma JJ, Geuze JJ, Heijnen HF. Morphology of the hemostatic plug in human skin wounds: transformation of the plug. *Lab Invest* 1979;41:182–92.

19. Monroe DM, Hoffman M. The clotting system: a major player in wound healing. *Haemophilia* 2012;18 Suppl 5:11–16.

20. Sixma JJ, Van den Berg A. The haemostatic plug in haemophilia A: a morphological study of haemostatic plug formation in bleeding time skin wounds of patients with severe haemophilia A. *Br J Haematol* 1984;58:741–53.

21. Moroi M, Jung SM, Okuma M, Shinmyozu K. A patient with platelets deficient in glycoprotein VI that lack both collagen-induced aggregation and adhesion. *J Clin Invest* 1989;84:1440–5.

22. Monković DD, Tracy PB. Functional characterization of human platelet-released factor V and its activation by factor Xa and thrombin. *J Biol Chem* 1990;265: 17132–40.

23. Drake TA, Morrissey JH, Edgington TS. Selective cellular expression of tissue factor in human tissues: implications for disorders of hemostasis and thrombosis. *Am J Pathol* 1989;134:1087–97.

24. Hoffman M, Colina CM, McDonald AG, et al. Tissue factor around dermal vessels has bound factor VII in the absence of injury. *J Thromb Haemost* 2007;5:1403–8.

25. Bajaj SP, Rapaport SI, Brown SF. Isolation and characterization of human factor VII: activation of factor VII by factor Xa. *J Biol Chem* 1981;256:253–9.

26. Nakagaki T, Foster DC, Berkner KL, Kisiel W. Initiation of the extrinsic pathway of blood coagulation: evidence for the tissue factor dependent autoactivation of human coagulation factor VII. *Biochemistry* 1991;30:10819–24.

27. Østerud B, Rapaport SI. Activation of 125I-factor IX and 125I-factor X: effect of tissue factor and factor VII, factor Xa and thrombin. *Scand J Haematol* 1980; 24:213–26.

28. Broze GJ Jr, Warren LA, Novotny WF, et al. The lipoprotein-associated coagulation inhibitor that inhibits the factor VII-tissue factor complex also inhibits factor Xa: insight into its possible mechanism of action. *Blood* 1988;71:335–43.

29. Rao LV, Rapaport SI. Studies of a mechanism inhibiting the initiation of the extrinsic pathway of coagulation. *Blood* 1987;69:645–51.

30. Jamieson GA, Okumura T, Hasitz M. Structure and function of platelet glycocalicin. *Thromb Haemost* 1980;42:1673–8.

31. Vu TK, Hung DT, Wheaton VI, Coughlin SR. Molecular cloning of a functional thrombin receptor reveals a novel proteolytic mechanism of receptor activation. *Cell* 1991;64:1057–68.

32. Kahn ML, Nakanishi-Matsui M, Shapiro MJ, et al. Protease-activated receptors 1 and 4 mediate activation of human platelets by thrombin. *J Clin Invest* 1999; 103:879–87.

33. Coller BS, Peerschke EI, Scudder LE, Sullivan CA. A murine monoclonal antibody that completely blocks the binding of fibrinogen to platelets produces a thrombasthenic-like state in normal platelets and binds to glycoproteins IIb and/or IIIa. *J Clin Invest* 1983;72:325–38.

34. Maynard DM, Heijnen HFG, Horne MK, et al. Proteomic analysis of platelet alpha-granules using mass spectrometry. *J Thromb Haemost* 2007;5:1945–55.

35. Morrissey JH, Choi SH, Smith SA. Polyphosphate: an ancient molecule that links platelets, coagulation, and inflammation. *Blood* 2012;119:5972–9.

36. De Candia E, Hall SW, Rutella S, et al. Binding of thrombin to glycoprotein Ib accelerates the hydrolysis of PAR-1 on intact platelets. *J Biol Chem* 2001; 276:4692–8.

37. Owen WG, Wagner RH. Antihemophilic factor: separation of an active fragment following dissociation by salts or detergents. *Thromb Diath Haemorrh* 1972;27: 502–15.

38. Heemskerk JW, Vuist WM, Feijge MA, et al. Collagen but not fibrinogen surfaces induce bleb formation, exposure of phosphatidylserine, and procoagulant activity of adherent platelets: evidence for regulation by protein tyrosine kinase-dependent Ca2+ responses. *Blood* 1997;90:2615–25.

39. Alberio L, Safa O, Clemetson KJ, et al. Surface expression and functional characterization of alpha-granule factor V in human platelets: effects of ionophore A23187, thrombin, collagen, and convulxin. *Blood* 2000;95:1694–702.

40. Van Dieijen G, Van Rijn JL, Govers-Riemslag JW, et al. Assembly of the intrinsic factor X activating complex–interactions between factor IXa, factor VIIIa and phospholipid. *Thromb Haemost* 1985;53:396–400.

41. Ahmad SS, Rawala-Sheikh R, Walsh PN. Comparative interactions of factor IX and factor IXa with human platelets. *J Biol Chem* 1989;264:3244–51.

42. Hoffman M, Monroe DM, Oliver JA, Roberts HR. Factors IXa and Xa play distinct roles in tissue factor-dependent initiation of coagulation. *Blood* 1995;86:1794–801.

43. Monroe DM, Hoffman M, Oliver JA, Roberts HR. A possible mechanism of action of activated factor VII independent of tissue factor. *Blood Coagul Fibrinolysis* 1998;9 (suppl 1):S15–20.

44. Maroney SA, Cooley BC, Ferrel JP, et al. Absence of hematopoietic tissue factor pathway inhibitor mitigates bleeding in mice with hemophilia. *Proc Natl Acad Sci USA* 2012;109:3927–31.

45. Oliver JA, Monroe DM, Roberts HR, Hoffman M. Thrombin activates factor XI on activated platelets in the absence of factor XII. *Arterioscler Thromb Vasc Biol* 1999;19:170–7.

46. Kravtsov DV, Matafonov A, Tucker EI, et al. Factor XI contributes to thrombin generation in the absence of factor XII. *Blood* 2009;114:452–8.

47. Giesen PL, Rauch U, Bohrmann B, et al. Blood-borne tissue factor: another view of thrombosis. *Proc Natl Acad Sci USA* 1999;96:2311–15.

48. Butenas S, Bouchard BA, Brummel-Ziedins KE, et al. Tissue factor activity in whole blood. *Blood* 2005;105:2764–70.

49. Delluc A, Rousseau A, Delluc C, et al. Venous thromboembolism in patients with pancreatic cancer: implications of circulating tissue factor. *Blood Coagul Fibrinolysis* 2011;22:295–300.

50. Falati S, Liu Q, Gross P, et al. Accumulation of tissue factor into developing thrombi in vivo is dependent upon microparticle P-selectin glycoprotein ligand 1 and platelet P-selectin. *J Exp Med* 2003;197:1585–98.

51. Orfeo T, Brummel-Ziedins KE, Gissel M, et al. The nature of the stable blood clot procoagulant activities. *J Biol Chem* 2008;283:9776–86.

52. Seegers WH, Johnson JF, Fell C. An antithrombin reaction to prothrombin activation. *Am J Physiol* 1954;176:97–103.

53. De Agostini AI, Watkins SC, Slayter HS, et al. Localization of anticoagulantly active heparan sulfate proteoglycans in vascular endothelium: antithrombin binding on cultured endothelial cells and perfused rat aorta. *J Cell Biol* 1990;111:1293–304.

54. Zhang J, Piro O, Lu L, Broze GJ Jr. Glycosyl phosphatidylinositol anchorage of tissue factor pathway inhibitor. *Circulation* 2003;108:623–7.

55. Heemskerk JW, Siljander P, Vuist WM, et al. Function of glycoprotein VI and integrin alpha2beta1 in the procoagulant response of single, collagen-adherent platelets. *Thromb Haemost* 1999;81:782–92.

56. Heemskerk JWM, Mattheij NJA, Cosemans JMEM. Platelet-based coagulation: different populations, different functions. *J Thromb Haemost* 2013;11:2–16.

57. Esmon NL, Owen WG, Esmon CT. Isolation of a membrane-bound cofactor for thrombin-catalyzed activation of protein C. *J Biol Chem* 1982;257:859–64.

58. Esmon CT, Esmon NL, Harris KW. Complex formation between thrombin and thrombomodulin inhibits both thrombin-catalyzed fibrin formation and factor V activation. *J Biol Chem* 1982;257:7944–7.

59. Fukudome K, Esmon CT. Identification, cloning, and regulation of a novel endothelial cell protein C/activated protein C receptor. *J Biol Chem* 1994;269:26486–91.

60. Dahlbäck B, Villoutreix BO. Molecular recognition in the protein C anticoagulant pathway. *J Thromb Haemost* 2003;1:1525–34.

61. Oliver JA, Monroe DM, Church FC, et al. Activated protein C cleaves factor Va more efficiently on endothelium than on platelet surfaces. *Blood* 2002;100:539–46.

62. Bertina RM, Koeleman BP, Koster T, et al. Mutation in blood coagulation factor V associated with resistance to activated protein C. *Nature* 1994;369:64–7.

63. Hemker HC, Wielders S, Kessels H, Béguin S. Continuous registration of thrombin generation in plasma, its use for the determination of the thrombin potential. *Thromb Haemost* 1993;70:617–24.

64. Hartert H. Blutgerinnungsstudien mit der Thrombelastographie, einem neuen Untersuchungsverfahren. *Klin Wochenschr* 1948;26:577–83.

65. Bouma BN, Griffin JH. Human blood coagulation factor XI: purification, properties, and mechanism of activation by activated factor XII. *J Biol Chem* 1977;252: 6432–7.

66. Seligsohn U. Factor XI in haemostasis and thrombosis: past, present and future. *Thromb Haemost* 2007;98:84–9.

67. Endler G, Marsik C, Jilma B, et al. Evidence of a U-shaped association between factor XII activity and overall survival. *J Thromb Haemost* 2007;5:1143–8.

CHAPTER 2

Vascular Endothelium, Influence on Hemostasis: Past and Present

Hussain I. Saba[1] and Sabiha R. Saba[2]

[1] Hematology/Hemophilia/Hemostasis & Thrombosis Center, USF College of Medicine, Tampa, FL, USA
[2] Department of Pathology and Cell Biology, USF College of Medicine, Tampa, FL, USA

Introduction

William Harvey was the first scientist to offer a new radical concept of blood circulation, in the year 1628 [1]. It led to immediate controversy in the medical community at that time, as it contradicted the usually unquestioned teaching of the Greek philosopher, Galen, regarding the theory and concept of blood movement. Galen's theory was based on the ideas that blood was formed in the liver, absorbed by the body, and flowed through the septum of the heart (dividing walls). Although Harvey's contradicting concept was based upon human and animal experiments, his findings were ridiculed and not well accepted. Later in the year 1661, Marcello Malpighi published his discovery of capillaries which then gave unwavering, factual evidence to support Harvey's concept of blood and circulation [2]. By the year 1800, Von Recklinghausen established that blood vessels were not merely a tunnel-like membrane structure similar in shape of cellophane tube, but had primary and important function of maintaining the vascular permeability [3]. Heidenhain (1891) introduced the concept that endothelium possessed an active secretory system [4]. In 1959, Gowans described the interaction between lymphocytes and endothelium at postcapillary venules. By 1959, electron microscopic studies by Palade [5] and the physical studies by Gowans [6] led to the current concept that endothelium is a dynamic heterogeneous disseminated organ which possesses vital secretory, metabolic, and immunologic activities.

In adult human subjects, the total endothelial surface consists of approximately $1–6 \times 10^{13}$ cells, weighing about 1 kg and covering an area of approximately $4–7 \times 10^3$ square meters. Endothelial cells line the blood

---

vessel of every inner human organ, are responsible for regulation of the flow of nutrients, and possess diverse biologically active molecules such as hormones, growth factors, coagulant and anticoagulant proteins, lipid transporting particles (LDL), and metabolites such as nitrous oxide. Protective and receptive endothelium also governs cell and cell matrix interaction. Endothelial cells that make up the lining of the inner surface of blood vessels wall are called vascular endothelial cells. These cells line the entire circulatory system from the heart to the smallest capillaries, and have very distinct and unique functions that are of importance to the vascular biology. Their functions include fluid filtration, such as that seen in the glomeri of the kidney. They maintain vascular tone and are, therefore, involved in the maintenance of blood pressure. The cells are also involved in mediation of hemostatic responses and trafficking of the neutrophil in and out of the lumen of the blood vessel to the tissue space. Endothelial cells are involved in many aspects of vascular biology. These are biologically of paramount importance. Their role has included the development of early and late stages of atherosclerosis. One of the very important functions of endothelial cells is their role in the maintenance of a non-thrombogenic surface apparently due to the presence of heparan sulfate, which works as a cofactor for activating antithrombin, a protease that inactivates several factors in the clotting cascades.

Function of endothelial cells

Endothelial cells are involved in many aspects of vascular biology, and play a role in the development of atherosclerosis. They also function as a selective barrier between blood cells and surrounding tissue, controlling the passage of material and the transit of white cells in and out of the bloodstream. Excessive and prolonged increase in the permeability of the endothelial cells monolayer such as that seen in cases of chronic inflammatory process may lead to accumulation of inflammatory fluid in the tissue space. Endothelial cells are involved in maintaining a nonthrombogenic and thromboresistant surface. This physiologic activity inhibits platelets and other cells from sticking to endothelium and is related to the presence of heparan sulfate on the endothelial surface, which works as a cofactor for activating antithrombin, a protease that inactivates several factors responsible for activating the clotting cascades. Vascular endothelium, because of its strategic location interfering between tissue and blood, is in an ideal situation to modulate and influence functions of various organs. Endothelial cell function includes transport of nutrients and solutes across the endothelium, maintenance of vascular tone and maintenance of the thromboresistant surface, and the activation and inactivation of various vasoactive hormones. Under normal conditions the endothelial cells provide a nonthrombogenic surface which does not allow platelets and other blood cells to adhere and to stick to the surface of endothelium. This nonthrombogenic nature of endothelium is unique for the flow of the blood as well as for the flow of blood cells.

The mechanism of the thromboresistance of endothelium has not been fully understood but is considered to be related to the interaction of anti-coagulant, fibrinolytic, and antiplatelet factors. The endothelium confers strong defense mechanisms against these insults by expressing a series of molecules. With successful culture of the endothelial cells, a myriad of molecules have been identified and characterized. The accepted view at this stage is that the main function of endothelial cells is to produce vaso-protective and thromboresistant molecules. Some molecules are constitu-tively expressed, while others are produced and respond to stimuli. Some are expressed on the interior endothelial surface and others are released. Molecules physiologically important in suppressing platelet activation and platelet vessel wall interaction include prostacyclin (PGI_2), nitric oxide (NO), and ecto-adenosine diphosphatase (ADPase). Molecules involved in controlling coagulation include the surface-expressed thrombomodulin (a heparin-like molecule), von Willebrand factor (VWF), protein S, and tissue factor pathway inhibitor (TFPI). Endothelial cells synthesize and secrete tissue plasminogen activator (TPA) and urokinase-type plasminogen acti-vator to promote fibrinolysis. To control TPA activity, the endothelium produces plasminogen activator inhibitor-1 (PAI-1), which serves to neu-tralize the TPA activity.

Antiplatelet factors

Prostacyclin
Prostacyclin (PGI_2) is a multifunctional molecule it is an important inhibi-tor of platelet activation, aggregation, and secretion [7–10]. It induces vascular smooth muscle relaxation and blocks monocyte endothelial cell interaction. It also reduces lipid accumulation in smooth muscles. Its platelet inhibitory activity is mediated via guanosine nucleotide-binding receptor with subsequent activation of adenylate cyclase and elevation of platelet adenosine monophosphate (cAMP).

cAMP levels will result in inhibition of platelet activation. Its actions on other cells are thought to be mediated by a similar receptor-mediated signal transduction pathway. Prostacyclin is primarily synthesized by vas-cular endothelial cells and smooth muscle cells. Its synthesis is catalyzed by a series of enzymes. When stimulated by diverse physiologic agonists including thrombin, histamine, and bradykinin, endothelial cell cytosolic phospholipase (PLA-2) is activated. Activated PLA-2 catalyzes the liberation of arachidonic acid (AA) primarily from phosphatidylcholine. The released free AA serves as a substrate for prostaglandin H synthase (PGHS), also known as cyclooxygenase.

PGHS is a bifunctional enzyme with two distinct enzymatic activities. Cyclooxygenase catalyzes the oxygenation of AA from prostaglandin to prostaglandin G2 (PGG_2) and peroxidase catalyzes the reduction of PGG_2 to prostaglandin H_2 (PGH_2). PGH_2 is a common precursor for the synthesis of prostaglandin, prostacyclin, and thromboxane. In endothelial cells, PGH_2 is primarily converted to PGI_2 by the specific enzyme PGI_2 synthase. PGI_2 synthesis is regulated at each enzymatic step. The exact regulatory mechanisms are not entirely clear, but it is generally believed that PGHS is the key step due to autoactivation of this enzyme during catalysis. Several studies have shown that PGI_2 synthesis by arterial segments of cultured endothelial cell stimulated with thrombin or histamine has a short duration of activity of 15–30 minutes. Overexpression of PGHS type 1 in an endothelial cell line by retrovirus-mediated transfer of the human PGHS-1 gene is accompanied by a 10- to 100-fold increase in PGI_2 synthesis. Two isoforms of PGHS have been identified in human endothelial cells. PGHS-1 is constitutively expressed and its synthesis may be augmented by shear stress, cytokines, and mitogenic factors. PGHS is thought to be primarily responsible for synthesizing the vasoprotective PGI_2 under physiologic conditions. Endothelial cells possess type 2 PGHS (PGHS-2) which is expressed in smaller quantities in resting cells but is highly inducible by mitogenic factors and cytokines. The inducible PGHS-2 is present on both inflammatory and neoplastic cells. This PGHS isoform has been considered to be primarily involved in cell inflammation and cell proliferation. However, there is suggestive evidence that PGHS-2 may play an important role in producing vasoprotective PGI_2 when the endothelium is under severe stress and cellular PGHS-1 levels are depleted because of autoactivation. Human PGHS-1 and PGHS-2 genes have been mapped to chromosomes 9 and 1 respectively; the structure and promoter activities of both genes have been characterized.

Prostacyclin synthase provides a final enzymatic step for this specific PGI_2 synthesis. This enzyme is membrane bound to cytochrome P450 enzymes [11]. Its complementary DNA has recently been cloned [12,13]. One report reveals that this enzyme is inducible and hence may play a role in determining the extent and duration of PGI_2 synthesis. Furthermore, PGI_2 synthesis, like PGHS-1, is autoactivated during catalysis. It is likely that this enzyme plays a major role in controlling the extent of PGI_2 production as well. PGI_2 may also be synthesized by a transcellular mechanism [14]. Hence the production of PGI_2 is tightly regulated and an alternate synthesis pathway exists to ensure a sufficient PGI_2 level for vasoprotection when the vessel is under stress.

Nitric oxide

Nitric oxide (NO) is elaborated as hetero atomic radical production guaranteed through the oxidation of L-arginine and L-citrulline by nitric oxide synthetase. NO is the mediator of vasorelaxation, immunomodulation, cytotoxicity, and neurotransmission [15]. NO also inhibits platelet activation. The role of NO in vasorelaxation was discovered by Furchgott and Zawadzki. [16] These investigators noted that blood vessels depleted of endothelium failed to relax when treated with acetylcholine [16]. They postulated that endothelium elaborates the factor(s) endothelium-dependent relaxing factor (EDRF) which is responsible for acetylcholine-induced vasorelaxation. The major component of EDRF was subsequently found to be nitrous oxide.

Biosynthesis of nitrous oxide is catalyzed by nitric oxide synthase (NOS). NOS converts L-arginine to L-citrulline and NO. NO is diffusible and is thought to be released primarily into the albuminal side where it activates smooth muscle cell guanylate cyclase and increases cytosolic cyclic guanosine monophosphate. NO may also diffuse into the luminal side where it enters into the platelets and inhibits platelet adhesion, activation, and aggregation via activation of guanylate cyclase. Nitrous oxide and prostacyclin act synergistically not only to inhibit platelet adhesion and aggregation, but also to reverse platelet aggregation [17]. The synergistic inhibition of platelet activation by these two molecules has been considered to be of importance in maintaining blood fluidity and controlling thrombus formation. Three isoforms of NOS have been identified and characterized. Vascular endothelium possesses a constitutive NOS (NOS-III), which shares about 50–60% of amino acid sequences identified with neuronal constitutive NOS (NOS-I) and inducible NOS (NOS-II).

Like NOS-I and NOS-II, NOS-III is a bifunctional enzyme containing a reductase domain and an oxygenase domain [5]. Although NOS-III is constitutively expressed in endothelial cells, the enzyme is inactive in resting cells and little NO is synthesized. When endothelial cells are activated by physiologic agonists, elevated cellular calcium binds to calmodulin (CaM) and the Ca^{2+}/CaM complex binds to CAM, binding sites on NOS thereby activating the enzyme. An elevated cytosolic calcium is also pivotal in PGI_2 synthesis. PGI_2 and NO are produced simultaneously during endothelial cell activation via calcium elevation.

The human NOS-III gene has been mapped to chromosome 7q35-36. Its 5′ flanking region lacks canonical TATA or CAAT and is guanine plus cytosine (G+C) rich, consistent with the feature of "housekeeping" gene [18]. However, this gene is regulated at the transcriptional level. It has been shown that high shear stress and lysophosphatidylcholine produced during minimal low density lipoprotein oxidation augment NOS-III transcription [19] and increase NOS-III enzyme activity in endothelial cells. NOS-III levels and activity may, hence, be regulated tightly at multiple steps transcriptionally and post-transcriptionally.

Basal production of PGI$_2$ and nitric oxide in vivo

Normal endothelium probably produces a constant basal level of PGI$_2$, as evidenced by urinary excretion of its metabolite, 2,3-dinor-6-keto-PGF$_{1a}$ [20]. The evidence of basal production of NO is less clear, but inhibitor studies do suggest a basal level of NO production. The stimulating factors responsible for maintaining constitutive PGI$_2$ and NO synthesis are probably multiple, including thrombin, histamine, shear stress, mechanical force, and lipid mediators. It should be noted that the endothelium may be stimulated by shear stress via two separate mechanisms: 1) activations of endothelium with resultant intracellular calcium elevation and, consequently, PLA2 and NOS activation leading to PGI$_2$, and NO synthesis; and 2) inductions of PGHS-1 and NOS-111 transcription. The 5′ flanking region of both genes contains putative shear stress response elements. However, binding of nuclear transcription activators to this element to promote PGHS-1 and NOS-III gene expression under controlled shear stress is a major, if not the only, factor responsible for sustained PGI$_2$ and NO synthesis. The levels of PGI$_2$ and NO production evoked by different levels of shear stress are considered to play an important role in defending against excessive thrombus formation.

Ecto-ADPase

The endothelial surface possesses an enzyme activity that degrades ADP to AMP. This enzyme is termed ecto-ADPase. As ADP released from activated platelets is an important mediator for recruiting and amplifying platelet aggregation, ecto-ADPase may play a physiologic role in limiting the extent of platelet aggregation [21]. However, endothelial ecto-ADPase has not been purified and characterized. As of this time, it is unclear whether it is identical to ecto-ADPase present on the surface of other cell types.

Anticoagulant factors

Thrombomodulin

The endothelial cell surface membrane provides an effective catalytic surface for the generation of activated protein C. Protein C is synthesized in the liver and, when activated, cleaves and inactivates factors Va and

VIIIa. Thrombin is the only enzyme capable of activating protein C. It binds to thrombomodulin (TM) at the endothelial cell surface where it undergoes conformational changes resulting in an enhancement of its affinity for protein C [22]. TM is an integral membrane protein with a molecular weight of 75. There are about 30,000–100,000 TM molecules on the endothelial surface. It has a membrane-spanning domain in the N-terminus with a short cytoplasmic sequence. The extracellular domain has six endothelial growth factor-like repeats and has extensive intramolecular disulfide bridging. The C-terminus has a lectin-like domain. Human recombinant TM has chondroitin sulfate attached to it. TM is present in all endothelial cells and is particularly prominent in the microvessels of the lung. By competing for thrombin, TM inhibits a number of procoagulant activities of thrombin, such as clotting of fibrinogen, activation of factors V and XIII, inactivation of protein S, and platelet aggregation. In addition, TM binds factor Xa and inhibits its activation of prothrombin [23]. The thrombin/TM complex is internalized by endocytosis whereby thrombin is degraded and TM is recycled to the surface. Furthermore, the glycosaminoglycan bound to TM accelerates inactivation of thrombin by antithrombin III [24]. A soluble form of TM, present in the plasma and excreted in the urine, has been used as a marker of endothelial cell activation. These soluble TMs are probably derived from the proteolytic modification of TM by leukocyte elastase. TM is transcribed from a single intronless gene. Multiple regulatory elements in the 3′ untranslated region have been characterized. In cultured endothelial cells, TM synthesis is downregulated transcriptionally by tumor necrosis factor, interleukin-1, and endotoxin. This may be relevant to activation of the coagulation system during inflammation.

Protein S

Protein S is a vitamin K-dependent glycoprotein that enhances the inactivation of factor Va by activated protein C. Unlike other vitamin K-dependent factors, it does not contain an active serine to function as a serine protease. It is synthesized by endothelium as well as by liver and megakaryocytes. Approximately 60% of plasma protein S is bound to C4b-binding protein, and this fraction does not have cofactor activity [25]. Protein S binds to the endothelial surface and activated protein C to form a complex. Recently, a protein S-independent cell surface receptor for activated protein C has been cloned and characterized [26].

Endothelial surface heparan sulfate

Proteoglycans are present on endothelial cells and in the subendothelial matrix [27]. Recent studies have demonstrated the presence of anticoagulant-active heparan sulfate proteoglycan on the surface of endothelium, which functions as a cofactor for antithrombin. Heparin-like molecules with anticoagulant activity are isolated from cloned endothelial cells, and treatment with heparinase abolishes this anticoagulant activity. Antithrombin III is a major serine protease inhibitor that is present in the plasma. It forms a 1:1 stoichiometric complex with thrombin and other serine proteases, such as factors Xa, IXa, and XIIa. This complex formation between antithrombin III and thrombin occurs at a relatively slow rate. Heparin accelerates this interaction dramatically. Heparin is a complex, highly sulfated proteoglycan. It is the only proteoglycan capable of activating antithrombin III. The binding site for antithrombin III on heparin contains a highly sulfated pentasaccharide structure. The nature of the critical groups that accelerate antithrombin III inactivation of serine proteases has been elucidated recently. They consist of at least two domains. One domain, containing eight or more oligosaccharide sequences, binds to a discrete region in antithrombin III and accelerates factor Xa–antithrombin III interactions. A larger domain, consisting of polysaccharides of 16 or more residues, is required for inactivation of thrombin. These larger segments are also required to accelerate factor XIa and factor IXa inactivation. A small fraction of plasma antithrombin III is bound to endothelial cell surface heparan sulfate and thus is located in a strategic locus to inactivate thrombin formed locally. In addition, much larger quantities of heparan sulfate proteoglycan are formed in the subendothelium, which may be exposed during vessel wall injury. Heparin activates another plasma protease inhibitor, heparin cofactor II. Other proteoglycans, especially dermatan sulfate, are able to accelerate the inhibitory effect of heparin cofactor II dramatically but have little effect on antithrombin III [28].

Tissue factor pathway inhibitor

Tissue factor pathway inhibitor (TFPI) is a protease inhibitor present in low concentrations in plasma. The factor VIIa–tissue factor complex is inhibited by TFPI in the presence of factor Xa [29,30]. TFPI is synthesized primarily in the liver but is also synthesized by endothelial cells. However, TFPI levels are normal in severe liver disease but decreased in severe disseminated intravascular coagulation (DIC), suggesting that endothelial cells may be the primary source of TFPI. Recombinant TFPI has been shown to be effective in preventing reocclusion after tPA infusion in an experimental canine femoral artery thrombosis [31]. However, no deficiency of TFPI is reported so far and so the physiologic role of this inhibitor remains to be ascertained.

Fibrinolytic factors

Endothelial cells are the major site of synthesis of tPA. Thrombin, shear stress, and phorbol myristate acetate have been shown to induce the synthesis and release of tPA. The mature protein, a 68-kDa glycoprotein, contains a finger domain, an epidermal growth factor domain, two kringle domains, and a catalytic domain. Both the single-chain and a plasmin-cleaved two-chain form are physiologically active. A variety of stimuli, such as exercise, an increase in venous pressure, acidosis, and hypoxia, can release tPA. Free tPA can bind to the surface of endothelial cells, and endothelial cell-bound tPA is protected from its physiologic inhibitor, plasminogen activator inhibitor-1 (PAI-1). tPA is inefficient in activating plasminogen in solution but, in the presence of fibrin, becomes effective as a result of the assembly of tPA and plasminogen on the surface of fibrin. Receptors for plasminogen and tPA have also been identified on the endothelial cell surface, allowing an efficient and regulated generation of fibrinolytic activity. Although the cultured endothelial cell can synthesize urokinase, the latter's in vivo synthesis and physiologic significance are not known at the present time. Endothelial cells also synthesize fibrinolytic inhibitors. PAI-1 is the major inhibitor of tPA in plasma. PAI-1 belongs to the family of serpins. In addition to endothelial cells, liver, megakaryocytes, and monocytes can synthesize PAI-1. In plasma, there is a molar excess of PAI-1 compared to tPA, and the expression of PAI-1 is also highly regulated. The expression of PAI-1 is stimulated by inflammation, hormones, and cytokines. PAI-1 is also present in the subendothelial matrix, where it may function to inhibit degradation of the matrix. Both plasma and subendothelial PAI-1 form a complex with vitronectin, a major cell adhesion protein.

Contribution of endothelium in hemostasis

Disruption of vascular integrity due to trauma or surgery leads to a chain of rapid reactions that induces vascular constriction, formation of hemostatic plugs, and vascular repair. The molecular basis for these processes is not entirely clear, but it is reasonable to presume that endothelial cells play a major role in all these processes. For example, endothelial cells produce endothelins which are active vasoconstrictors and may be involved in hemostatic vasoconstriction. Endothelial cells elaborate several growth factors, such as vascular endothelial growth factor, which may be responsible for endothelial cell generation and vascular repair. However, their roles in hemostasis are not well established. On the other hand, von

Willebrand factor (VWF), produced by endothelial cells and megakaryocytes, clearly plays a major role in hemostatic plug formation. VWF is a multimeric molecule with a nascent molecular weight of about 20×10^6. The VWF gene produces a monomer of about 250 kDa. Extensive posttranslational modification and multimerization are required for formation of functional VWF. VWF is constitutively secreted and is also stored in intraendothelial Weibel–Palade granules [32].

Constitutive synthesis and secretion of VWF appear to be under tight regulation as the plasma VWF level is fairly constant in healthy subjects. In plasma, VWF is degraded by proteolytic enzymes. The plasma VWF molecules are composed of intact and degraded multimers with molecular weights of $1–20 \times 10^6$. VWF is pivotal in hemostasis and thrombosis [33]. It serves as a ligand for platelet adhesion to denuded vascular wall, and as a bridge molecule for platelet aggregation, particularly when aggregation is induced by high shear stress [34]. It possesses binding sites for coagulation factor VIII, thereby stabilizing its activity. Platelet adhesion absolutely requires VWF; VWF binds concurrently to both subendothelial collagen and platelet glycoprotein (GP) Ib–IX [35]. VWF also binds to platelet GP-IIb–IIIa to support agonist-induced platelet aggregation. Under high shear stress, binding of VWF to GP-IIb–IIIa is the primary mechanism underlying shear stress-induced platelet aggregation.

The importance of VWF in hemostasis is attested to by the severe bleeding disorders which are a consequence of total absence of VWF (type III VWD, a homozygous defect in VWF synthesis resulting from mutations in the VWF gene). Types I and II VWD are also associated with mucocutaneous bleeding, although the bleeding is milder and variable because of the presence of various amounts of functional VWF in the plasma and the subendothelial matrix. VWF release from the Weibel–Palade granules is stimulated by desmopressin (DDAVP) and estrogen. DDAVP is efficacious in treating mild VWD (type I and type IIa).

Contribution of endothelium in thrombosis

Endothelial cell injuries and resultant endothelial loss and/or dysfunction play a key role in all types of thrombotic disorders. Loss of endothelial cell protective properties coupled with the expressions of procoagulant and prothrombotic molecules in the subendothelial matrix and or on the dysfunctional endothelium tilts the hemostatic balance toward thrombosis. The perturbation allows platelets to adhere to the subendothelial surface. The adhered platelets are activated, thereby releasing ADP and thromboxane A_2. These molecules recruit additional platelets and amplify platelet activation and aggregation.

In addition, platelet membrane GP-IIb–IIIa is conformationally changed to facilitate fibrinogen binding. Fibrinogen binding is the fundamental mechanism by which platelet aggregation occurs in response to agonists. Platelet surface membrane phospholipids undergo conformational rearrangements to facilitate the binding of coagulation cofactors such as factor Va and factor VIIIa to the platelet surface. Binding of these two cofactors is critical for coagulation. Binding of factor VIIIa allows for VIIIa/IXa/X/Ca^{2+} complex (Xase) assembly, which leads to the rapid catalytic conversion of factor X to Xa. Factor Xa then binds to factor Va on the platelet surface, and a Va/Xa/II/Ca^{2+} complex (prothrombinase) is assembled. This complex assembly facilitates the conversion of prothrombin to thrombin.

Thrombin is a multifunctional protease. Its prothrombotic activities include induction of platelet aggregation, fibrin formation, and conversion of coagulation factors, notably V, VIII, and XIII, into their active forms. Thrombin coordinates augmentation of platelet and coagulation activation, thereby amplifying platelet-fibrin thrombus formation. Thrombin also possesses antithrombotic properties. The antithrombotic properties of thrombin depend almost entirely on healthy endothelial cells; thus, thrombin stimulates prostacyclin and NO synthesis. In addition, thrombin must bind to endothelial TM to activate protein C, which triggers anticoagulant activity. Healthy endothelial cells are capable of inactivating thrombin by at least two mechanisms. First, endothelial cell surface heparin-like molecules serve as a cofactor for antithrombin to neutralize thrombin. Second, thrombin bound to TM is internalized and neutralized. Hence, endothelial cells provide a multitude of mechanisms against thrombus formation, and endothelial loss or dysfunction leaves the prothrombotic properties of thrombin unopposed, creating a very strong prothrombotic environment.

Endothelial cells also play a critical role in defense against thrombosis and atherosclerosis induced by high shear stress. High shear stress induces platelet aggregation primarily through binding of VWF (in contrast to fibrinogen binding to platelets during chemical-induced aggregation). Binding of VWF to GP-IIb–IIIa can activate platelets and trigger a series of chemical and cellular reactions. High shear stress has also been shown to stimulate prostacyclin and NO synthesis. These two antiplatelet molecules reduce the shear stress-induced thrombotic potential. In the event of endothelial cell loss or dysfunction, the thrombotic potential becomes fully manifested.

Studies indicate that oxidized low density lipoprotein, despite its well-recognized ability to damage endothelial cells and cause vascular lesions, can stimulate vasoprotective NO and PGI$_2$ [19,36]. Its ability to damage vasculature becomes rampant following loss of endothelial cell PGI$_2$ and

NO synthetic abilities due to endothelial cell dysfunction or loss. Clinical and pathologic manifestations of vascular thrombotic disorders following vascular injury differ according to blood vessels, types of insults, blood flow, and shear stress. Common human thrombotic disorders are divided into: 1) arterial thrombosis, including coronary arterial, cerebrovascular, and peripheral arterial thrombosis; 2) deep venous thrombosis; and 3) thrombotic microangiopathy, including thrombotic thrombocytopenic purpura (TTP), hemolytic uremic syndrome, thrombotic microangiopathy in toxemia of pregnancy, and transplant rejection.

The following are general salient features of these disorders as related to endothelial function. In arterial thrombotic disorders, medium-size arteries are chronically injured by dietary lipids, cigarette smoking, hypertension, diabetes mellitus, and viral and immunologic agents. There is an emerging view that, during the early phase of injury, endothelial cells respond to most insulting agents by accelerating the production of vasoprotective molecules, thereby protecting the blood vessel from damage. However, when insults are chronic and severe, endothelial damage occurs and its vasoprotective properties dwindle. Furthermore, the dysfunctional endothelium may manifest procoagulant activity. Interactions among lipoproteins, platelets and monocytes, and the vascular wall cells and proteins lead to complex changes that result in atherosclerosis, intimal hyperplasia, and acute thrombosis.

In deep vein thrombosis, coagulation activation is the initial event triggered by stasis of blood flow at the venous valvular junction. Thrombin generation causes fibrin formation and platelet aggregation, leading to the formation of fibrin-rich clots. The role of endothelial cells in deep venous thrombosis is considered to be less important than in arterial thrombosis. There is evidence for endothelial damage in venous thrombosis, but the damage appears reversible. Chronic injury to venous endothelium has not been observed in humans. However, when venous segments are used as a graft in coronary artery bypass surgery, severe stenosis and thrombosis can occur in the venous graft, suggesting that resistance of veins to chronic injury may not be entirely due to the veins per se but may be related to blood flow, shear stress, and mechanical stress.

Thrombotic microangiopathy is thought to be closely associated with endothelial cell dysfunction and damage. In TTP, for example, there is evidence in plasma levels of abnormally high molecular-weight VWF, possibly reflecting endothelial dysfunction during acute TTP attacks. As plasma exchange therapy has been efficacious in treating TTP and related thrombotic microangiopathies, with resultant correction of VWF abnormalities, endothelial dysfunction in TTP is probably reversible. Thrombotic microcytopathy can be a result of endothelial cell injury and its alteration. Under normal conditions, endothelium provides a nonthermogenic surface that does not allow platelet and other cellular counterparts of circulating blood to adhere and stick to the surface of the endothelial cells.

The prevailing view has therefore been that the major function of endothelial cells has been of vasoprotection and thromboresistance. Besides being a structural barrier between circulation and surrounding tissue, endothelial cells secrete substances influencing vascular hemodynamics. Hence endothelial cells contribute to the regulation of blood pressure and blood flow. These agents include nitrous oxide (NO), prostaglandins (PGI_2) as vasodilators, and vasoconstricter substance(s) such as endothelin and platelet-activating factor (PAF). These substance(s) are not stored in intracellular granules but their major biologic effects are regulated by localizations of specific receptors on vascular cells.

Endothelial cell dysfunction: pathophysiology and biology

Excessive stimulation of endothelial cells by a variety of stimuli, notably cytokines, microbial toxins, lipid mediators, and immunologic agents, may lead to a state of endothelial cell dysfunction. Most evidence has been provided by in vitro experiments. Although it is likely that endothelial dysfunction occurs in a variety of human diseases as a result of excessive stimulation of endothelium by a host of factors, detection of in vivo endothelial dysfunction remains quite difficult, primarily because of a lack of specific markers or tests.

Some studies have measured vascular tone in response to acetylcholine as a test of endothelial function and dysfunction. Others have measured plasma levels of soluble forms of TM, vascular cell adhesion molecule (VCAM)-1, intercellular adhesion molecule (ICAM)-1, and E-selectin. The utility of these measurements for accurately detecting endothelial dysfunction remains uncertain. Exposure of cultured endothelial cells to a variety of stimulants in vitro leads to the suppression of anticoagulant activity and expression of procoagulant activity. There is decreased expression of thrombomodulin and increased expression of tissue factor activity. Such perturbation of endothelial cells has been induced by endotoxin, tumor necrosis factor, interleukin 1, advanced glycosylation end products, viral infections, and hypoxia [37–40]. Resting endothelial cells in culture have also been shown to possess specific cell surface receptors for factors IX and IXa, promoting the assembly of factor IXa/VIII/X complex and leading to the generation of factor Xa. In addition, prothrombinase complex can also assemble on the surface of endothelial cells. Thus, a pathway for thrombin generation exists on the surface of endothelial cells.

Enhancement of endothelial procoagulant activity by cytokines has been proposed as a possible mechanism for initiation of coagulation in inflammatory conditions such as the Shwartzman phenomenon and in the pathogenesis of vascular lesions in diabetes. However, studies on intact vessels using in situ hybridization and immunofluorescent techniques consistently failed to show the expression of tissue factor by endothelial cells, whereas its expression could be readily demonstrated in the subendothelium and in other tissues [41,42].

Following an infusion of a lethal dose of *Escherichia coli* to induce sepsis in baboons, tissue factor expression could be seen only weakly in splenic vascular beds whereas remaining endothelial cells did not express tissue factor [43]. The expression of thrombomodulin and E-selectin could readily be demonstrated in this model. Thus, tissue factor expression, though readily demonstrated in vitro, may be under stricter control in vivo. Manipulations involving isolation of arterial segments in physiologic studies could lead to release of tissue factor from the subendothelium to the lumen [44]. The capacity of intact endothelial cells to initiate coagulation reactions in vivo remains to be established.

The Schwartzman phenomenon in rabbits, elicited by two sequential injections of endotoxin, is characterized by diffuse capillary thrombosis, renal cortical necrosis, DIC, and leukocyte infiltration. This reaction can effectively be prevented by rendering the animal leukopenic, suggesting the central role of leukocyte procoagulant activity rather than endothelial cells in the Shwartzman phenomenon. Endothelial dysfunction induced by cytokines and microbial toxins is accompanied by the expression of a series of membrane adhesive molecules, including P-selectin, E-selectin, ICAM-1, and VCAM-1, which serve as receptors and ligands for leukocyte ligands or receptors [45,46]. Expression of these molecules results in leukocyte–endothelial cell interactions, characterized first by leukocyte rolling on the endothelial surface, followed by irreversible adherence and then emigration.

References

1. Harvey W. *On the Motion of the Heart and Blood in Animals*. Vol XXXVIII Part 3. The Harvard Classics. New York: P.F. Collier & Son, 2001.
2. Pearce JM. Malpighi and the discovery of capillaries. *Eur Neurol* 2007;58:253–5.
3. Cines DB, Pollak ES, Buck CA, et al. Endothelial cells in physiology and in the pathophysiology of vascular disorders. *Blood Journal* 1998;9:3527–61.
4. Michel CC. One hundred years of Starling's hypothesis. *News Physiol Sci* 1996; 11:229–37.
5. Palade GE. Fine structure of blood capillaries. *J Applied Sci* 1953;24:1424.
6. Gowans JL. The recirculation of lymphocytes from blood to lymph in the rat. *J Physiol* 1959;146:54–69.

7. Saba, SR, Zucker WH, Mason, RG. Some properties of endothelial cells isolated from human umbilical cord vein. *Am J Haematol* 1973;6:456–86.
8. Saba SR, Mason RG. Studies of activity from endothelial cells that inhibits platelet aggregation, serotonin release and clot retraction. *Thromb Res* 1974;5:747–57.
9. Weksler BB, Marcus AJ, Jaffe EA. Synthesis of prostaglandin I$_2$ (prostacyclin) by cultured human endothelial cells. *Proc Natl Acad Sci USA* 1977;74:3922–3926.
10. Wu KK, Thiagarajan P. Role of endothelium in thrombosis and hemostasis. *Annu Rev Med* 1996;47:315–31.
11. DeWitt DL, Smith WL. Purification of prostacyclin synthase from bovine aorta by immunoaffinity chromatography. *J Biol Chem* 1983;258:3285–93.
12. Hara S, Miyata A, Yokoyama C, et al. Isolation and molecular cloning of prostacyclin synthase from bovine endothelial cells. *J Biol Chem* 1994;269:19897–903.
13. Pereira B, Wu KK, Wang L-H. Molecular cloning and characterization of bovine prostacyclin synthase. *Biochem Biophys Res Comm* 1994;203:59–66.
14. Wu KK, Papp AC. Interaction between platelets and lymphocytes in biosynthesis of prostacyclin. *Methods Enzymol* 1990;187:578–84.
15. Moncada S, Palmer RMJ, Higgs EA. Nitric oxide: physiology, pathophysiology and pharmacology. *Pharmacol Rev* 1991;43:109–42.
16. Furchgott RF, Zawadzki JV. The obligatory role of endothelial cells in the relaxation of arterial smooth muscle by acetylcholine. *Nature* 1980;288:687–92.
17. Radomski MW, Palmer PMJ, Moncada S. The anti-aggregating properties of vascular endothelium interactions between prostacyclin and nitric oxide. *Br J Pharmacol* 1987;92:639–46.
18. Marsden PA, Hing HHQ, Scherer SW, et al. Structure and chromosomal localization of human endothelial nitric oxide synthase. *J Biol Chem* 1993;268:17478–88.
19. Zembowicz A, Tang J-L, Wu KK. Transcriptional induction of endothelial nitric oxide synthase by lysophosphatidylcholine. *J Biol Chem* 1995;270:17006–10.
20. FitzGerald GA, Pedersen AK, Patrono C. Analysis of prostacyclin and thromboxane biosynthesis in cardiovascular disease. *Circulation* 1984;67:1174–77.
21. Marcus AJ, Safier LB, Haffar KA, et al. Inhibition of platelet function by an aspirin-insensitive endothelial cell ADPase. *J Clin Invest* 1990;88:1690–6.
22. Esmon CT. Molecular events that control the protein C anticoagulant pathway. *Thromb Haemost* 1993;70:29–35.
23. Thompson EA, Salem HH. Inhibition of human thrombomodulin of factor Xa mediated cleavage of prothrombin. *J Clin Invest* 1986;78:13–17.
24. Preissner KT, Delvos U, Muller-Bergaus G. Binding of thrombin to thrombomodulin accelerates inhibition of the enzyme by antithrombin III: evidence for heparin-independent mechanism. *Biochemistry* 1987;26:2521–8.
25. Dahlback B. Interaction between vitamin K-dependent protein S and complement protein, C4b-binding protein. *Semin Thromb Hemost* 1984;10:139–45.
26. Fukudome K, Esmon CT. Molecular cloning and expression of murine and bovine endothelial cell protein C/activated protein C receptor (EPCR). *J Biol Chem* 1995;270:5571–76.
27. Rosenberg RD, Bauer KA. The heparin-antithrombin system: a natural anticoagulant mechanism. In Coleman RW, Hirsch J, Marder VJ, Salmon EW (eds), *Hemostasis and Thrombosis*. Philadelphia, PA: Lippincott, 1994;837–60.
28. Tollefsen DM, Marrone MM, McGuire EA, et al. Heparin cofactor II activation by dermatan sulfate. *Ann NY Acad Sci* 1989; 556:116–22.
29. Rappaport SI, Rao LV. Initiation and regulation of tissue factor-dependent blood coagulation. *Arterioscler Thromb* 1991;12:1111–21.

30. Girard TJ, Broze GJ Jr. Tissue factor pathway inhibitor. *Methods Enzymol* 1993; 222:195–209.
31. Haskel EF, Torr, SR, Day KC, et al. Prevention of arterial reocclusion after thrombolysis with recombinant lipoprotein-associated with coagulation inhibitor. *Circulation* 1991;84:821–27.
32. Handin RI, Wagner DD. Molecular and cellular biology of vonWillebrand factor. *Prog Haemost Thromb* 1989;9:233–45.
33. Ruggeri ZM. Glycoprotein Ib and von Willebrand factor in the process of thrombus formation. *Ann NY Acad Sci* 1994;714:200–10.
34. Moake JL, Turner NA, Stathopoulos NA, et al. Involvement of large plasma VWF multimers in shear-stress induced platelet aggregation. *J Clin Invest* 1986; 78:1456–61.
35. Lopez JA. The platelet glycoprotein Ib–IXcomplex. *Blood Coagul Fibrinolysis* 1994; 5:97–119.
36. Zembowicz A, Jones SL, Wu KK. Induction of cyclooxygenase-2 in human umbilical vein endothelial cells by lysophosphatidylcholine. *J Clin Invest* 1995;96:1688–92.
37. Stern DM, Kaiser E, Nawroth PP. Regulation of the coagulation system by vascular endothelial cells. *Haemostasis* 1988;18:202–14.
38. Ryan J, Brett J, Tijburg P, et al. Tumor necrosis factor-induced endothelial tissue factor is associated with subendothelial matrix vesicles but is not expressed on the apical surface. *Blood* 1994;80:966–74.
39. Ogawa S, Shreeniwas R, Butura C, et al. Modulation of endothelial function by hypoxia: perturbation of barrier and anticoagulant function, and induction of a novel factor X activator. *Adv Exp Med Biol* 1990;281:303–12.
40. Key NS, Vercellotti GM, Winkelmann JC, et al. Infection of vascular endothelial cells with herpes simplex virus enhances tissue factor activity and reduces thrombomodulin expression. *Proc Natl Acad Sci USA* 1991;87:7095–99.
41. Wilcox JN, Smith KM, Schwartz SM, et al. Localization of tissue factor in normal vessel wall in atherosclerotic plague. *Proc Natl Acad Sci USA* 1989;86:2839–43.
42. Fleck RA, Rao LV, Rapaport SI, et al. Localization of human tissue factor antigen by immunostaining with monospecific, polyclonal anti-human tissue factor antibody. *Thromb Res* 1990;59:421–37.
43. Drake TA, Cheng J, Chang A, et al. Expression of tissue factor, thrombomodulin, and E-selectin in baboons with lethal Escherichia coli sepsis. *Am J Physiol* 1993; 143:1458–70.
44. Weiss HJ, Hoffmann T, Turitto VT, et al. Further studies on the presence of functional tissue factor activity on the subendothelium of normal human and rabbit arteries. *Thromb Res* 1994;73:313–26.
45. Bevilacqua MP. Endothelial-leukocyte adhesion molecules. *Annu Rev Immunol* 1993;11:767–804.
46. Springer TA. Traffic signals for lymphocyte recirculation and leukocyte emigration: the multistop paradigm. *Cell* 1994;76:301–14.

CHAPTER 3

Coagulation Testing: Basic and Advanced Clinical Laboratory Tests

Nils Egberg and Margareta Blombäck

Department of Molecular Medicine and Surgery, Division of Clinical Chemistry and Blood Coagulation, Karolinska Institutet, Stockholm, Sweden

Introduction

It is practical to divide hemostatic disorders into those leading to bleeding diatheses or those leading to thrombotic events. A number of screening tests for bleeding disorders have been developed, with the results suggesting in which part of the coagulation process a defect is to be suspected. Guided by the outcome of the screening tests, specific hemostatic assays may then be selected. Generally, severe bleeding disorders caused by a coagulation factor defect can be easily diagnosed. On the other hand, the majority of mild bleeding disorders are most likely caused by mild forms of von Willebrand disease (VWD) or mild platelet function defects, making their diagnosis more difficult. Unfortunately, many functional platelet defects are very difficult if not impossible to identify. There are few screening tests for thrombotic disorders. However, there are a number of specific assays that could be run, especially in younger patients who have suffered thrombotic events. In about 50% of patients with thrombotic manifestations, a likely cause can be found by laboratory testing.

Blood sampling for diagnosis of hemostatic disorders

Some facts should be considered about the variation of hemostatic components in patients and controls in order to better advise the clinicians [1].

Hemostasis and Thrombosis: Practical Guidelines in Clinical Management, First Edition.
Hussain I. Saba and Harold R. Roberts.
© 2014 John Wiley & Sons, Ltd. Published 2014 by John Wiley & Sons, Ltd.

Prior to blood draw, the patient should sit at rest for about 15 minutes in order to stabilize the orthostatic blood pressure. Both mental and physical stress before the drawing can influence the results; factor VIII (FVIII) and von Willebrand factor (VWF) can increase many times over in a stressful situation. Diurnal variations occur for several factors but are described in more detail for plasminogen activator inhibitor 1, PAI-1 (highest levels late at night).

Inflammation, infection, and surgery lead to increased levels, often for several weeks, of FVIII, VWF, PAI-1, and fibrinogen – all considered acute phase proteins. Smoking and age affect the levels of several factors (e.g., VWF and fibrinogen levels increase). Estrogen and high-dose contraceptives affect coagulation and fibrinolysis (e.g., FVIII, VWF, and fibrinogen are increased while antithrombin, protein C, and FVII are lowered). During normal pregnancy the levels of the inhibitors antithrombin and protein C remain within normal levels, while protein S decreases. At the same time, the thrombin markers (such as soluble fibrin and thrombin–antithrombin complexes) are increased, as are the plasminogen activator inhibitors 1 and 2.

Blood groups also influence the levels of FVIII and, to a greater degree, VWF, which are about 30% lower in blood group O. Thus, at the lower reference limit it is difficult to decide if the patient is healthy or has a mild form of VWD.

Other variables to consider

For most analyses of plasma samples, the patient should be fat-fasting for at least 6 hours; if testing for a bleeding diathesis, acetylsalicylic acid (ASA) and clopidogrel should be discontinued 7–10 days and NSAIDs 1–3 days prior to testing after consultation with and concurrence from the physician in charge of the patient. In fertile women, samples ought to be drawn on days 1–4 after the start of menstruation. Contraceptives and other hormone-containing drugs should be withdrawn at least 2 months before the blood draw. After pregnancy it is best to wait until breastfeeding has finished and menstrual cycles have been re-established. After a thromboembolic event, testing should be done at least 3 months after the last event, if possible, to avoid acute phase interaction. Testing in patients receiving heparin or vitamin K antagonist (VKA) drugs should be carried out in consultation with a hematologist specializing in blood coagulation.

It is preferable that most screening assays are performed on fresh plasma samples. The (activated) partial thromboplastin time [(a)PTT] is most sensitive to storage at room temperature and testing should be done within one hour after sampling. For other assays, the samples could be maintained at room temperature for a few hours without adversely affecting results. Samples for determination of fibrinogen should not be placed in

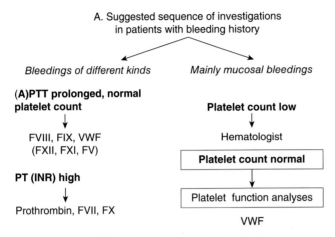

A. Suggested sequence of investigations
in patients with bleeding history

Bleedings of different kinds   *Mainly mucosal bleedings*

**(A)PTT prolonged, normal
platelet count**
↓   **Platelet count low**
                                         ↓
FVIII, FIX, VWF   Hematologist
(FXII, FXI, FV)
                                         Platelet count normal

PT (INR) high   ↓
↓   Platelet function analyses
Prothrombin, FVII, FX   VWF

B. Suggested sequence of investigations
in patients with history of thromboembolism

• Investigation of APC resistance/factor V Leiden mutation
• Determination of antithrombin, protein C, and protein S
• Global assay – indications of increased thrombin generation

Figure 3.1 (A) Suggested sequence of investigations in patients with bleeding history. (B) Suggested sequence of investigations in patients with history of thromboembolism.

the refrigerator, as there is a risk for cold precipitation of fibrinogen. Most specific hemostatic factors can be tested on plasma frozen within one hour of sampling. Most of the clotting assays mentioned below could give false pathological values if the samples are contaminated with heparin.

Figure 3.1 provides a summary of suggested sequence of investigations in patients with (a) bleeding history and (b) history of thromboembolism.

Screening for bleeding disorders

(Activated) partial thromboplastin time, (a)PTT

In a citrated plasma sample, coagulation is initiated by contact activation by means of addition of silica, kaolin, etc. After 1–5 minutes of contact activation calcium chloride is added to start the sequence of reactions leading to generation of thrombin and a final clot formation. Clot formation can be recorded photometrically or visually, and the time from addition of calcium to clot formation is measured. Clot formation can also be detected by mechanical means, and several types of widely used analyzers use the mechanical method. To obtain a normal PTT all reactions from initiation to fibrin formation should work normally. Experience has shown that most prolonged PTTs result from deficiencies of factors XII, XI, IX, and VIII. In patients developing circulating anticoagulants, prolonged PTTs are often the first signs of this complication. Lupus anticoagulants also often cause prolongation of PTT.

Prothrombin time, PT

Coagulation in a citrated whole blood or plasma sample is initiated by addition of tissue factor (TF), phospholipid, and calcium, leading to generation of thrombin and formation of a fibrin clot. Currently, recombinant tissue factor (rTF) is often used but many reagents include thromboplastin (TF plus phospolipid) extracted from human placenta or animal brain (ox or rabbit).

There are two types of PT assays, Quick and Owren types. The former uses plain and the latter combined thromboplastin reagents. The Owren reagent is supplemented with animal plasma (usually ox) adsorbed for factors VII, X, and prothrombin, and is, therefore, only sensitive to factors VII, X, and prothrombin; Quick assays are also sensitive to reduced levels of factor V and fibrinogen. The Quick assay should and the Owren assay could be calibrated according to a World Health Organization protocol or modifications thereof (international standards are available from the WHO) [2]. The Owren assay is however more easily calibrated by means of pooled normal plasma or certified calibrators [3].

It is of vital importance that the local reagent–instrument combination is properly calibrated, and results should be expressed as INR (international normalized ratio) in order to obtain reproducible results comparable between laboratories. Strictly, INR should only be used when monitoring coumarin/warfarin treatment, but INR is often also used for screening for factors VII, X, and prothrombin defects as well as for impaired liver synthesis. Results expressed as clotting times are sometimes used locally instead of the calculated INR. Circulating anticoagulants and lupus anticoagulants may also prolong the clotting time.

Fibrinogen

Plasma fibrinogen is most commonly measured in a clotting system where the thrombin-induced clotting time is inversely correlated to the fibrinogen concentration (Clauss assay). The assay ought to be standardized against an international standard. Fibrinogen can also be measured using commercial immunochemical methods. It may sometimes be of value to assess the level with an immunological method since the Clauss method can be influenced by fibrinolytic split products.

Hereditary fibrinogen deficiency is rare. Abnormal fibrinogens are sometimes revealed by a low plasma fibrinogen level, but are even more scarce than afibrinogenemia or hypofibrinogenemia.

Low plasma fibrinogen levels can also be seen in cases of consumption coagulopathies (e.g., disseminated intravascular coagulation; DIC) as well as after dramatic per- and postoperative bleeding or at post-traumatic bleeding.

The normal plasma level of fibrinogen is 2–4 g/L. It was, until recently, considered that 1 g/L was enough to maintain hemostasis. Optimal levels for different conditions cannot be stated. However, at least the lowest reference level ought to be attained.

Antithrombin

Antithrombin (AT) is the major inhibitor of thrombin but it also, to some extent, inhibits all other coagulation proteases except factor VIIa.

The concentration of antithrombin in plasma samples is generally measured after addition of a small amount of heparin in order to increase the reaction rate. Thrombin or factor Xa is usually added in excess and the residual enzymatic activity measured using a thrombin (or Xa) specific synthetic peptide substrate. There is an inverse relationship between antithrombin concentration and remaining thrombin activity.

Hereditary antithrombin deficiency is a relatively rare cause of thrombosis; the frequency of AT deficiency in thrombotic patient samples is 2–3%. Both arterial and venous thrombosis have been described.

AT is often consumed in DIC and the test is usually included among tests used for the diagnosis of DIC.

Fibrin D-dimer

Fibrin D-dimer is a fibrinolytic cleavage product that is immunochemically measured. It is liberated when plasmin cleaves fibrin wherever it is formed within the vascular network. All thrombotic episodes are supposedly accompanied by liberation of D-dimers but, since other deposits of fibrin generate D-dimers, the presence of D-dimers is not indicative of an ongoing thrombotic process. Consequently, the clinical relevance of measuring D-dimers is mostly to exclude the possibility of current thrombosis. A negative test practically excludes thrombosis. In case of a positive test there is reason for further investigation as to whether thrombosis could be the cause or not. Some investigators also find D-dimer a good test to include in a test battery for the diagnosis of DIC.

Screening for circulating anticoagulants

Circulating anticoagulants are commonly found in previously healthy individuals who unexpectedly develop bleeding that may be severe. An initial finding could be a clearly prolonged (a)PTT. A simple test for circulating anticoagulants would be to make a series of dilutions of patient plasma in normal plasma (e.g., 1 + 2, 1 + 4, 1 + 9 of patient to normal plasma, respectively). After dilution, (a)PTT assays are performed on these plasma mixtures. If there is an anticoagulant present the 1 + 9 dilution mostly gives a clearly prolonged clotting time. If only the 1 + 2 dilution gives a prolonged clotting time there are generally other causes for the prolonged (a)PTT.

Lupus anticoagulant

There are extensive international guidelines for the diagnosis of lupus anticoagulant (antibodies to protein–phospholipid complexes) [4]. A moderately or sometimes clearly prolonged (a)PTT is often the initial finding. Since these patients often have had thrombotic symptoms, it is essential to rule out heparin or coumarin treatment as a cause.

Platelet count

A platelet count should always be performed to rule out the possibility of thrombocytopenia as the cause of bleeding symptoms. A low platelet count should be further investigated by a hematologist.

Bleeding time

If there is a normal platelet count, a bleeding time (BT) could reveal a functional platelet disorder. Template bleeding time ("Ivy bleeding time") is the most commonly used technique, and commercial devices are available. However, bleeding times are difficult to standardize and several studies show inconsistent results.

Many argue that bleeding time should be avoided and replaced by other methods, but at present there are no simple methods available that have proven to give a relevant screening evaluation of the hemostatic function of platelets.

Specific blood coagulation factor analyses for diagnosis of bleeding disorders

Coagulation factor deficiencies

Hereditary, severe bleeding disorders are usually detected early (before 1 year of age) for hemophilia A (FVIII deficiency), hemophilia B (FIX deficiency), and severe VWD; more seldom for FV, FX and FXI deficiencies. Severe hereditary forms of FVII, prothrombin (FII), and fibrinogen deficiencies are seldom found. The severe form of FXIII deficiency is often observed neonatally as bleeding from the umbilical cord. FXI and FV deficiencies are normally detected later in life, unless a family history exists. Combined FV and FVIII deficiencies can result in neonatal bleeding. Hereditary deficiency of factor XII (Hageman factor) or factor XI, which initiate the intrinsic pathway of coagulation, may impair thrombus formation and protect from vascular events while having minimal impact on hemostasis [5].

Laboratory analyses of coagulation factor deficiencies

Factor deficiencies other than fibrinogen or FXIII deficiencies are investigated by utilizing an adapted PT (for factors II, V, VII, or X) or aPTT assay (for factors VIII, IX, XI, and XII). A so called one stage factor assay is essentially performed as follows: Serial dilutions of standard reference citrated plasma are made in plasma deficient in the factor being tested but with normal levels of other factors; this results in a standard curve of clotting time versus factor concentration. By replacing standard plasma with citrated plasma sample of the patient the resulting clotting times can be used to obtain the amount of factor present. Testing can be done manually or in a specially designed coagulation instrument. One, however, should be aware that the accuracy of this assay system decreases at very low factor concentrations (<1% of normal or <1 kIU/L) and more specialized analyses should be made. This is especially important for diagnosing severe hemophilia A, B, or VWD, as a small change in percentage at the low levels may indicate a requirement for different treatment regimes.

Laboratory analyses of von Willebrand disease

Von Willebrand disease (VWD) may be caused by quantitative (types 1 and 3) or qualitative (type 2) deficiencies of the von Willebrand factor (VWF). Type 2 can be divided into subtypes 2A ,2B, 2M, and 2N. Type 3 is a very severe disorder characterized by a prolonged bleeding time, very low VWF, and very low FVIII since VWF is a carrier protein for FVIII. Type 3 VWD is common in some fairly isolated parts of the world where intermarriage between relatives occurs. They are homozygous or compound heterozygous for different mutations. Type 1 patients are very common in several countries (1–2% of the population, mostly undiagnosed). Type 1 patients often have insignificant bleeding symptoms except for menorrhagia, bleeding postpartum, and bleeding with major surgery. The bleeding time is normal or only slightly prolonged. Studies indicate that patients with type 3 deficiency originate from two parents with type 1 VWD. A choice of various assays are employed in order to diagnose VWD.

Recommended analyses for von Willebrand disease

1. Bleeding time analysis (requires skilled personnel): This assay might have some relevance in revealing severe cases. However, it generally does not work in mild cases.
2. VWF:antigen can be measured by several immunological assays, such as electroimmunoassay, enzyme-linked immunosorbent assay (ELISA) and latex immunoassay (LIA). Antigen levels are undetectable in type 3 disease, decreased in type 1, decreased or normal in 2A, 2B, and 2M, but normal in type 2N disease.
3. Collagen binding assay (CBA) [6] measures the interaction of VWF and collagen and is based on a more physiological function. The levels are decreased in all types of VWD except type 2N.
4. The ristocetin cofactor (RCo) assay [6] measures VWF mediated agglutination of platelets in the presence of the antibiotic ristocetin, and has long been used to diagnose VWD.
5. However, a new assay has been introduced to replace the ristocetin cofactor assay. VWF binds to and agglutinates latex particles carrying antibodies to GP-Ibα coupled with recombinant GP-Ibα (the receptor for VWF on platelets). VWF present in the patient sample induces particle agglutination which is measured by turbidimetry [7].
6. VWF multimeric analysis is a method for analyzing the distribution and the structure of the VWF multimers in plasma. High-molecular-weight multimers have the greatest hemostatic capacity. The method is used to differentiate VWD type 1 and the different forms of VWD type 2. The analysis is carried out by electrophoresis of plasma samples using non-reducing agarose gels in the presence of sodium dodecyl sulfate (SDS); visualization of the VWF multimer pattern (see Figure 3.2) is accomplished by means of enzyme-linked antibodies against VWF [8].

Factor XIII

Factor XIII is a tetrameric zymogen (FXIII-A(2)B(2)) which is converted to an active transglutaminase (FXIIIa) by thrombin in the terminal phase of the clotting cascade. By cross-linking fibrin monomers with gamma-glutamyl-epsilon-lysyl amide bonds to fibrin polymers FXIIIa mechanically stabilizes fibrin and protects it from fibrinolysis. Severe deficiency is rare and characterized by delayed umbilical stump bleeding, spontaneous intracranial bleeding, as well as decreased fertility and increased frequency of abortions. FXIII is important for wound healing. Acquired FXIII deficiency has been observed in chronic inflammatory intestinal disorders. During recent years decreased FXIII levels have been found to be a reason for severe bleeding in trauma patients (often at the same time as a

medium resolution gel

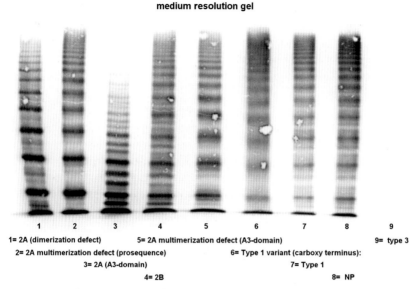

1 2 3 4 5 6 7 8 9

1= 2A (dimerization defect)   5= 2A multimerization defect (A3-domain)   9= type 3

2= 2A multimerization defect (prosequence)   6= Type 1 variant (carboxy terminus):

3= 2A (A3-domain)   7= Type 1

4= 2B   8= NP

Figure 3.2 Multimeric patterns of VWF. Source: Professor Ulrich Budde, Hamburg, Germany. Reproduced with permission of Professor Budde.

decreased fibrinogen level). A quantitative FXIII activity assay (e.g., chromogenic assay) is developed for the assay of FXIII activity [9].

Platelet aggregation

Though calcium is essential for normal platelet function, platelet aggregation can be induced and assessed by the addition of various agonists in citrated plasma. A platelet-rich plasma (PRP) sample is obtained by centrifuging whole blood at low g forces. A sample is spun at high speed in order to produce a platelet-poor plasma (PPP) sample. PRP is diluted with the PPP to a standardized platelet count, usually around 250×10^9/L. After calibrating the photometer/aggregometer – 100% light transmission with the PPP and 0% with the PRP – the response of the platelets to various agonists can be assessed. The most commonly used aggregating agents are adenosine diphosphate (ADP), epinephrine, collagen, arachidonic acid, and ristocetin. Often a reduced response to epinephrine can be seen, but such an isolated defect does not result in bleeding problems. In Glanzmann's thrombasthenia (absence of the GP-IIb/IIIa fibrinogen receptors), no aggregation response is seen to any of the aggregating agents. In Bernard–Soulier syndrome (absence of the GP-IbA/IX VWF receptors), no ristocetin-induced agglutination is seen. An absent response to arachidonic acid may indicate a defect in the metabolic pathway leading to generation of thromboxane.

For many years, platelet aggregation has also been evaluated by imped-ance aggregometry performed on whole blood. A few years ago a mul-tichannel instrument that could be used bedside was introduced under the trade name Multiplate. It has been found useful for the diagnosis of VWD as well as for evaluating the effects of various drugs interfering with plate-let function [10].

Formation of platelet aggregates can also be detected by assembling platelet aggregates on a filter. The number of aggregates formed is reflected by an increase in flow resistance through the filter (platelet function studied at high shear). This device, the Platelet Function Analyzer (PFA-100) has been found to be pretty useful for evaluating the platelet defect associated with VWD, both in diagnosis and in monitoring treatment [11].

Screening for thrombotic disorders

Protein C and protein S
In vivo, protein C is activated to activated protein C (APC) by thrombomodulin–thrombin complexes. However, the copperhead snake venom enzyme can also be used in vitro to activate protein C. APC is then measured by means of a chromogenic substrate. Monoclonal antibodies against protein C can be used for immunological assays of protein C, often using an enzyme-linked immunosorbent assay (ELISA).

Protein S acts as a cofactor to APC in its cleavage of factors V and VIII. Protein S circulates in blood both as a free, physiologically active entity and bound to C4b-binding protein. Some activity methods have been designed to evaluate the plasma level of free functional protein S. The cofactor function with regard to the APC degradation of factor V has been measured. However, the assays have not been easy to handle. ELISA-type assays are available where C4b binding protein has been bound to the plastic surface in order to catch free protein S in the sample. An enzyme-linked detecting antibody is then added. Free, functional protein S is easily measured in this way.

Activated protein C resistance
Resistance to activated protein C, APC-R, caused by the Leiden factor V mutation G1691A, was initially assessed by measuring the prolongation of an aPTT. However, these tests were found to be somewhat unreliable. Chromogenic assessments and genetic tests were then introduced. Various tests are available today in order to rapidly disclose whether the mutation in question is present or not. Among Caucasians the frequency of this mutation is 5–15%. Other mutations leading to APC-R have been found but are relatively rare.

However, acquired APC-R (often seen during pregnancy and treatment with estrogens) cannot, of course, be discovered with genetic testing. A functional test is necessary.

Thrombosis in rare disorders

Thrombotic phenomena have been described particularly in patients with afibrinogenemia, FXI and FVII deficiency. Congenital FVII deficiency has often given rise to thromboembolism; the mechanism still unclear.

Tissue factor pathway inhibitor

Tissue factor pathway inhibitor (TFPI) is a FXa-dependent inhibitor of the FVIIa–tissue factor complex that can be assessed by ELISA. Its role in thromboembolism is still uncertain.

Platelet-derived microparticles

During platelet activation or apoptosis microparticles, also known as microvesicles, are released from the cell membrane by a blebbing or shedding process, resulting in the generation of microparticles of 0.1–1.0 μm in diameter. Platelet-derived microparticles (PDMPs) are generally measured by means of flow fluorocytometry [12] and in order to differentiate PDMPs from other types of vesicles, platelet-specific membrane structures like GP-Ib (CD 42b) are identified with fluorochrome labeled monoclonal antibodies. PDMPs can thus be measured in blood as a marker of increased platelet activation. The function of PDMPs is still somewhat obscure but they certainly contribute to offer an extended phospholipid surface for coagulation enzymes to interact on. There are also reports that PDMPs can carry tissue factor most likely originating from other cell types such as monocytes and thereby stimulate blood coagulation.

Synthetic peptide chromogenic substrates for hemostatic assays

Chromogenic substrates for various hemostatic enzymes were developed in the 1970s. Most of them were constructed as oligopeptides (2–4 amino acids) coupled with para-nitroanilide (p-NA). Fluorogenic groups have also been used. All these synthetic substrates had high selectivity for their respective enzyme and high sensitivity. However, there were no assays like PT and (a)PTT constructed for chromogenic substrates and instruments for clotting assays were improving, which led to a limited use of the chromogenic assays. Anyhow, today there are a number chromogenic assays available and methods for antithrombin, protein C, α_2-plasmin inhibitor, factor VIII, heparins, and pentasaccharides [13,14] are in use. With the introduction of new specific enzyme inhibitors like thrombin and factor Xa inhibitors, one might expect an increased use of chromogenic substrates for evaluation of the functional plasma levels of these inhibitors.

Global assays

Assays for single coagulation factors and inhibitors can sometimes not reliably estimate the risk of bleeding. In some situations global assays are of help, for example, when there is a need for monitoring therapy for bleeding complications after major surgery or severe trauma.

Blood viscosity increases as the fibrin network forms; the elasticity of the clot depends on the contractile force exerted by the platelets, platelet function and concentration, the hematocrit, the fibrinogen concentration, and the thrombin generation during coagulation. Different methods and instruments have been described for the measurement of these functions. Whole blood thromboelastography (TEG) and thromboelastometry (ROTEM) provide global information on the dynamics of clot development, stabilization, and dissolution that reflect in vivo hemostasis. These methods seem to be useful in reducing blood component therapy and blood loss. The movement of the blood is initiated either from a cup (TEG) or a pin (ROTEM). Different triggers, for example, tissue factor, can be used depending on the aim of measurement. Free oscillation rheometry, a new technology, can measure both viscosity (in contrast to TEG and ROTEM) and elasticity in whole blood and in dissolving clots. In the instrument ReoRox oscillation is initiated by a forced turn of the sample cup and, after a short time, the sample cup is released, allowing rotational oscillation with very low friction around the longitudinal axis. The frequency and amplitude will be influenced by the viscoelastic properties of the sample. Gold-plated reaction chambers are used to avoid detachment from the cup wall due to clot retraction when determining the coagulum elasticity [15].

A very interesting method to assess whether a hypercoagulable or hypocoagulable state exists has been developed by the Hemker group. Thrombin is measured as it develops and disappears in clotting plasma by the conversion of an added fluorogenic thrombin-specific substrate. The thrombin concentrations are obtained by comparison to a fixed known thrombin activity in a parallel experiment (calibrated automated thrombinography; CAT). The main parameters of the thrombin curve are: lag-time (time needed to obtain thrombin detected), thrombin peak, and area under the curve (i.e., the endogenous thrombin potential; ETP). The method has been proven to be useful in determining thrombotic risk, the risk of bleeding, and in measuring the effect of antithrombotics [16].

A global assay for evaluation of the coagulation and the fibrinolytic capacity in a patient plasma sample was developed at our laboratory. We calculate the overall hemostatic potential, OHP, as the area under the curve after initiating coagulation with a small amount of thrombin; by adding a small amount of tPA the fibrinolytic capacity can be evaluated [17]. The method was refined by adding TF and purified phospholipids instead of thrombin, in order to make it more physiologic; a coagulation and a fibrinolytic profile were determined [18].

The fibrinolytic system

The fibrinolytic system clears the vascular tree from obstructive thrombotic material. However, necessary fibrin networks protecting leakage from the vascular bed must be preserved in order to provide a framework into which cells can grow in order to heal the damaged area. Consequently, the fibrinolytic system has to be strictly regulated by effective enzyme inhibitors.

Plasminogen
Plasminogen is the key proenzyme in the fibrinolytic system. Tissue plasminogen activator (tPA) is the enzyme that activates plasminogen to plasmin. Plasminogen and tPA both have lysine binding sites that bind them to fibrin (clots) whereby the enzyme and its substrate come into proximity. Activation can take place. The fibrin-bound plasmin is, to some extent, protected from being inhibited by α_2-plasmin inhibitor, a fast reacting enzyme inhibitor. Plasminogen in plasma is easily determined by means of plasmin-sensitive chromogenic substrates after activation of plasmin by, for example, streptokinase.

α_2-Plasmin inhibitor
α_2-Plasmin inhibitor is also determined by chromogenic assays where excess plasmin is added to the sample and residual plasmin activity measured.

Tissue plasminogen activator
Tissue plasminogen activator (tPA) is a blood protein involved in the breakdown of blood clots. To assess the tPA levels, tPA in the sample is allowed to activate plasminogen added to the system in the presence of fibrin monomers. The assay measures the ability of tPA to activate plas-

minogen to plasmin by quantifying it using a chromogenic plasmin-sensitive substrate.

Tissue plasminogen activator inhibitor, PAI-1

Tissue plasminogen activator inhibitor, PAI-1 is the most important inhibitor of the fibrinolytic system. It is usually measured in a semi-immunological assay where tPA has been bound to a plastic surface and, thereafter, PAI-1 from the sample is allowed to react with the bound tPA. After washing, a monoclonal enzyme-linked antibody against PAI-1 is added and, after subsequent addition of a suitable enzyme substrate, the concentration of PAI-1 is estimated. This type of assay gives a good view of the available functional PAI-1 level in plasma. (There are also latent and inactive forms of PAI-1 in plasma.)

Thrombin activatable fibrinolytic inhibitor

Thrombin activatable fibrinolytic inhibitor (TAFI) is an enzyme (carboxypeptidase) described as an inhibitor to fibrinolysis; it can be regarded as a link between coagulation and fibrinolysis. It is decreased in hemophilia, in liver cirrhosis, and in DIC, and increased in APC resistance. Methods to determine TAFI levels include immunochemical (ELISA) and functional assays (retardation of clot lysis).

References

1. Blombäck M, Konkle BA, Manco-Johnson MJ, et al. ISTH SSC Subcommittee on Women's Health Issues. Preanalytical conditions that affect coagulation testing, including hormonal status and therapy. *J Thromb Haemost* 2007;5:855–8.
2. Ibrahim SA, Jespersen J, Pattison A, et al. Evaluation of European Concerted Action on Anticoagulation lyophilized plasmas for INR derivation using the PT/INR line. *Am J Clin Pathol* 2011;135:732–40.
3. Lindahl TL, Egberg N, Hillarp A, et al. INR calibration of Owren-type prothrombin time based on the relationship between PT% and INR utilizing normal plasma samples. *Thromb Haemost* 2004;91:1223–31.
4. Pengo V, Tripodi A, Reber G, et al. Update of the guidelines for lupus anticoagulant detection. Subcommittee on Lupus Anticoagulant/Antiphospholipid Antibody of the Scientific and Standardisation Committee of the International Society on Thrombosis and Haemostasis. *J Thromb Haemost* 2009;7:1737–40.
5. Müller F, Gailani D, Renné T. Factor XI and XII as antithrombotic agents. *Curr Opin Hematol* 2011;18:349–55.
6. Turecek PL, Siekmann J, Schwarz HP. Comparative study on collagen-binding enzyme-linked immunosorbent assay and ristocetin cofactor activity assays for detection of functional activity of von Willebrand factor. *Semin Thromb Hemost* 2002;28:149–60.
7. Patzke J, Schneppenheim R. Laboratory diagnosis of von Willebrand disease. *Hamostaseologie* 2010;30:204–6 (*see* reference #24).

8. Budde U, Schneppenheim R, Eikenboom J, et al. Detailed von Willebrand factor multimer analysis in patients with von Willebrand disease in the European study, Molecular and Clinical Markers for the Diagnosis and Management of Type 1 von Willebrand disease (MCMDM-1VWD). *J Thromb Haemost* 2008;6:762–71.

9. Karpati K, Penke B, Katona E, et al. A modified, optimized kinetic photometric assay for the determination of blood coagulation factor XIII activity in plasma. *Clin Chem* 2000;46:1946–55.

10. Valarche V, Desconclois C, Boutekedjiret T, et al. Multiplate whole blood impedance aggregometry: a new tool for von Willebrand disease. *J Thromb Haemost* 2011;9: 1645–7.

11. Cattaneo M, Federici AB, Lecchi A, et al. Evaluation of the PFA 100 system in the diagnosis and therapeutic monitoring of patients with von Willebrand disease. *Thromb Haemost* 1999;82:35–9.

12. Mobarrez F, Antovic J, Egberg N, et al. A multicolor flow cytometric assay for measurement of platelet-derived microparticles. *Thromb Res* 2010;125:110–6.

13. Blombäck M, Egberg N. *Chromogenic peptide substrates in the laboratory diagnosis of clotting disorders*. In Bloom A, Thomas D (eds), *Haemostasis and Thrombosis*. Edinburgh: Churchill Livingstone, 1986/1987;967–81.

14. Rosén S. Chromogenic methods in coagulation diagnostics. *Hämostaseologie* 2005;25:259–66.

15. Lindahl TL, Ramström S. Methods for evaluation of platelet function. *Trans Apher Sci* 2009;41:121–5.

16. Hemker HC, Al Dieri R, Béguin S. Thrombin generation assays: accruing clinical relevance. *Curr Opin Hematol* 2004;11:170–5.

17. He S, Antovic A, Blombäck M. A simple and rapid laboratory method for determination of haemostasis potential in plasma. II. Modifications for use in routine laboratories and research work. *Thromb Res* 2001;103:355–61.

18. Leander K, Blombäck M, Wallen H, He S. Impaired fibrinolytic capacity and increased fibrin formation associate with myocardial infarction. *Thromb Haemost* 2012; 107:1092–9.

CHAPTER 4

Factor VIII Deficiency or Hemophilia A: Clinical Bleeding and Management

Pier Mannuccio Mannucci[1] and Massimo Franchini[2]
[1] Scientific Direction, IRCCS Cà Granda Foundation Maggiore Policlinico Hospital, Milan, Italy
[2] Department of Transfusion Medicine and Hematology, C. Poma Hospital, Mantova, Italy

Introduction

Hemophilia A is an X-chromosome-linked coagulation disorder included among the rare diseases and caused by mutations in the factor VIII (FVIII) gene [1–3], an essential component of the intrinsic pathway of blood coagulation. The incidence of hemophilia A is 1 in 5000 male live births and affected individuals have severe, moderate, and mild forms of the disease, defined by FVIII plasma levels of less than 1%, 1 to 5%, and 6 to 30%, respectively [1,2].

Hemophilia was recognized in ancient times. The *Talmud*, a collection of Jewish rabbinical writings from the second century AD, stated that male boys should not be circumcised if two brothers had already died owing to excessive bleeding from the procedure. The Arabic physician Albucasis, who lived in the 12th century, described a family where males died from bleeding after trivial injury [3]. The first modern description of hemophilia is that by John Conrad Otto, a physician from Philadelphia, who in 1803 published a treatise entitled "An account of an hemorrhagic disposition existing in certain families" [4]. He clearly appreciated the three cardinal features of hemophilia (i.e., an inherited tendency of males to bleed). However, the first use of the word "hemophilia" appears in a description of the condition written in 1828 by Hopff from the University of Zurich.

Although clinically indistinguishable from hemophilia A and also transmitted by X-chromosome inheritance, hemophilia B (Christmas disease) is differentiated from the former disease since it is the result of deficiency

Hemostasis and Thrombosis: Practical Guidelines in Clinical Management, First Edition.
Hussain I. Saba and Harold R. Roberts.
© 2014 John Wiley & Sons, Ltd. Published 2014 by John Wiley & Sons, Ltd.

of factor IX, another component of the intrinsic coagulation pathway [2]. Hemophilia B was distinguished from the more common hemophilia A only in 1952 [5], and it has been recently demonstrated that Victoria, Queen of England from 1837 to 1901, was a hemophilia B carrier and thus was instrumental in transmitting the disease on to the British, Spanish, German, and Russian royal families [6].

Factor VIII is a plasma glycoprotein consisting of six domains, A1-A2-B-A3-C1-C2. The encoding gene is located on the long arm of the X chromosome (Xq28). The mature protein is a heterodimer with a light chain consisting of domains A3-C1-C2 and a heavy chain with the domains A1-A2-B. The majority of FVIII is thought to be synthesized in liver sinusoidal cells. Multiple mutations leading to hemophilia A have been described on the FVIII gene: the most common genetic defect, affecting about 45% of individuals with severe disease, is a large inversion and translocation of exons 1 or 22 (together with introns), which completely disrupts the gene. Patients with mutations that severely truncate or prevent production of FVIII (intron 1 and 22 inversions, large deletions, non-sense mutations) are more susceptible to the development of FVIII alloantibodies than those carrying missense mutations and small deletions [7].

The diagnosis of hemophilia A should be suspected whenever unusual bleeding occurs in a male and is supported by the results of screening laboratory tests, including a prolonged partial thromboplastin time (aPTT), contrasting with a normal platelet count, prothrombin time (PT), and bleeding time, but the definitive diagnosis relies on the assay for FVIII coagulant activity.

Clinical manifestations of hemophilia A

It is not surprising that the large number of different molecular defects in the FVIII gene responsible for hemophilia A account for the clinical heterogeneity of this hemorrhagic disorder. It can be generally assumed that the clinical features of hemophilia A correlate with FVIII levels. Thus, patients with a mild form of the disease (6–30% of the normal FVIII activity) rarely have unprovoked hemorrhages and usually experience major bleeding only with trauma or surgery. By contrast, patients with moderate disease (1–5% of the normal FVIII activity) will occasionally have spontaneous hemorrhages, and patients with severe disease (<1% of the normal FVIII activity) will develop spontaneous hemorrhages since early infancy, usually at the time of starting to walk (Table 4.1). The clinical hallmarks of hemophilia A are joint and muscle hemorrhages, easy

Table 4.1 Clinical classification of hemophilia: correlation with factor VIII activity.

Coagulation factor activity (%)	Clinical manifestations
<1 (severe disease)	Recurrent spontaneous bleeding episodes
	Frequent spontaneous hemarthroses
1–5 (moderate disease)	Occasional spontaneous bleeding
	Post-surgical or post-traumatic bleeding
6–30 (mild disease)	Post-surgical or post-traumatic bleeding

bruising, and prolonged and potentially fatal hemorrhage after trauma or surgery. The joints most frequently involved are the knees, elbows, ankles, shoulders, and hips [2]. Hemarthroses usually begin with mild discomfort and a slight limitation of the joint motion, followed by pain, swelling, and cutaneous warmth. If untreated, joint hemorrhage will usually lead to severe limitation of motion. Unfortunately, the pathologic processes continue after bleeding stops, because inflammation causes damage to the blood-filled joints leading to synovitis, which in turn increases the likelihood of more frequent hemarthroses in target joints. The final step of this vicious circle that characterizes hemophilic arthropathy is the narrowing of the joint space due to loss of cartilage, development of bone cysts, and limitation of motion resulting in permanent disability. Intramuscular hematomas can cause severe problems by compressing vital structures [3]. Closed-space bleeding is especially dangerous, since it can lead to nerve paralysis or to vascular or airway obstruction. Bleeding into the iliopsoas muscle is a typical complication of hemophilia. Hematomas in this muscle may lead to contracture, nerve palsies, and atrophy. Hemorrhage into the central nervous system is the most dangerous hemorrhagic event in these patients, requiring urgent management. Intracranial bleeding may be unprovoked, but in approximately half of cases a previous trauma can be recognized [8]. Symptoms often occur soon after trauma, but sometimes bleeding is delayed as, for example, in the case of a subdural hematoma. Thus, hemophilic patients with unexplained and persistent headaches should always be suspected of hemorrhage in the brain parenchyma, or a subdural or an epidural hematoma. Almost all severely affected hemophilic patients experience during their life at least one episode of spontaneous hematuria that is usually episodic and painless unless intraureteral clots produce renal colic. Finally, carrier females with low FVIII levels in the range of mild hemophilia may experience bleeding symptoms such as menorrhagia, oral bleeding, and surgical and trauma-related bleeding.

Management of hemophilia A

Replacement therapy with intravenously delivered FVIII concentrates aimed at correcting the coagulation factor deficiency is the cornerstone of hemophilia A management. In addition, the administration of desmopressin (DDAVP) may be useful in milder forms.

Desmopressin

Desmopressin (1-deamino-8-D-arginine vasopressin) is a synthetic analogue of the antidiuretic hormone vasopressin, which was originally developed for the treatment of diabetes insipidus [9,10]. DDAVP has been successfully used for more than 25 years in patients with mild hemophilia A to prevent or treat bleeding episodes [9]. However, its clinical usefulness is highly correlated with the postinfusion plasma levels of FVIII, which in turn depends on the patient's basal FVIII. Hence, mild hemophilia A patients should undergo a test infusion with DDAVP prior to therapeutic use. This is particularly true for children where a lower response rate to DDAVP may be evident when compared with adults [11]. It is generally agreed that a FVIII postinfusion level of at least 30% should be sufficient for the treatment of minor bleeding or for minor surgery, such as dental extractions. On the other hand, a level higher than 50% post-administration is required for treatment of major surgery. Unfortunately, repeated administrations of DDAVP over a short time period may induce tachyphylaxis and hamper its clinical efficacy. The optimal dose of DDAVP to achieve maximum FVIII response is $0.3 \mu g/kg$ intravenously, giving a 2–4 times increase of FVIII levels over baseline within one hour after completion of the infusion, the circulating FVIII half-life being approximately 5–8 hours. Doses can be repeated at 12- to 24-hour intervals if needed, though tachyphylaxis may occur, but a single dose may be sufficient for the management of minor surgical interventions [9]. Subcutaneous injection at the same dose ($0.3 \mu g/kg$) produces a similar, although more delayed, FVIII response to that seen with intravenous infusion. Intranasal DDAVP can also be used, although this product is not available in all countries [12]. DDAVP usage has a few, self-limited and minor side-effects including facial flushing, headache, a small decrease in blood pressure, and an increase in heart rate. Furthermore, the drug should be administered cautiously in young children due to their increased risk of hyponatremia [12]. There are some concerns regarding the use of DDAVP in pregnant symptomatic hemophilia A carriers as it may cause placental insufficiency because of vasoconstriction, miscarriage due to an oxytocic effect, and maternal/neonatal hyponatremia. However, the results of a survey on the use of DDAVP in 32 pregnant

FVIII-deficient women indicate that DDAVP can be safely used during the first two trimesters of pregnancy [13].

Factor VIII replacement therapy

The modern management of hemophilia started in the 1970s, when the increased availability of lyophilized plasma concentrates of coagulation factors and the widespread adoption of home replacement therapy led to the early control of hemorrhages and the reduction of the musculoskeletal damage typical until then of untreated or poorly treated patients. Primary prophylaxis (i.e., the regular infusion of factor concentrate) was successfully pioneered in Sweden and then adopted in other countries, achieving the goal of preventing the majority of bleeding episodes and further reducing the impact of arthropathy [14]. Specialized hemophilia centers became less overwhelmed by the burden of providing emergency treatment and could develop programs of comprehensive care, with the involvement of such specialists as orthopedic surgeons, physiotherapists, dentists, and social workers. Elective surgery, particularly orthopedic operations, became possible and safe, and helped to correct or minimize the musculoskeletal abnormalities that had developed as a consequence of untreated or inadequately treated bleeding episodes into joints and muscles.

This optimistic perception of hemophilia changed dramatically in the early 1980s, at a time when 60–70% of patients with severe disease became infected with the human immunodeficiency virus (HIV) that had contaminated coagulation factor concentrates. Almost all treated hemophilic patients were also infected with the hepatitis C virus (HCV) (at that time called the non-A, non-B hepatitis virus) that was transmitted by factor concentrates manufactured from plasma pooled from thousands of donors [15]. As a consequence of the devastating sequelae of the acquired immunodeficiency syndrome (AIDS) and hepatitis epidemics, the need for a safe treatment became crucial for the hemophilia community. The implementation of purification (cryoprecipitation, ion exchange, gel permeation, or monoclonal antibody immunoaffinity chromatography), viral inactivation (solvent detergent, heat treatment/pasteurization) or removal (ultrafiltration) techniques for the production of plasma-derived factor concentrates, as well as the adoption of new methods to screen viruses in blood donation (i.e., nucleic acid testing; NAT), greatly improved the safety of plasma-derived products, as shown by the fact that blood-borne transmission of hepatitis viruses or HIV has not occurred during the last 20–25 years [16]. According to the techniques of purification, plasma-derived FVIII concentrates are classified as high purity or intermediate purity. As the latter also contain von Willebrand factor (VWF), they may be useful for the treatment of von Willebrand disease (VWD).

However, the most important advance in this field was represented by the rapid progress in DNA technology (following the cloning in 1984 of the FVIII gene), which allowed the industrial production of recombinant FVIII, culminating with the publication in 1989 of the first report of clinical efficacy of this product in two patients with hemophilia A [17]. Three different generations of recombinant FVIII products were produced. The first generation of full-length recombinant FVIII products used animal-derived proteins in the cell culture medium, and had human serum albumin added to stabilize the final formulation. Second-generation products used human-derived proteins in the culture medium but had no albumin added to the final formulation, and the production process included a solvent/detergent viral inactivation step to further enhance the safety of recombinant FVIII replacement therapy. Finally, third-generation recombinant FVIII products have now been developed that are manufactured without albumin in either the culture medium or the final formulation [18]. Second- and third-generation recombinant FVIII products may be full-length or lacking in the B-domain, which is disposable for the coagulant activity of the FVIII molecule. Table 4.2 reports the main characteristics of plasma-derived and recombinant FVIII products.

The availability of replacement therapy of high-quality factor concentrates has been important not only for reducing the likelihood of death from hemorrhage but also for the broad implementation of prophylactic treatment regimens in order to prevent bleeding and resultant joint damage, that ultimately allows patients to maintain a near normal lifestyle [19]. This fact, together with progress in the management of the blood-borne viral infections through surveillance of patients with chronic hepatitis (especially with respect to the development of hepatocellular carcinoma and liver failure), the availability of newer treatment options such as antiviral treatment against HIV (highly active antiretroviral therapy; HAART) and HCV (combined therapy with α-interferon,d riba-virin, and liver transplantation), has greatly contributed to the improved quality of life and reduced morbidity in the hemophilia population [20]. Thus, the last 10–15 years represent a "golden era" in hemophilia treatment, with a life expectancy for these patients that progressively approaches that of males in the general population, at least in high- and middle-income countries [20].

Whether purified from human donor plasma or from recombinant DNA expression systems, the primary indication for the administration of FVIII products is the prevention of bleeding episodes. Short-term prophylaxis encompasses the infusion of FVIII concentrate to assure adequate hemostasis during surgical or invasive procedures. According to the current

Table 4.2 Main characteristics of licensed plasma-derived and recombinant factor VIII concentrates.

Plasma-derived factor VIII concentrates			
Product	Manufacturer	Fractionation method	Viral inactivation
Alphanate	Alpha Therapeutics	Heparin ligand chromatography	SD + dry heat (80°C, 72 h)
Beriate	CSL Behring	IE chromatography	Pasteurization (60°C, 10 h)
Biostate	CSL Bioplasma	Heparin/glycine precipitation + gel filtration	SD + dry heat (80°C, 72 h)
Emoclot	Kedrion	IE chromatography	SD + dry heat (100°C, 30 m)
Fanhdi	Grifols	Heparin ligand chromatography	SD + dry heat (80°C, 72 h)
Haemate P	CSL Behring	Multiple precipitation	Pasteurization (60°C, 10 h)
Haemoctin SDH	Biotest	IE chromatography	SD + dry heat (100°C, 30 m)
Hemofil M	Baxter	IA chromatography	SD
Immunate	Baxter	IE chromatography	SD + vapor heat (60°C, 10 h)
Koate-DVI	Talecris	Multiple precipitation + size exclusion	SD + dry heat (80°C, 72 h)
Wilate	Octapharma	IE + size exclusion chromatography	SD + dry heat (100°C, 2 h)

Recombinant factor VIII concentrates					
Product	Manufacturer	Host cell line	FVIII molecule	FVIII stabilizer	Purification/ viral inactivation
First generation					
Recombinate	Baxter Healthcare	CHO	Full-length	Human albumin	IA/IE
Second generation					
Kogenate FS/ Helixate FS	Bayer Healthcare CSL Behring	BHK	Full-length	Sucrose	IA/IE/SD/UF
Refacto	Wyeth Pharmaceuticals	CHO	BDD	Sucrose	IA/IE/SD
Third generation					
Advate	Baxter Healthcare	CHO	Full-length	Trehalose	IA/IE/SD
Xyntha/ Refacto AF	Pfizer	CHO	BDD	Sucrose	IA/IE/SD/NF

BDD, B-domain-deleted; BHK, baby hamster kidney; CHO, Chinese hamster ovary; IA, immunoaffinity; IE, ion exchange; NF, nanofiltration; rFVIII, recombinant factor VIII; SD, solvent/ detergent treatment; UF, ultrafiltration.

Table 4.3 Recommended dosages of factor VIII concentrates for the treatment and prevention of bleeding episodes in hemophilia A patients.

Type of hemorrhage	Factor VIII dose (U/kg)
Mild/moderate hemarthroses or hematomas	20–30
Severe hemarthroses or hematomas; external bleeding with anemia; moderate post-traumatic bleeding	30–50
Cranial trauma; cerebral hemorrhage	50–100
Surgery prophylaxis	50–100 (maintain FVIII levels above 50% for 7–15 days after surgery)

definitions and with the aim of preserving joint structure and function, primary prophylaxis is intended as a regular continuous long-term treatment (at a dose of 25–30 U/kg three times/week), started before the age of 2 years and/or after no more than one joint bleed, whereas secondary prophylaxis includes all long-term regular treatments not fulfilling these criteria [21]. While primary prophylaxis is recommended as the first choice of treatment of severe hemophilia by the World Health Organization (WHO) and the World Federation of Hemophilia (WFH) [22], there is increasing evidence of the benefits of secondary prophylaxis in improving quality of life [23,24].

Table 4.3 summarizes the recommended dosages of FVIII concentrates for the treatment and prevention of bleeding episodes in hemophilia A patients.

Management of factor VIII inhibitors

The development of inhibitory alloantibodies against FVIII is actually the most challenging complication of therapy. Indeed, these inhibitors, which develop in approximately 25–30% of severe hemophilia A patients, render replacement therapies ineffective, limit patient access to a safe and effective standard of care, and predispose them to an increased risk of morbidity and mortality [25]. In addition, the management of hemophilia complicated by inhibitors requires high amounts of resources [26]. A number of studies have revealed the importance of genetic (e.g,, ethnicity, FVIII gene mutations, major histocompatibility complex genotype, polymorphisms of immune response genes) and circumstantial (e.g., number of FVIII exposure-days, age at first exposure to FVIII concentrate, type of FVIII concentrate administered, and modality of treatment) risk factors in the development of inhibitors, confirming that inhibitor formation in hemophilia is a complex multifactorial process [27].

The introduction of bypassing agents, such as activated prothrombin complex concentrates (APCC) first (Factor Eight Inhibitor Bypassing Activity – FEIBA, administered at a dose of 70–100 U/kg every 8–12 hours) and recombinant activated factor VII (rFVIIa, NovoSeven, administered at a dose of 90–120 µg/kg every 2–3 hours), has dramatically improved the management of acute bleeding in inhibitor patients, allowing home treatment and a substantial amelioration of their quality of life. Both products have been found to be quite effective in the control of bleeding episodes in patients with inhibitors [28]. Increasing evidence suggests that a single dose of 270 µg/kg rFVIIa may be a convenient, safe, and effective alternative to the repeat-dose regimen for hemophilia patients with inhibitors, reducing, especially in children, the difficulties caused by the need for repeated venous access [29,30].

Immune tolerance induction (ITI) through the long-term intensive treatment of patients with replacement therapy with large doses of coagulation factors is actually the best method to eradicate inhibitors. In the last few years, a number of large-scale prospective randomized trials have been launched with the aim of resolving one of the unanswered questions on ITI, namely the optimal ITI regimen. However, the International Immune Tolerance Induction (I-ITI) study [31], aimed at evaluating the success rate and time to success in 150 patients with good prognostic profile (historical peak titer ≥ 5 BU and ≤ 200 BU; starting titer < 10 BU) randomized to receive FVIII doses of 50 IU/kg three times weekly or 200 IU/kg daily, was interrupted prematurely because of safety concerns. Indeed, a significantly greater cumulative number of bleeding episodes in joint and non-joint sites was indeed observed in the low-dose arm than in the high-dose arm, at all stages of ITI, but particularly in the first ITI phase, when inhibitors were still detectable [32]. At study termination, although ITI success rates were not different in the two treatment arms, median time to achieve negative inhibitor titer and normal FVIII recovery were significantly shorter (about 50%) in patients receiving the high-dose regimen. Thus, the earlier attainment of tolerance with the higher dosage (and hence of measurable FVIII levels in plasma) perhaps explains the difference in the number of bleeding episodes between the two arms. A number of clinical studies have also explored the role of the FVIII source in ITI, and some clinical experience in Europe and the United States suggests that FVIII products rich in VWF may increase the likelihood of successful ITI [33,34].

The future of treatment

The most likely progress in this field will be in the availability of FVIII molecules with longer half-lives. This would be a significant step forward, considering that, in countries that can afford primary prophylaxis, the main obstacles to its widespread adoption are problems related to venous access. Several pharmaceutical companies are currently developing factors with a longer half-life to obviate frequent administration [35,36]. The main strategies being applied to FVIII include modifications of the molecule, such as the addition of polyethylene glycol (PEG) polymers or polysialic acids. Improved pharmacokinetic properties of recombinant clotting factors have also been obtained through genetic engineering modification by fusion with carrier proteins such as albumin and Fc region of immunoglobulin G.

Finally, studies in hemophilia B patients using gene therapy, the definitive cure for hemophilia, recently resumed after an initial halt due to concerns regarding the safety of this procedure [37].

References

1. Mannucci PM, Tuddenham EGD. The hemophiliac – from royal genes to gene therapy. *N Engl J Med* 2001;344:1773–9.
2. Bolton-Maggs PH, Pasi KJ. Hemophilias A and B. *Lancet* 2003;361:1801–9.
3. Hoyer LH. Hemophilia A. *N Engl J Med* 1994;330:38–47.
4. Otto JC. An account of an hemorrhagic disposition existing in certain families. *Med Repos* 1803;6:1–4.
5. Biggs R, Douglas AS, Macfarlane RG, et al. Christmas disease: a condition previously mistaken for haemophilia. *Br Med J* 1952;ii:1378–82.
6. Rogaev EI, Grigorenko AP, Faskhutdinova G, et al. Genotype analysis identifies the cause of the "royal disease". *Science* 2009;326:817.
7. Oldenburg J, Schwaab R. Molecular biology of blood coagulation. *Semin Thromb Hemost* 2001;27:313–24.
8. Martinowitz U, Heim M, Tadmor R, et al. Intracranial hemorrhage in patients with hemophilia. *Neurosurgery* 1986;18:538–41.
9. Mannucci PM. Desmopressin (DDAVP) in the treatment of bleeding disorders: the first twenty years. *Haemophilia* 2000;6(suppl.1):60–7.
10. Franchini M. The use of desmopressin as a hemostatic agent. *Am J Hematol* 2007;82:731–5.
11. Revel-Vilk S, Blanchette VS, Sparling C, et al. DDAVP challenge tests in boys with mild/moderate haemophilia A. *Br J Haematol* 2002;117:947–51.
12. Lethagen S. Desmopressin in mild hemophilia A: indications, limitations, efficacy, and safety. *Semin Thromb Hemost* 2003;29:101–6.
13. Mannucci PM. Use of desmopressin (DDAVP) during early pregnancy in FVIII-deficient women. *Blood* 2005;105:3382.
14. Nilsson IM. Experience with prophylaxis in Sweden. *Semin Hematol* 1993; 30:16–19.

15. Mannucci PM. Hemophilia: treatment options on the twenty-first century. *J Thromb Haemost* 2005;1:1349–55.
16. Mannucci PM. Back to the future: a recent history of haemophilia treatment. *Haemophilia* 2008;14:10–18.
17. White GC, McMillan CW, Kingdon HS, Shoemaker CB. Use of recombinant antihemophilic factor in the treatment of two patients with classic hemophilia. *N Engl J Med* 1989;320:166–70.
18. Franchini M, Lippi G. Recombinant FVIII products. *Semin Thromb Hemost* 2010; 36:537–49.
19. Franchini M, Mannucci PM. Co-morbidities and quality of life in elderly persons with haemophilia. *Br J Haematol* 2010;148:522–33.
20. Tagliaferri A, Rivolta GF, Iorio A, et al. Italian Association of Hemophilia Centers: Mortality and causes of death in Italian persons with haemophilia, 1990–2007. *Haemophilia* 2010;16:437–46.
21. Berntorp E, Astermark J, Bjorkman S, et al. Consensus perspectives on prophylaxis therapy for haemophilia: summary statement. *Haemophilia* 2003;9:1–4.
22. Berntorp E, Boulyjenkov V, Brettler D, et al. Modern treatment of haemophilia. *Bull World Health Organ* 1995;73:691–701.
23. Coppola A, Franchini M, Tagliaferri A. Prophylaxis in people with hemophilia. *Thromb Haemost* 2009;101:674–81.
24. Gringeri A, Lundin B, Von Mackensen S, et al. The ESPRIT Study Group. A randomized clinical trial of prophylaxis in children with hemophilia A (the ESPRIT Study). *J Thromb Haemost* 2011;9:700–10.
25. Franchini M, Mannucci PM. Inhibitors of propagation of coagulation (factors VIII, IX and XI): a review of current therapeutic practice. *Br J Clin Pharmacol* 2011;72: 553–62.
26. Gringeri A, Mantovani LG, Scalone L, Mannucci PM. COCIS Study Group. Cost of care and quality of life for patients with hemophilia complicated by inhibitors: the COCIS Study Group. *Blood* 2003;102:2358–63.
27. Astermark J. Overview of inhibitors. *Semin Hematol* 2006;43:S3–7.
28. Franchini M, Mannucci PM. Past, present and future of hemophilia treatment: a narrative review. *Orphanet J Rare Dis* 2012;7:24.
29. Santagostino E, Mancuso ME, Rocino A, et al. A prospective randomized trial of high and standard dosages of recombinant factor VIIa for treatment of hemarthroses in hemophiliacs with inhibitors. *J Thromb Haemost* 2006;4:367–71.
30. Kavakli K, Makris M, Zulfikar B, et al. NovoSeven trial (F7HAEM-1510) investigators. Home treatment of haemarthroses using a single dose regimen of recombinant activated factor VII in patients with haemophilia and inhibitors: a multi-centre, randomised, double-blind, cross-over trial. *Thromb Haemost* 2006;95:600–5.
31. DiMichele DM, Hay CR. The international immune tolerance study: a multicenter prospective randomized trial in progress. *J Thromb Haemost* 2006;4:2271–3.
32. DiMichele DM, Goldberg I, Foulkes M, Hay CRM, on behalf of the International Immune Tolerance Study Group. International prospective randomized immune tolerance (ITI) study: preliminary results of therapeutic efficacy and safety [abstract 07S03]. *Haemophilia* 2010;16:29.
33. Kaveri S, Mannucci PM, Kurth MH, et al. Von Willebrand factor: what is its role in the immune response in haemophilia? *Haemophilia* 2011;17:e235–8.
34. Mannucci PM. Plasma-derived versus recombinant factor VIII concentrates for the treatment of haemophilia A: plasma-derived is better. *Blood Transfus* 2010;8: 288–91.

35. Mannucci PM, Mancuso ME, Santagostino E. How we choose factor VIII to treat hemophilia. *Blood* 2012;119:4108–14.

36. Mannucci PM, Mancuso ME. Investigational drugs for coagulation disorders. *Expert Opin Investig Drugs* 2013;22:945–53.

37. Nathwani AC, Tuddenham EG, Rangarajan S, et al. Adenovirus-associated virus vector-mediated gene transfer in hemophilia B. *N Engl J Med* 2011;365:2357–65.

CHAPTER 5

Factor IX Deficiency or Hemophilia B: Clinical Manifestations and Management

Raj S. Kasthuri,[1] Harold R. Roberts,[1] and Paul E. Monahan[2]

[1]Department of Medicine, Division of Hematology/Oncology, University of North Carolina at Chapel Hill, Chapel Hill, NC, USA
[2]Department of Pediatrics, Division of Hematology/Oncology, University of North Carolina at Chapel Hill, Chapel Hill, NC, USA

Introduction

Factor IX is one of the vitamin K-dependent coagulation factors and consists of 415 amino acids. All vitamin K-dependent coagulation factors contain gamma carboxyl glutamic acid residues, which in factor IX consist of 12 amino terminal glutamic acid residues that have been post-translationally converted to carboxyl glutamic (Gla) acid, and are necessary for the normal functioning of the molecule by virtue of its interaction with calcium ions and activated platelet surfaces as well as with other activators and substrates including the vascular endothelium [1,2].

Factor IX was first described in 1952 by Dr. Paul Aggeler and colleagues [3]. They identified a factor distinct from factor VIII and called it "plasma thromboplastin component" or PTC. Shortly thereafter a deficiency of a similar factor was described by Biggs, Douglas, and McFarland and this factor was later designated factor IX [4]. Factor IX deficiency leads to a bleeding disorder called hemophilia B that is clinically indistinguishable from that caused by a deficiency of factor VIII (classical hemophilia or hemophilia A). Another name for Factor IX deficiency is Christmas disease, named after the initial patient described by Biggs and colleagues [4]. The incidence of factor IX deficiency is 1/25,000–30,000 in males; thus hemophilia B is less common than classical hemophilia.

In humans, factor IX is necessary for the normal generation of thrombin. The factor IX zymogen must be activated by release of an activation

Hemostasis and Thrombosis: Practical Guidelines in Clinical Management, First Edition.
Hussain I. Saba and Harold R. Roberts.

peptide that leads to the formation of an enzymatic form of factor IX called factor IXa. Factor IXa can be generated by the proteolytic cleavage of factor IX by factor XIa/Ca^{2+} or by the tissue factor–factor VIIa complex. On the surface of activated platelets, factor IXa enhances the capacity of the Tenase complex to rapidly convert prothrombin to thrombin. A lack of adequate amounts of factor IX results in thrombin generation below that required for normal hemostasis. In fact, deficient thrombin generation is a hallmark of all hemophilic conditions.

On a historical note, the descendants of Queen Victoria, many of whom ended up in the royal houses of Europe, were initially believed to have hemophilia A. However, recent DNA analysis of the remains of Czarevitch Alexis, the son of Nicholas II, indicate that he had hemophilia B and suggest that all hemophilic descendants of Queen Victoria had hemophilia B rather than classic hemophilia, thus making Queen Victoria a carrier for hemophilia B [5].

Genetics and molecular biology of factor IX deficiency

The gene for factor IX is located on the long arm of the X chromosome. Factor IX deficiency is thus transmitted as a sex-linked recessive disorder, similar to factor VIII deficiency. The severity of factor IX deficiency depends on the mutation in the factor IX gene. The factor IX gene has been more extensively studied than factor VIII, likely because it is smaller in size (33 kb) and less complex. Large deletions, stop codons, and splice junction defects may result in severe disease, whereas missense mutations result in milder forms. Polymorphisms that do not seem to affect function have also been described, most of which are found in non-coding regions of the factor IX gene [6]. To date, over a thousand mutations have been identified in the factor IX gene. As with hemophilia A, approximately 30% of hemophilia B is the result of de novo mutations. A database of known factor IX mutations can be accessed at http://www.factorix.org (updated database based on the factor IX mutation database previously maintained at King's College, London). Unlike hemophilia A, certain special or variant forms of hemophilia B have been described and some of these are discussed below.

Hemophilia B$_{Leyden}$
One of the first variant forms to be recognized is hemophilia B$_{Leyden}$ [7]. This is characterized by severe hemophilia B at birth which gradually improves as the patient reaches puberty, correlating with an increase in factor IX production. Sometimes the level of factor IX will increase from

less than 1% to normal. Both androgen-responsive and growth hormone-responsive transcriptional regulatory elements have been described in the factor IX promoter and flanking sequences, and mutations in these regions are believed to account for the age-related changes in factor IX expression in this variant.

Hemophilia B$_M$

Another variant form of hemophilia B is hemophilia B$_M$ where the "M" stands for the surname of the initial patient in which this variant was identified. This is a hemophilia B variant where the prothrombin time (PT) is also prolonged. This was first described in PT assays where ox-brain thromboplastin was used as the source of tissue factor (TF). The same has since been reported with use of both rabbit and human sources of thromboplastin, albeit with milder prolongations in the PT. The abnormal factor IX interaction with ox-brain thromboplastin can be caused by a number of missense mutations at amino acid position 180-182 [8]. Of note, ox-brain thromboplastin is no longer used in the United States.

Congenital combined deficiency of vitamin K-dependent clotting factors

Factor IX deficiency may be severe in a rare autosomal recessive condition in which all the vitamin K-dependent factors are deficient. This was first described by McMillan and Roberts, and has subsequently been confirmed in several other laboratories [9]. The defect in some of these patients has been in the hepatic γ-glutamyl carboxylase (GGCX) with ineffective carboxylation of the factor IX molecule as well as the other vitamin K-dependent factors [10]. In other cases there have been defects in vitamin K-dependent epoxide reductase (VKORC1) [11,12]. Affected individuals have prolongation of both the PT and the partial thromboplastin time (PTT).

Clinical manifestations of hemophilia B

The bleeding defects and manifestations in factors VIII and IX deficiency are similar and the two disorders are clinically indistinguishable. The severity of the disease depends on the severity of factor IX deficiency and affected individuals are classified as having mild (>5% factor IX), moderate (1–5% factor IX) or severe (<1% factor IX) disease, as with hemophilia A. As the bleeding symptoms in hemophilia B are similar to those described in hemophilia A, these will only be discussed briefly in this section.

Bleeding into joints (hemarthrosis) and muscle (soft tissue) account for the vast majority of bleeding episodes in patients with factor IX deficiency, with the joints most frequently involved being knees, elbows, and ankles in that order. Breakdown of red blood cells within the joint space following a bleeding episode results in deposition of iron within the joints. Over time, recurrent hemarthroses lead to synovial hyperplasia and the development of hemophilic arthropathy. In addition, hemorrhages into muscles and soft tissues also occur and may be quite frequent. Intracranial hemorrhage may occur during birth or later in life – either spontaneously or following trauma. Subdural bleeding is often delayed, sometimes for weeks, and one must always be careful to treat unusual headaches in patients with hemophilia and be suspicious for intracranial events. This type of bleeding must be treated promptly with factor IX concentrates. Serious bleeding other than intracranial bleeding includes hemorrhage at or around the airway, hemorrhage from the kidneys, and hemorrhage in or around vital organs. Mucocutaneous bleeding, such as epistaxis and bleeding from the gastrointestinal tract can also occur in patients with factor IX deficiency. The bleeding that occurs in hemophilia B_{Leyden} and hemophilia B_M can also be severe or mild, depending upon the factor IX mutation. Treatment of hemophilia will be discussed later in this chapter.

Women who are carriers of factor IX deficiency may also be symptomatic. This can range from easy bruising to menorrhagia to significant bleeding following surgical procedures or trauma. In the case of symptomatic carriers, the factor IX levels are usually significantly below 50%. Such patients may benefit from administration of factor IX prior to elective surgical procedures and at the time of delivery to prevent peri/postpartum hemorrhage. Severe bleeding may occur in some carriers who have Turner's syndrome or extreme lyonization.

Carrier detection and prenatal diagnosis

The factor IX defect can be found in families and yet may not be expressed, depending on genetics of the patients and the carriers of the disease. If a carrier marries a normal male and she has daughters, 50% of them will be carriers themselves and may not be aware of it. By the same token, she may have normal sons, depending on whether they inherit the abnormal X chromosome containing the factor IX gene from the mother. Thus the factor IX defect can be hidden for more than one generation. Therefore, testing for carrier status should be considered even in women with a distant family history of factor IX deficiency. Screening for carrier status can be performed by measurement of factor IX levels as in hemophilia A. However, this approach can miss about 30% of hemophilia B carriers and alternate approaches should be considered [13]. These include restriction fragment length polymorphism (RFLP) analysis and direct gene mutation analysis. It should be remembered that about 30% of cases of factor IX deficiency are the result of de novo mutations.

Prenatal genetic counseling should be offered to all carriers. Prenatal testing can be performed using chorionic villus sampling at 12 weeks' gestation or by amniocentesis after 16 weeks' gestation [14]. Direct measurement of fetal factor IX plasma levels by fetoscopy can be performed after 20 weeks' gestation but this approach is less useful in factor IX deficiency, given the physiologically low levels of factor IX in the fetus and newborn.

Laboratory findings

Factor IX deficiency is characterized by an abnormal PTT, which may be severely prolonged in cases of severe factor IX deficiency and only mildly prolonged in mild to moderate forms of the disorder. The bleeding time is normal, as are PT and the thrombin time, although the PT may be prolonged in patients with hemophilia B_M as discussed previously. A PTT mixing study combining the patient's plasma with normal plasma (1:1) will typically normalize the prolonged PTT. The diagnosis can be confirmed by direct measurement of factor IX activity.

Differential diagnosis

Factor IX deficiency has to be distinguished from hemophilia A since the clinical symptoms can be virtually identical. Known family history of hemophilia B in a newborn with excessive bleeding or a prolonged PTT virtually confirms that the child in question also has hemophilia B. It is important to note that not uncommonly factor IX levels may be low in early infancy as infantile hepatocytes may be delayed in producing fully carboxylated factor IX. Factor IX levels may be low in patients with the rare combined deficiency of vitamin K-dependent clotting factors. In such cases, in addition to factor IX, the levels of factors II, VII, and X will also be low. Further, these patients will have significant prolongations of the PT in addition to the PTT. Factor IX levels can be low in patients who are on treatment with vitamin K antagonists (warfarin) or in the setting of liver disease. Again, these situations will be associated with decreased levels of other clotting factors. Inhibitors to factor IX occur in hemophilia B as discussed below but spontaneous inhibitors to factor IX occurring in otherwise normal patients are rare.

Inhibitors to factor IX

Alloantibodies to factor IX occur in about 3% of severely affected patients, significantly less than is seen in patients with hemophilia A [15]. A sudden lack of responsiveness to factor IX concentrates is the typical manifestation of inhibitor development in a patient with severe hemophilia B. Some of these patients may experience anaphylaxis upon exposure to factor IX [16]. Treatment is usually with bypassing agents, as in patients with factor VIII alloantibodies. Repeated factor IX challenge for immune tolerance induction may result in nephrotic syndrome, which is usually reversible.

Specific treatment of factor IX deficiency

There are now purified factor IX concentrates that contain ample quantities of factor IX such that the factor IX level can be raised to 100% without danger of associated volume overload or thromboembolic episodes. An alternate choice is the use of intermediate-purity factor IX concentrates or prothrombin complex concentrates, which have varying levels of factors II, X, and VII in addition to factor IX. There is concern that chronic use of these concentrates will increase the risk of thrombotic complications. Therefore, purified concentrates containing only factor IX are the treatment of choice in patients with hemophilia B [17]. These can be derived from plasma purification or recombinant DNA technology. Recombinant factor IX is used most widely, but it is important to remember that the initial factor IX recovery is at least 30% lower than plasma-derived factor IX in adults, and even lower in children, as has been extensively reviewed [18]. Currently available recombinant and plasma-derived factor IX products, and prothrombin complex concentrates for the treatment of factor IX deficiency, are listed in Table 5.1.

Bleeding episodes are treated with prompt infusion of high-purity factor IX concentrates immediately after onset of symptoms. The dose and duration of treatment depend on the severity of the bleeding episode. Typically, increasing factor IX levels to 30–50% will serve to stop mild to moderate bleeding episodes (uncomplicated musculoskeletal and mucocutaneous hemorrhages). One to three once-daily infusions should be sufficient in this case. In the case of severe bleeding (e.g., intracranial, gastrointestinal, iliopsoas, compartment syndrome bleeding), the goal is to increase factor

Table 5.1 Currently available factor IX containing products.* Adapted from [19–21].

Plasma-derived factor IX concentrates		
Product [manufacturer]	Fractionation method	Viral inactivation
Aimafix [Kedrion]	Anion exchange; DEAE sephadex/ sepharose; affinity chromatography	TNBP/polysorbate 80; dry heat; nanofiltration
AlphaNine SD [Grifols]	Ion exchange; dual polysaccharide ligand chromatography	Solvent/detergent; nanofiltration
Berinin P [CSL Behring]	Multiple precipitation and adsorption; DEAE-sephadex; affinity chromatography	Pasteurization
BETAFACT [LFB]	Ion exchange chromatography; affinity chromatography	TNBP/polysorbate 80; nanofiltration
Factor IX Grifols [Grifols]	Precipitation and multiple chromatography	Solvent/detergent; nanofiltration
Haemonine [Biotest]	Anion exchange; immunoaffinity chromatography; hydrophobic interaction chromatography	TNBP/polysorbate 80; nanofiltration
Hemo-B-RAAS [Shangai-RAAS]	Ion exchange and affinity chromatography	Solvent/detergent; dry heat; nanofiltration
Immunine [Baxter]	Ion exchange; hydrophobic interaction chromatography	Polysorbate 80 and vapor heat; sodium thiocyanate
Mononine [CSL Behring]	Immunoaffinity chromatography	Sodium thiocyanate; ultrafiltration
Nanotiv [Octapharma]	Ion exchange and affinity chromatography	TNBP/Triton X 100; nanofiltration
Nonafact [Sanquin]	Immunoaffinity and hydrophobic interaction chromatography	TNBP/polysorbate 80; nanofiltration
Octanine F [Octapharma]	Ion exchange and affinity chromatography	TNBP/polysorbate 80; nanofiltration
Replenine-VF [BioProducts Lab.]	Metal chelate chromatography	Solvent detergent; nanofiltration
TBSF FIX [CSL Biotherapies]	Ion exchange and affinity chromatography	TNBP/polysorbate 80; nanofiltration
Recombinant factor IX concentrates		
Product [manufacturer]	Host cell	Purification/viral inactivation
BeneFIX [Pfizer]	Chinese hamster ovary cell	Affinity chromatography; nanofiltration

(Continued)

Table 5.1 (*Continued*)

Prothrombin complex concentrates (PCCs)		
Product [manufacturer]	Three (or) four factor concentrate	Purification/viral inactivation
Bebulin [Baxter]	3-factor (very low amounts of factor VII)	Vapor heat; nanofiltration
Beriplex P/N [CSL Behring]	4-factor concentrate	Pasteurization; nanofiltration
Cofact [Sanquin]	4-factor concentrate	Solvent/detergent; nanofiltration
Haemosolvex Factor IX [National Bioproducts]	4-factor concentrate	TNBP/polysorbate 80
HT DEFIX [SNBTS]	3-factor (no factor VII)	Dry heat
KASKADIL [LFB]	4-factor concentrate	Solvent/detergent
Octaplex [Octapharma]	4-factor concentrate	Solvent/detergent; nanofiltration
Profilnine SD [Grifols]	3-factor (very low amounts of factor VII)	Solvent/detergent
Prothrombinex VF [CSL Bioplasma]	3-factor (no factor VII)	Dry heat; nanofiltration
Prothromplex T [Baxter]	4-factor concentrate	Vapor heat; nanofiltration
Prothroraas [Shanghai RAAS]	4-factor concentrate	Solvent/detergent; nanofiltration
Uman Complex D.I. [Kedrion]	3-factor (no factor VII)	Solvent/detergent; dry heat

*This list is not intended to include every available product.

IX levels to 80–100%. In the case of elective surgical procedures, patients are given prophylactic factor IX infusions to maintain hemostatic levels of factor IX. Again, the duration of prophylaxis depends on the severity of the surgery.

Prophylactic factor IX infusions given twice a week or every three days are widely used in developed countries to prevent the development or progression of joint disease in children with hemophilia B. When begun in the early preschool years and maintained through childhood (primary prophylaxis), children with hemophilia B should be able to enter adulthood without significant joint disease, and primary prophylaxis must be considered the standard of care in developed countries [22]. In addition, intracranial hemorrhage is reduced in individuals with severe hemophilia receiving prophylaxis [23,24]. The dose of factor IX used for primary prophylaxis ranges from 30 to 80 IU/kg/dose [25,26]. Breakthrough bleeding episodes should be treated with factor IX replacement to achieve hemostatic levels appropriate to the severity of hemorrhage [17].

The rare hemophilia B patient who develops high-titer inhibitory alloantibodies to factor IX is unlikely to achieve hemostasis using purified factor IX concentrates. Further, exposure of such a patient to factor IX may lead to anamnestic increase of the inhibitor titer in addition to increasing the risk for hypersensitivity reactions [15]. For this reason, bypassing agent therapy with either activated prothrombin complex concentrates (aPCCs, e.g., FEIBA) or with recombinant activated factor VII (rFVIIa) is the preferred approach in hemophilia B patients with inhibitors. Recombinant FVIIa is the preferred therapy in order to avoid exposure to the substantial amounts of factor IX in aPCCs.

Therapies in development

Protein therapies: engineered factor IX to extend plasma survival

The best long-term outcomes using factor IX prophylaxis are seen when prophylaxis is begun very early in the preschool years. Nevertheless, decades of adherence with the demands of prophylaxis can be extremely burdensome, and the repeated need for venous access is especially challenging in small boys and older gentlemen. Prelicensure clinical trials of several factor IX therapies modified to increase the circulating survival of factor IX are advancing, and it is likely that one or more extended half-life factor IX proteins will be authorized for clinical use. The current approaches to prolonging the survival of factor IX fall into two categories: chemical modification of factor IX or creation of factor IX fusion proteins using recombinant DNA technology. The addition of bulky, charged polyethylene glycol (PEG) moieties to recombinant proteins is increasingly commonly employed to decrease the plasma clearance, with licensed drugs in the areas of hematology, oncology, and inflammation. A first human dose trial of a factor IX modified via glycopegylation of the activation peptide has now been completed [27]. The half-life of the glycopegylated factor IX was five times improved in the study subjects, as compared to the unmodified factor IX product currently in use. These results indicate a favorable pharmacokinetic advantage, although trials need to be conducted to determine the effect on bleed prevention in humans.

Two recombinant factor IX fusion proteins are also in prelicensure testing. One is a recombinant factor IX-Fc fusion protein that has the factor IX covalently fused to the human IgG_1 Fc domain. An endothelial cell receptor, the neonatal Fc receptor, reportedly protects IgG_1 Fc-fusion proteins from lysosomal degradation, and instead recycles Fc-fused proteins in the circulation. A human clinical trial reports that, across a wide range of doses, the rFIXFc product improves the factor IX mean residence time approximately threefold [28]. A related approach has been taken by another group, creating a fusion protein linking factor IX with human albumin [29]. A first human pharmacokinetic trial has been completed and demonstrated favorable pharmacokinetics. These included a mean incremental recovery that was improved relative to unmodified plasma-derived or recombinant factor IX and a more than 5 times prolongation of half-life when compared to the individual subject's previous factor IX replacement product [30]. One important unknown for all of these products is whether prolongation of plasma circulation alone will ultimately be associated with reduced breakthrough bleeding. Unmodified factor IX has a significant degree of extravascular binding and partitions into tissues to some extent. It is possible that protein modifications that create physical or charge changes may alter the in vivo hemostatic properties by sequestering the factor IX from extracirculatory sites of action. Hemostatic efficacy in animal models suggests that these modified proteins will permit extended bleed-free intervals between factor IX doses. Nevertheless, rates of breakthrough bleeding in larger human trials and in post-marketing surveillance will determine the acceptance of these modified proteins as the standard of care for reducing long-term morbidity.

Gene therapy

Gene therapy includes any treatment approach in which a nucleic acid is delivered as therapy. Hemophilia and hemophilia B in particular, has long been considered an ideal model condition to test the potential of gene addition or gene correction strategies. The factor IX gene and its regulation, the structure/function properties of the factor IX protein's domains and the protein's post-translational modifications are all well characterized, as are the effects of modifications and mutations throughout each domain of the protein. Gene correction can be measured using assays of factor IX activity that are in widespread clinical use, which facilitates direct interpretation in translational research. Both small animal (mouse) and large animal (dog) hemophilia B models closely mimic pathophysiologic features of human factor IX deficiency and have contributed to decades of investigation of hemophilia B pathogenesis and therapy [31].

Gene therapy usually involves either delivery of DNA or RNA in vivo or ex vivo. The body naturally defends against incorporating nucleic acids that originate outside the self. For this reason in vivo gene delivery usually involves some sort of vector (e.g., a virus vector used to deliver the gene) or at the least some chemical conjugation (e.g., DNA formulated with lipid vesicles) to protect the gene of interest from degradation while delivering its therapeutic message. Genes can alternatively be inserted into cells ex vivo (that is to say, outside of the body). After confirmation that the gene is functional in the cells that have been targeted ex vivo, the cells are returned to the patient to express the gene that the patient otherwise lacks. Both in vivo vector-mediated gene therapy and ex vivo cell-based approaches have been attempted in human clinical trials for hemophilia A; however, persistent correction of factor VIII deficiency has never been achieved in a human clinical trial [32].

Proof of principle for the use of a virus to deliver factor IX to the liver and correct the hemophilia B bleeding phenotype was demonstrated as early as 1993 [33]. Dogs with hemophilia B from the colony maintained at the University of North Carolina demonstrated low levels of circulating factor IX activity and partial correction of bleeding for several months after delivery of a recombinant retrovirus factor IX vector into the portal circulation. Subsequent investigations took advantage of the relatively small size of the cDNA for factor IX (especially as compared to the enormous size of the factor VIII gene) and used a non-pathogenic virus called the adeno-associated virus (AAV) for in vivo vector-mediated delivery. Although the AAV vector is derived from a virus in the Parvoviridae family, and despite the fact that most humans are exposed to AAV in early childhood and may develop antibodies against the virus, AAV is not associated with any human disease. In fact, wild-type AAV is not capable of independently replicating its DNA, suggesting a good safety profile for the use of AAV vectors to express genes in a variety of tissues that have relatively low cell turnover (e.g., liver, skeletal muscle).

An initial human clinical trial of AAV delivery to the liver resulted in clinical safety and transient circulating plasma factor IX activity [34]. The factor IX expression was lost after a few weeks, however, apparently due to reactivation of memory immune cells that recognized the AAV virus as a result of prior environmental exposure, with a cytotoxic lymphocyte response eliminating the successfully treated hepatocytes. Subsequent engineering of the AAV factor IX vectors have improved their efficiency, and in 2011 the first definitive success in a human clinical trial of hemophilia gene therapy was reported [35,36]. All individuals in this trial persistently expressed plasma factor IX levels of 1–7% with follow-up of up to two years, associated with decreased bleeding and decreased need for factor IX protein infusions. At the highest doses in this trial, vector-associated immune response targeting the liver was again measurable, although no study subjects were symptomatic. Ongoing efforts seek to further improve the efficiency of AAV factor IX vectors so that correction of hemophilia B to very mildly deficient (10–40%) or normal factor IX levels may be achieved without triggering immune responses including hepatitis. It remains unknown how long factor IX expression from AAV will persist in humans; ongoing expression has been shown for at least 6–10 years in dogs, rhesus macaques, and in skeletal muscle in humans [37–39]. Additional areas of development address the needs that are not met by the current AAV factor IX vectors. Most important are the need for approaches to treat individuals who have pre-existing antibodies that neutralize AAV as well as individuals who have inhibitors. Cell-based approaches, such as expression of factor IX from ex vivo transduced platelet progenitors, may prove useful as a strategy for individuals with pre-existing immunity to viral vectors [40]. For the first time, the translation of gene therapy to larger clinical trials for hemophilia B appears to be likely and the potential that cure could become a standard of care demands consideration.

References

1. Fryklund L, Borg H, Andersson LO. Amino-terminal sequence of human factor IX: presence of gamma-carboxyl glumatic acid residues. *FEBS Lett* 1976;65: 187–9.
2. Morita T, Isaacs BS, Esmon CT, Johnson AE. Derivatives of blood coagulation factor IX contain a high affinity Ca2+-binding site that lacks gamma-carboxyglutamic acid. *J Biol Chem* 1984;259:5698–704.
3. Aggeler PM, White SG, Glendening MB, Page EW, et al. Plasma thromboplastin component (PTC) deficiency; a new disease resembling hemophilia. *Proc Soc Exp Biol Med* 1952;79:692–4.
4. Biggs R, Douglas AS, Macfarlane RG, et al. Christmas disease: a condition previously mistaken for haemophilia. *Br Med J* 1952;2(4799):1378–82.
5. Rogaev EI, Grigorenko AP, Faskhutdinova G, et al. Genotype analysis identifies the cause of the "royal disease". *Science* 2009;326(5954):817.
6. Wallmark A, Kunkel G, Mouhli H, et al. Population genetics of the Malmo polymorphism of coagulation factor IX. *Hum Hered* 1991;41:391–6.
7. Briet E, Bertina RM, van Tilburg NH, Veltkamp JJ. Hemophilia B Leyden: a sex-linked hereditary disorder that improves after puberty. *N Engl J Med* 1982;306: 788–90.
8. Hamaguchi N, Roberts H, Stafford DW. Mutations in the catalytic domain of factor IX that are related to the subclass hemophilia Bm. *Biochemistry* 1993;32:6324–9.
9. McMillan CW, Roberts HR. Congenital combined deficiency of coagulation factors II, VII, IX and X. Report of a case. *N Engl J Med* 1966;274:1313–15.
10. Brenner B, Sanchez-Vega B, Wu SM, et al. A missense mutation in gamma-glutamyl carboxylase gene causes combined deficiency of all vitamin K-dependent blood coagulation factors. *Blood* 1998;92:4554–9.
11. Li T, Chang CY, Jin DY, et al. Identification of the gene for vitamin K epoxide reductase. *Nature* 2004;427(6974):541–4.
12. Rost S, Fregin A, Ivaskevicius V, et al. Mutations in VKORC1 cause warfarin resistance and multiple coagulation factor deficiency type 2. *Nature* 2004;427(6974): 537–41.
13. Graham JB. Genotype assignment (carrier detection) in the haemophilias. *Clin Haematol* 1979;8:115–45.
14. Gitschier J, Lawn RM, Rotblat F, et al. Antenatal diagnosis and carrier detection of haemophilia A using factor VIII gene probe. *Lancet* 1985;1(8437):1093–4.

15. DiMichele D. Inhibitor development in haemophilia B: an orphan disease in need of attention. *Br J Haematol* 2007;138:305–15.
16. Chitlur M, Warrier I, Rajpurkar M, Lusher JM. Inhibitors in factor IX deficiency a report of the ISTH-SSC international FIX inhibitor registry (1997–2006). *Haemophilia* 2009;15:1027–31.
17. Srivastava A, Brewer AK, Mauser-Bunschoten EP, et al. Guidelines for the management of hemophilia. *Haemophilia* 2013;19:e1–47.
18. Monahan PE, Di Paola J. Recombinant factor IX for clinical and research use. *Semin Thromb Hemost* 2010;36:498–509.
19. Sorensen B, Spahn DR, Innerhofer P, et al. Clinical review: Prothrombin complex concentrates – evaluation of safety and thrombogenicity. *Critical Care* 2011;15:201.
20. Franchini M, Frattini F, Crestani S, Bonfanti C. Haemophilia B: Current pharmacotherapy and future directions. *Expert Opin Pharmacother* 2012;13:2053–63.
21. World Federation of Hemophilia. *Registry of Clotting Factor Concentrates* (ninth edition, 2012). http://www1.wfh.org/publications/files/pdf-1227.pdf.
22. Astermark J, Petrini P, Tengborn L. Primary prophylaxis in severe haemophilia should be started at an early age but can be individualized. *Br J Haematol* 1999;105:1109–13.
23. Aledort LM, Haschmeyer RH, Pettersson H. A longitudinal study of orthopaedic outcomes for severe factor-VIII-deficient haemophiliacs. The Orthopaedic Outcome Study Group. *J Intern Med* 1994;236:391–9.
24. Witmer C, Presley R, Kulkarni R, et al. Associations between intracranial haemorrhage and prescribed prophylaxis in a large cohort of haemophilia patients in the United States. *Br J Haematol* 2010;152:211–16.
25. Blanchette VS, Manco-Johnson M, Santagostino E, Ljung R. Optimizing factor prophylaxis for the haemophilia population: where do we stand? *Haemophilia* 2004;10(suppl 4):97–104.
26. Monahan PE, Liesner R, Sullivan ST, et al. Safety and efficacy of investigator-prescribed BeneFIX prophylaxis in children less than 6 years of age with severe haemophilia B. *Haemophilia* 2010;16:460–8.
27. Negrier C, Knobe K, Tiede A, et al. Enhanced pharmacokinetic properties of a glycoPEGylated recombinant factor IX: a first human dose trial in patients with hemophilia B. *Blood* 2011;118:2695–701.
28. Shapiro AD, Ragni MV, Valentino LA, et al. Recombinant factor IX-Fc fusion protein (rFIXFc) demonstrates safety and prolonged activity in a phase 1/2a study in hemophilia B patients. *Blood* 2012;119:666–72.
29. Metzner HJ, Weimer T, Kronthaler U, et al. Genetic fusion to albumin improves the pharmacokinetic properties of factor IX. *Thromb Haemost* 2009;102:634–44.
30. Santagostino E, Negrier C, Klamroth R, et al. Safety and pharmacokinetics of a novel recombinant fusion protein linking coagulation factor IX with albumin (rIX-FP) in hemophilia B patients. *Blood* 2012;120:2405–11.
31. Sabatino DE, Nichols TC, Merricks E, et al. Animal models of hemophilia. *Prog Mol Biol Transl Sci* 2012;105:151–209.
32. High KA. Gene therapy for haemophilia: a long and winding road. *J Thromb Haemost* 2011;9(suppl 1):2–11.
33. Kay MA, Rothenberg S, Landen CN, et al. In vivo gene therapy of hemophilia B: sustained partial correction in factor IX-deficient dogs. *Science* 1993;262(5130):117–19.
34. Manno CS, Pierce GF, Arruda VR et al. Successful transduction of liver in hemophilia by AAV-Factor IX and limitations imposed by the host immune response. *Nat Med* 2006;12:342–7.

35. Nathwani AC, Tuddenham EG, Rangarajan S, et al. Adenovirus-associated virus vector-mediated gene transfer in hemophilia B. *N Engl J Med* 2011;365:2357–65.

36. Wu Z, Sun J, Zhang T et al. Optimization of self-complementary AAV vectors for liver-directed expression results in sustained correction of hemophilia B at low vector dose. *Mol Ther* 2008;16:280–9.

37. Buchlis G, Podsakoff GM, Radu A, et al. Factor IX expression in skeletal muscle of a severe hemophilia B patient 10 years after AAV-mediated gene transfer. *Blood* 2012;119:3038–41.

38. Nathwani AC, Rosales C, McIntosh J, et al. Long-term safety and efficacy following systemic administration of a self-complementary AAV vector encoding human FIX pseudotyped with serotype 5 and 8 capsid proteins. *Mol Ther* 2011;19:876–85.

39. Niemeyer GP, Herzog RW, Mount J, et al. Long-term correction of inhibitor-prone hemophilia B dogs treated with liver-directed AAV2-mediated factor IX gene therapy. *Blood* 2009;113:797–806.

40. Zhang G, Shi Q, Fahs SA, et al. Factor IX ectopically expressed in platelets can be stored in alpha-granules and corrects the phenotype of hemophilia B mice. *Blood* 2010;116:1235–43.

CHAPTER 6

Factor XI Deficiency or Hemophilia C

Charles E. Bane,[1] Anne T. Neff,[1,2] and David Gailani[1,2]

[1] Department of Pathology, Microbiology, and Immunology, Vanderbilt University, Nashville, TN, USA

[2] Division of Hematology/Oncology, Vanderbilt University, Nashville, TN, USA

History

In 1953, Rosenthal and coworkers described three members of a Jewish family (two sisters and their maternal uncle) who bled excessively after tooth extraction or tonsillectomy [1,2]. The plasmas of these individuals clotted slowly in a glass tube (a predecessor of the activated partial thromboplastin time [aPTT] assay), similar to plasmas from patients with hemophilia A or B (factor VIII or IX deficiency). However, bleeding was milder than with the X-linked hemophilias, and affected females and males. The missing plasma factor was called plasma thromboplastin antecedent (PTA), and was subsequently designated factor XI (FXI). FXI deficiency is sometimes referred to as hemophilia C, and in the past was also called PTA deficiency or Rosenthal syndrome.

Factor XI structure and function

FXI is a 160-kDa plasma glycoprotein that is the precursor of the trypsin-like protease factor XIa (FXIa) [3–6]. From an evolutionary perspective, it is the most recent addition to the blood coagulation cascade, appearing during the course of mammalian evolution as the result of a duplication of the gene for the protease zymogen prekallikrein (PK) [5]. FXI is synthesized primarily by hepatocytes and circulates in plasma in a complex with the glycoprotein high-molecular-weight kininogen (HK) at a concentration of ~30 nM (normal range 15–45 nM). The plasma half-life of FXI is 45–52 hours. Each FXI molecule consists of two identical 80-kDa

Hemostasis and Thrombosis: Practical Guidelines in Clinical Management, First Edition.
Hussain I. Saba and Harold R. Roberts.
© 2014 John Wiley & Sons, Ltd. Published 2014 by John Wiley & Sons, Ltd.

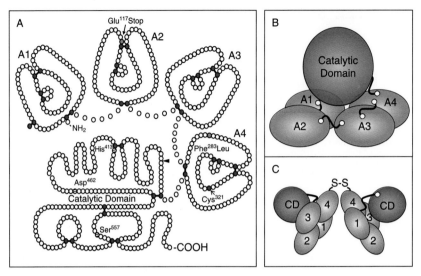

Figure 6.1 Factor XI structure. (A) Schematic diagram showing the domain and disulfide bond organization of a human FXI subunit. Each circle represents one amino acid. Red Circles indicate positions of Cysteine residues. (B) Ball-and-stick model of a FXI subunit showing the relative positions of the apple domains and the catalytic domain. (C) Model of the FXI dimer. Models in panels B and C are based on the crystal structure of human FXI [4].

subunits (Figure 6.1) [3–6]. The dimeric structure, which is unique among coagulation proteases, is conserved across species; however, its functional importance has not been definitively established. Each subunit contains four 90–91 amino acid repeats called apple domains (designated A1 to A4) and a catalytic domain at the C-terminus (Figure 6.1A and 6.1B) [3,4]. The apple domains form a platform (Figure 6.1B) to which other macromolecules involved in coagulation bind [4–6]. For example, the FXIa substrate factor IX binds to the A3 domain, while HK binds to the side of the apple domain platform opposite the catalytic domain in a groove formed by A1, A2, and A4 [6]. The two subunits of a FXI dimer interact through a hydrophobic interface between the A4 domains (Figure 6.1C) and a disulfide bond involving Cys321 (Figures 6.1A and 6.1C) [4]. FXI lacks the calcium-binding Gla-domain found at the N-terminus of vitamin K-dependent coagulation proteases. FXI synthesis, therefore, does not require vitamin K, and plasma FXI levels are not affected by therapy with vitamin K antagonists such as warfarin. Conversion of a FXI subunit to the active protease FXIa involves proteolytic cleavage of the peptide bond between Arg369 and Ile370 (indicated by the black arrowhead in Figure 6.1A). Forms of FXIa in which one or both subunits are activated have been described [5,6]. Each FXIa catalytic domain contains a triad of histidine (His413), aspartic acid (Asp462), and serine

(Ser557) residues (indicated by the cross-hatched circles in Figure 6.1A) that is required for protease activity.

In the original cascade/waterfall model of coagulation, the process of thrombin generation is initiated by conversion of factor XII to the protease factor XIIa when blood comes into contact with a negatively charged surface in a process called *contact activation* (discussed in Chapter 9) [5]. Contact activation also requires PK and HK. Factor XIIa activates FXI, and FXIa in turn activates the next protein in the cascade, factor IX. This process ultimately leads to thrombin generation and a fibrin clot. In the cascade model, FXI is an important part of a mechanism for *initiating* coagulation. However, the well-established observation that patients lacking factor XII, PK, or HK do not have a bleeding disorder suggests, at the very least, that other mechanisms must exist to activate FXI during hemostasis in vivo. Contact activation is no longer considered to be an important trigger for thrombin generation (at least during normal hemostasis), and FXI has been assigned a role in the propagation phase of thrombin generation during certain types of hemostatic challenges (Chapter 1). FXI can be converted to FXIa by various forms of thrombin [5], consistent with the hypotheses that: 1) factor XIIa is not required for FXI activation in vivo; and 2) that thrombin generation has already started prior to activation of FXI. This reinterpretation of FXI's role from an initiator to a sustainer of thrombin generation fits well with the patterns of abnormal bleeding seen in FXI deficiency that are discussed below.

Congenital factor XI deficiency: inheritance pattern

More than 250 FXI gene mutations have been identified in FXI-deficient patients (www.hgmd.org; www.med.unc.edu/isth; www.wienkav.at/kav/kar/texte_anzeigen.asp; www.FactorXI.org) [5–7]. The severe form of the disorder (FXI activity <20% of normal) is thought to be rare in the general population (~1 in a million) [8]; however, the true incidence may be higher as some patients do not experience bleeding episodes that would cause them to seek medical attention. Severe FXI deficiency is among the most common inherited disorders in Ashkenazi Jews, with an incidence of 1 in 450 persons [8–11]. Two mutations predominate in this ethnic group [10,11]. Glu117Stop (Figure 6.1A; also called the "type II" mutation) causes premature termination of the protein in the A2 domain. Homozygosity for nonsense mutations such as Glu117Stop would result in complete absence of FXI protein in plasma because they prevent synthesis of protein within the cell (Figure 6.2). Heterozygosity for such mutations would not affect the product of a normal FXI allele, resulting

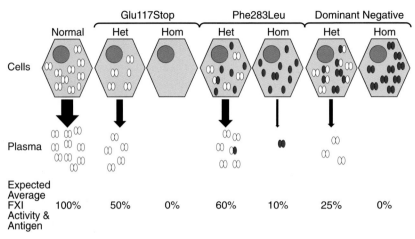

Figure 6.2 Mechanisms causing CRM-FXI deficiency. Hexagons represent hepatocytes (circles are nuclei). The smaller ovals represent FXI monomers (one oval) or dimers (two adjacent ovals). Arrows indicate relative amounts of secretion. The number of FXI dimers below the arrows indicates the relative amounts of protein in plasma. Het, heterozygote; Hom, homozygote for fXI gene mutation.

in ~50% of the normal FXI plasma level. Phe283Leu (Figure 6.1A; the "type III" mutation) is located in the A4 domain. This mutation does not prevent protein synthesis, but does interfere with dimer formation, and is associated with intracellular retention of monomeric protein (Figure 6.2). Heterozygosity for a mutation like Phe283Leu would have little effect on the product of the normal FXI allele, because mutant subunits would rarely form dimers with wild-type subunits. The relatively few heterodimers or mutant homodimers that do form are secreted and have normal activity.

Patients homozygous for Phe283Leu have ~10% of the normal FXI level in plasma. Compound heterozygotes for Glu117Stop and Phe283Leu have ~3% of the normal plasma FXI level, while patients heterozygous for only one of the mutations typically have half of the normal FXI plasma level (Figure 6.2). As heterozygotes do not usually exhibit a hemostatic defect, FXI deficiency in the Jewish population behaves as an autosomal recessive disorder [8,10,11].

The majority of FXI gene mutations causing FXI deficiency are associated with the absence of FXI protein in plasma (cross-reactive material [CRM] negative deficiency). In most cases, severe deficiency is probably due to homozygosity or compound heterozygosity for mutations that interfere with protein synthesis (e.g., Glu117Stop) or protein dimerization (e.g., Phe283Leu). As discussed above, severe deficiency caused by such mutations would likely be transmitted in an autosomal recessive manner, because the gene product of the mutant allele would not affect the normal allele product in a heterozygote. [5]. However, because FXI is a multimeric protein, there is a mechanism by which heterozygosity for certain types of mutations could cause severe deficiency and, therefore, behave as a dominant trait. A FXI subunit that contains a mutation that prevents it from being secreted from the cell, but that does not interfere with dimer formation, could form non-secretable heterodimers with normal FXI subunits, trapping the normal subunit within the cell (a dominant negative effect; Figure 6.2) [12]. A similar mechanism can lead to type I von Willebrand disease and hypofibrinogenemia, disorders that also involve multimeric proteins. Several FXI gene mutations have been identified that produce a dominant negative effect (e.g., Ser225Phe and Cys398Tyr), and it is possible that this is a relatively common mechanism for FXI deficiency in the general population.

Other congenital and acquired causes of factor XI deficiency

As with most coagulation factors, FXI levels may become low in patients with moderate to severe liver insufficiency or disseminated intravascular coagulation (DIC). Mild to moderate FXI deficiency (20–50% of the normal plasma level) is a common finding in patients with Noonan syndrome [13], and the carbohydrate deficient glycoprotein syndrome (a group of disorders associated with defects in glycosylation of secretory glycoproteins) [14]. It can also be seen in patients with the Prader–Willi syndrome. Acquired FXI deficiency due to autoantibody inhibitors has been reported, but is rare. Alloantibodies to FXI develop in up to one-third of patients with the most severe form of congenital FXI deficiency (<1% of the normal FXI plasma level, e.g., homozygotes for Glu117Stop) after exposure to FXI-containing plasma products [15].

Clinical presentation

Abnormal bleeding in severe factor XI deficiency is almost always injury-related, and is most frequent when the oral cavity, nasopharynx, or urinary tract are involved [5,8–10,16,17]. These areas have high intrinsic levels of fibrinolytic activity, and it is postulated that sustained thrombin generation through FXIa is required for both maintenance of the fibrin clot, and for enhanced clot resistance to fibrinolysis in these environments. Injury to these areas causes excessive bleeding in two-thirds of patients with severe deficiency, regardless of the genotype. Bleeding may start at the time of injury or be delayed by hours, and oozing from tooth extraction sites may persist for days. Injury at other locations is less frequently associated with excessive bleeding, and tends to occur in those with the lowest FXI levels (e.g., homozygotes for Glu117Stop would tend to bleed more than homozygotes for Phe283Leu) [8,10]. Excessive bleeding with skin laceration, circumcision, appendectomy, and orthopedic surgery is infrequent [16,17], and spontaneous bleeding, except for menorrhagia, is uncommon. Normal vaginal childbirth is associated with excessive bleeding in ∼20–30% of cases [18].

Bleeding correlates relatively poorly with plasma FXI levels. Not all patients with severe deficiency experience excessive bleeding, even with surgery, and a patient may exhibit a variable bleeding tendency over time [8,9]. In addition to variation in bleeding associated with injury to different parts of the body, other inherited or acquired hemostatic defects may contribute to bleeding variability. There are different opinions regarding the propensity of patients with mild deficiency (20–50% of normal) to bleed [8,9]. Some studies describe minimal bleeding with tooth extraction, tonsillectomy, nasal surgery, and urologic surgery, while others report difficulty distinguishing severe from mild deficiency on clinical grounds. In a study of 45 families with FXI deficiency (mostly due to Glu117Stop or Phe283Leu), the odds ratios for excessive bleeding were 13.0 for homozygotes or compound heterozygotes, and 2.6 for heterozygotes [19]. Thus, mild deficiency seems to confer, at most, a slightly increased bleeding risk, but substantially less than the risk with severe deficiency.

Factor XI deficiency has been described in the veterinary literature, and can cause an injury-related bleeding disorder in Holstein cattle, several varieties of domestic dogs (Kerry Blue Terriers, Weimaraners, Great Pyrenees dog, English Springer Spaniel), and in domestic cats.

Laboratory diagnosis

Patients with severe FXI deficiency inevitably have a prolonged activated partial thromboplastin time (aPTT) with a normal prothrombin time. Definitive diagnosis involves a modified aPTT in which the patient plasma is tested for its ability to correct the defect in FXI deficient plasma. Results are reported as % activity of a pooled normal plasma control. The normal range for FXI is typically 50–150% of the control activity. Mild FXI deficiency may not prolong the aPTT, and FXI activity should be measured directly if there is a high index of suspicion for the disorder.

Treatment

As bleeding in FXI-deficient patients is rarely spontaneous, treatment is primarily directed at stopping or preventing injury-related bleeding. During preparation of a FXI-deficient patient for an invasive procedure, it is important to recognize that the likelihood of bleeding varies depending on the procedure and tissue involved. Consequently, a negative bleeding history does not necessarily imply a low risk of bleeding with subsequent procedures [8,9,16–18]. In addition, patients with the most severe deficiency (<1% of normal plasma level) are at high risk of developing neutralizing anti-FXI antibodies, often after a single blood product exposure [15]. Based on these observations, treatment recommendations have been refined to limit exposure to FXI, with the understanding that some cases of milder deficiency (20–30% of normal) may require factor replacement in some situations. During preoperative evaluation, the prothrombin time and platelet count should be normal, and the possibility of hemostatic abnormalities unrelated to FXI deficiency should be addressed. Patients with FXI levels >40–45% of normal generally do not have symptoms [8,16–18]. A history of abnormal bleeding in such a patient suggests that another hemostatic abnormality (congenital or acquired) may be present. Antiplatelet therapy should be stopped one week before surgery. The possibility of a neutralizing FXI inhibitor should be considered in a FXI-deficient patient who has been recently exposed to blood products [15].

Factor replacement is recommended for most major surgery and should be initiated before the procedure. FXI replacement to keep the plasma level >40% of normal for at least 7 days is recommended for invasive procedures involving the orophayrynx, nasopharynx, or urinary tract [8,9,16–18]. A similar approach is appropriate for neurosurgery, head and neck surgery, cardiothoracic surgery, and major abdominal or pelvic surgery. In addition, antifibrinolytic therapy (ε-aminocaproic acid [Amicar] or tranexamic acid [IV – Cyklokapron, or oral – Lysteda]) should be strongly considered for surgery on the oropharynx. With surgery on the lower urinary tract, particularly prostatectomy, flushing the bladder with saline containing an antifibrinolytic agent can be beneficial. Minor procedures on vulnerable tissues may be treated with replacement to keep the FXI level >30% for 5 days. Patients with FXI levels >40–45% of normal do not require FXI replacement.

Replacement therapy for FXI deficiency is either with fresh frozen plasma (FFP) or FXI concentrate. Cryoprecipitate does not contain FXI. In the United States, almost all cases are currently covered with FFP. The long plasma half-life of FXI (45–52 hours) facilitates daily or every other day administration. In anticipation of surgery, plasma can be administered for several consecutive days prior to surgery with the expectation that the protein will accumulate in plasma. This approach may be preferable to a single administration of a large amount of FFP prior to surgery in patients who may not tolerate large volumes of intravenous fluid.

FXI concentrates (Hemoleven®, LFB Biomedicaments; or FXI concentrate, Bio Products Laboratory) facilitate administration of factor in relatively small volumes, and are effective at preventing bleeding during surgery [20,21]. Hemoleven® received orphan drug designation from the United States Food and Drug Administration in 2007, and should be available in the USA under an FDA Expanded Access Program in the near future. In the 1990s, use of FXI concentrates was associated with thrombosis and evidence of DIC, primarily in older patients with known cardiovascular disease receiving doses >30 U/kg. To reduce procoagulant potential, current concentrates contain antithrombin and heparin, with or without C1 inhibitor. The plasma FXI level should not be raised above 60% of the normal level with concentrates.

Circumcision, appendectomy, and orthopedic surgery are associated with low bleeding rates, and withholding factor replacement (unless bleeding occurs) has been advocated [17]. A "wait and see" approach is also used by some groups for vaginal deliveries [18], although this is not universally accepted [22]. However, there are insufficient data to conclude that epidural anesthesia is safe in the absence of coverage, and factor replacement is recommended. There are several other situations in which factor replacement can be safely withheld. Tooth extraction can be treated with antifibrinolytic therapy (ε-aminocaproic acid 5–6 g q6 hrs or tranexamic acid 1 g q6 hrs) beginning 12 hours before the procedure and continuing for 7 days [23]. Systemic antifibrinolytic therapy is also an option for treating menorrhagia and for skin biopsies. Prolonged therapy with antifibrinolytic agents must be undertaken with caution in patients who are not mobile, who have a history of thromboembolism, or who have significant urogenital bleeding. The drugs interfere with urokinase-mediated fibrinolytic activity in the genitourinary tract, and thrombotic occlusion of the ureter can lead to renal outflow obstruction. Dental procedures such as scaling or root canal treatment can be safely performed using ε-aminocaproic acid or tranexamic acid mouthwash prepared from the intravenous formulation three to four times daily, with or without systemic antifibrinolytic therapy. Fibrin glues can be used for skin biopsies and resections of skin lesions in place of antifibrinolytic therapy.

The effectiveness of DDAVP in mild FXI deficiency is not established, but there are reports that FXI levels increase modestly in response to this drug. FXI-deficient patients with inhibitors do not usually have spontaneous bleeding. Recombinant factor VIIa has been used successfully for major surgery in patients with inhibitors [8,9,16–18]. Factor VIIa has also been used in patients without inhibitors to cover surgery or epidural block during labor and delivery, and is a reasonable choice for situations in which exposure to plasma products needs to be limited.

Factor XI and thrombosis

Some patients with FXI deficiency do experience thromboembolic episodes. Aspirin or clopidogrel can be used in FXI-deficient patients with myocardial infarction or other manifestations of atherosclerosis. Atrial fibrillation or venous thromboembolism should be treated with warfarin, with the goal of not allowing the INR to exceed 2.5. There is no published information on the newer inhibitors of thrombin (dabigatran etixilate [Pradaxa]) and factor Xa (rivaroxaban [Xarelto] and apixaban (Eliquis]) in FXI-deficient patients.

Recent studies have implicated FXI in the pathogenesis of venous and arterial thrombosis [5,24]. A plasma FXI level that is at the upper end of the normal distribution (or greater than the upper limit of normal) is a modest independent risk factor for venous thromboembolism (VTE), stroke, and myocardial infarction. Similarly, patients with severe FXI deficiency appear to have lower incidences of VTE and stroke. The data are consistent with those from animal models that show FXI contributes to the growth and stability of a large pathologic thrombus. The possibility that FXIa may play a significant role in thrombosis has led to increased interest in the protease as a therapeutic target for treating or preventing thrombotic disorders. A treatment strategy targeting FXIa would presumably be associated with a lower risk of treatment-induced bleeding compared to current anticoagulants. FXI antisense oligonucleotides have been used to reduce FXI levels safely in humans, and a phase II trial is currently enrolling patients to test the effectiveness of this strategy in preventing perioperative venous thrombosis associated with knee replacement. Several small-molecule inhibitors of FXIa are at various stages of development.

References

1. Rosenthal RL, Dreskin OH, Rosenthal N. New hemophilia-like disease caused by deficiency of a third plasma thromboplastin factor. *Proc Soc Exper Biol Med* 1953;82:171–4.

2. Rosenthal RL, Dreskin OH, Rosenthal N. Plasma thromboplastin antecedent (PTA) deficiency; clinical, coagulation, therapeutic and hereditary aspects of a new hemophilia-like disease. *Blood* 1955;10:120–31.

3. McMullen BA, Fujikawa K, Davie EW. Location of the disulfide bonds in human coagulation factor XI: the presence of tandem apple domains. *Biochemistry* 1991;30:2056–60.

4. Papagrigoriou E, McEwan PA, Walsh PN, Emsley J. Crystal structure of the factor XI zymogen reveals a pathway for transactivation. *Nat Struct Mol Biol* 2006;13: 557–8.

5. Gailani D, Renne T, Emsley J. (2010) *Factor XI and the contact system*. In Valle D, Beaudet AL, Vogelstein B, et al. (eds), *The Online Metabolic and Molecular Basis of Inherited Disease*. Philadelphia, PA: Lippincott, Williams & Wilkins, 2010.

6. Emsley J, McEwan PA, Gailani D. Structure and function of factor XI. *Blood* 2010;115:2569–77.

7. Santoro R, Prejano S, Iannaccaro P. Factor XI deficiency: a description of 34 cases and literature review. *Blood Coagul Fibrinolysis* 2011;22:431–5.

8. Seligsohn U. (2009) Factor XI deficiency in humans. *J Thromb Haemost* 2009;7(suppl 1):84–7.

9. Bolton-Maggs PH. Factor XI deficiency-resolving the enigma? *Hematology Am Soc Hematol Educ Program* 2009:97–105.

10. Asakai R, Chung DW, Davie EW. Factor XI deficiency in Ashkenazi Jews in Israel. *N Engl J Med* 1991;325:153–8.

11. Peretz H, Mulai A, Usher S, et al. The two common mutations causing factor XI deficiency in Jews stem from distinct founders: one of ancient Middle Eastern origin and another of more recent European origin. *Blood* 1997;90:2654–9.

12. Kravtsov DV, Wu W, Meijers JC, et al. Dominant factor XI deficiency caused by mutations in the factor XI catalytic domain. *Blood* 2004;104:128–34.

13. Bertola DR, Carneiro JD, D'Amico EA, et al. Hematological findings in Noonan syndrome. *Revista do Hospital das Clinicas* 2003;58:5–8.

14. Young G, Driscoll MC. Coagulation abnormalities in the carbohydrate-deficient glycoprotein syndrome: case report and review of the literature. *Am J Hematol* 1999;60:66–9.

15. Salomon O, Zivelin A, Livnat T, et al. Prevalence, causes, and characterization of factor XI inhibitors in patients with inherited factor XI deficiency. *Blood* 2003;101:4783–8.

16. Duga S, Salomon O. Factor XI deficiency. *Sem Thromb Haemost* 2009;35:416–25.

17. Salomon O, Steinberg DM, Seligsohn U. Variable bleeding manifestations characterize different types of surgery in patients with severe factor XI deficiency enabling parsimonious use of replacement therapy. *Haemophilia* 2006;12:490–3.

18. Salomon O, Steinberg DM, Tamarin I, et al. Plasma replacement therapy during labor is not mandatory for women with severe factor XI deficiency. *Blood Coagul Fibrinolysis* 2005;16:37–41.

19. Brenner B, Laor A, Lupo H, et al. Bleeding predictors in factor-XI-deficient patients. *Blood Coagul Fibrinolysis* 1997;8:511–15.

20. Aledort LM, Goudemand J, Hemoleven Study Group. United States' factor XI-deficiency patients need a safer treatment. *Am J Hematol* 2005;80:301–2.

21. Santoro C, Goldberg I, Bridey F, et al. Successful hip arthroplasty in an adult male with severe factor XI deficiency using Hemoleven, a factor XI concentrate. *Haemophilia* 2011;17:777–82.

22. Kadir R, Chi C, Bolton-Maggs P. Pregnancy and rare bleeding disorders. *Haemophilia* 2009;15:990–1005.
23. Berliner S, Horowitz I, Martinowitz U, et al. Dental surgery in patients with severe factor XI deficiency without plasma replacement. *Blood Coag Fibrinol* 1992;3: 465–8.
24. Muller F, Gailani D, Renne T. Factor XI and XII as antithrombotic targets. *Curr Opin Hematol* 2011;18:349–55.

CHAPTER 7

Factor VIII and IX Inhibitors in Hemophilia

Meera Chitlur and Jeanne Lusher
Wayne State University, Children's Hospital of Michigan, Detroit, MI, USA

Introduction

The hallmark of severe hemophilia is bleeding into joints, muscles, and other soft tissues. Recurrent joint bleeding often leads to progressive joint damage and arthropathy. The introduction of factor VIII (FVIII) and factor IX (FIX) concentrates in the early 1970s revolutionized the management of hemophilia and dramatically improved quality of life. However, close upon the heels of this radical breakthrough came the epidemics of transfusion-related HIV infection and hepatitis. In response to these serious complications, recombinant factor VIII and IX concentrates were developed and, soon thereafter, home treatment and routine prophylaxis became the standard of care in prevention of hemophilic arthropathy. As viral safety, joint function, and overall quality of life improved for persons with hemophilia, inhibitor development became the major complication usually seen in patients with severe hemophilia. The development of such alloantibodies often precludes the use of factor replacement products. Patients with any clotting factor deficiency may develop inhibitory antibodies to the replacement products, but inhibitors to FVIII and FIX constitute the major proportion of cases encountered.

Definition of inhibitors

An inhibitor is a high-affinity polyclonal immunoglobulin G (IgG) antibody that specifically inactivates a particular clotting protein. Inhibitors are classified as high- or low-responding based on their peak activity (less than or greater than 5 Bethesda units, BU) by the Scientific and Standardization Committee of the International Society of Thrombosis and

Hemostasis and Thrombosis: Practical Guidelines in Clinical Management, First Edition.
Hussain I. Saba and Harold R. Roberts.
© 2014 John Wiley & Sons, Ltd. Published 2014 by John Wiley & Sons, Ltd.

Hemostasis (ISTH). The high-responding subtype is associated with an anamnestic increase in inhibitor titer with continued exposure to the offending protein. The low-responding type may be transient and may spontaneously resolve, or may continue to increase to become a high-titer inhibitor.

Rarely, non-neutralizing antibodies occur that target non-functional epitopes on the clotting proteins; these may not be clinically significant [1].

Laboratory diagnosis of inhibitors in hemophilia

As described in the chapter on laboratory diagnosis, mixing studies are commonly used to screen for the presence of inhibitors. The Bethesda assay, which is a specific assay for inhibitors, was first described by Kasper et al. in 1975 and is based on the observation that FVIII inhibitors will neutralize a known concentration of FVIII:C over a period of time at 37°C [2]. One Bethesda unit (BU) is defined as the amount of antibody that decreases the FVIII:C by 50%. Most laboratories use $\geq 0.6\,BU$ as the cut-off for a "positive" inhibitor assay. In 1995, the Nijmegen modification to the Bethesda assay was introduced to improve the specificity and reliability to detect low-titer inhibitors [3]. This modification involves adding an imidazole buffer to normal pooled plasma substrate and using a FVIII:C-deficient plasma in the place of buffer for the control.

Kinetics of factor VIII inactivation

The reaction kinetics of the FVIII inhibitor determines whether it is a type 1 or type 2 antibody. Type 1 inhibitors neutralize FVIII in linear dose-dependent manner, whereas the antibody can only be neutralized by repeated additions of FVIII that is a type 2 antibody. Most inhibitors which develop in persons with congenital hemophilia are type 1, while acquired inhibitors seen in non-hemophilic patients demonstrate type 2 kinetics.

Factor VIII gene and inhibitor characteristics

The FVIII gene has been localized to the long arm of the X-chromosome, Xq28. It is estimated to be 186 kb in length and has 26 exons [4]. While more than 900 mutations have been identified to cause hemophilia, the most common genetic defects involve intron 22 inversions, which occur in 45–50% of patients with severe hemophilia A [5,6]. Most cases of mild (FVIII:C = 5–30%) and moderate (FVIII:C = 1–5%) hemophilia A result from missense mutations [7]. The FVIII protein has 2,332 amino acids with a domain structure of A1-a1-A2-a2-B-a3-A3-C1-C2. The alloantibodies to FVIII belong to the IgG subclass with the majority being IgG4. The FVIII A2 domain inhibitors inhibit the formation of the Xase complex and anti-FVIII C2 domain inhibitors block the phospholipid and von Willebrand factor binding sites, thereby blocking amplification of clot formation [8].

Factor IX gene and inhibitor characteristics

The FIX gene is located on the long arm of the X-chromosome at Xp27.1 and spans 33 kbp. It has 8 exons from which a 415 amino acid protein is transcribed. Missense/nonsense mutations are the most common type of genetic mutation associated with hemophilia B (64% of all mutations) [9]. However, many patients who develop inhibitors have large gene deletions. Inhibitors to FIX bind to the γ-carboxyglutamic acid region and the serine protease domain and are mostly IgG4. IgG1 subclass antibodies have been noted in some patients with hemophilia B with inhibitors, who develop anaphylactic reactions with infusion of FIX-containing products [10,11].

Risk factors for inhibitor development

In children with severe hemophilia A, 25–30% develop inhibitors to the replacement products after a mean of 9–11 exposure days (ED). Many of these (approximately 40%) are low titer and transient despite continued exposure to FVIII-containing products. Interestingly, only 1–5% of patients with hemophilia B develop inhibitors. Both genetic and environmental risk factors play a role.

African-American or Latino race and family history of inhibitors are associated with an increased risk of inhibitor formation in hemophilia A [12]. A recent study showed that the former may be due to a discrepancy between the FVIII haplotype and the haplotype of the product used for treatment, but this study had a small sample size and did not take into consideration other confounding factors such as mutation type [13]. In hemophilia A, the highest incidence of inhibitors is seen in patients with splice site mutations followed by intron 1 or intron 22 inversion [14]. These indicate that mutations resulting in the absence of FVIII are associated with a higher risk of inhibitor formation. Similarly, in hemophilia B the inhibitor risk is significantly higher in patients with gross or complete deletions [15]. The Malmö International Brothers Study, and a North American study of brother pairs with inhibitors published by Gill in 1999, showed that the concordance of inhibitor occurrence was 50% in brothers and only 9% in the extended family members [16,17]. This indicates that the genetic mutation causing the disease alone does not determine the risk of inhibitor occurrence.

When the FVIII molecule is introduced into the body, it is endocytosed by the antigen-presenting cells (APC) and the processed protein is presented on the surface of the APC via the class II major histocompatability molecule to the CD4+ helper T-cells. These activated helper T-cells then stimulate the antigen-specific B-cells to proliferate and differentiate into secreting plasma cells and memory B-cells. This process also requires costimulatory pathways such as CD28 and B7 and CD40 and CD40L, and the effective synthesis of immunoglobulins and cytokine release by Th1 and Th2 cells, which then direct the B-cell to produce antibodies or inhibitors. Therefore, mutations in any of the immune response genes or cytokine expression genes may predispose to an increased risk of inhibitor formation by promoting the expansion of inhibitor-producing clones of B-cells.

Treatment-related risk factors include intensive treatment with FVIII products in the presence of "danger signals" (tissue damage or inflammation). The risk of inhibitor formation with exposure to FVIII concentrate is highest within the first 50 ED or days on which the patient received FVIII. The CANAL study showed that an increased intensity of exposure during the first 50 ED resulted in a three- to fourfold increase in the risk of inhibitor development [18] while there was no detectable difference in the inhibitor risk with plasma-derived versus recombinant FVIII products, and switching between different products did not show an increase in inhibitor risk [19]. The role of von Willebrand factor (VWF) in decreasing the immunogenicity of FVIII is currently a topic of discussion. While VWF in a product has been shown to be protective in in-vitro studies and animal models, there are no clinical data in persons with hemophilia A to support this theory [20]. Comparisons of the incidence of inhibitors between different recombinant products have shown no difference in the rates of inhibitor occurrence [21,22]. Retrospective studies in 2001 and 2003 showed a decrease in inhibitor incidence with delay in exposure to FVIII products, with few inhibitors seen in those who were <1.5 years of age at first exposure [23,24]. However, recent studies have shown that early and regular prophylaxis with a FVIII product may in fact be "protective" when administered in the absence of immunologic stimulus [25,26]. Traditionally, the factor is administered as a bolus injection, but in order to avoid the peaks and troughs seen in this method a continuous infusion is sometimes preferred and may be the choice of administration in the event of serious bleeding such as intracranial hemorrhage or major surgery. Although there have been some reports of an increased incidence of inhibitor formation with the use of continuous infusion, this has not been confirmed in large randomized controlled trials. Higher immunologic stimulation along with high intensity of treatment may play a role in this situation.

Inhibitors in mild and moderate hemophilia A

Patients with mild or moderate hemophilia are generally considered to be at a lower risk for inhibitor development, with a prevalence of 3–13% [27]. These inhibitors often appear later in life than in severe hemophilia A, and after an episode of intensive treatment. The Arg593→Cys mutation is the most common mutation associated with inhibitor formation in patients with mild hemophilia A [27].

Inhibitors in hemophilia B

Inhibitor development in patients with severe hemophilia B usually occurs early, after a median of 9–11 ED to any FIX-containing products. The risk factors for the development of inhibitors in hemophilia B patients are similar to hemophilia A. Large deletions and frame shift mutations resulting in loss of protein production are more likely to be associated with inhibitor development. Unlike hemophilia A, where a higher incidence of inhibitors is noted in the African-American population, there is no racial predilection for inhibitor development in hemophilia B. The roles of environmental factors, concurrent immune challenges, and immune response gene polymorphisms are being investigated. Unique complications associated with inhibitor formation in hemophilia B are the occurrence of anaphylaxis and nephrotic syndrome. An international registry on FIX inhibitors was established in 1997 by Dr. Warrier under the FVIII/IX subcommittee of the ISTH/SSC (Scientific and Standardization Committee) and anaphylaxis was reported in 56/94 (approx 60%) patients with hemophilia B with inhibitors. Nephrotic syndrome was reported in 13 patients, 11 of whom also had a history of anaphylaxis. All patients who developed nephrotic syndrome had been receiving high doses of FIX for immune tolerance induction therapy for approximately 6–8 months, and the edema and proteinuria resolved after discontinuation of the FIX product. In view of the risk of anaphylaxis, it is recommended that the first 20 infusions of a FIX product be performed in a healthcare facility where the patient can be closely monitored and treated for anaphylaxis if it develops [28].

Management of patients with factor VIII and factor IX inhibitors

The availability of bypassing agents has significantly improved the management of acute bleeding episodes in patients with inhibitors. In patients with low-responding or low-titer inhibitors, the use of higher doses of factor concentrate may be sufficient to achieve hemostasis. The increased dose can be given empirically if the dose of factor required to saturate the inhibitor can be calculated using the formula: number of units of factor to be infused = volume of plasma (mL) × inhibitor titer (BU/mL). In infants and young children who develop low-titer inhibitors, one can usually continue to use FVIII products on demand and monitor them to see if the titer increases or disappears, as long as clinical response to treatment is noted. By continuing to use FVIII, the patient may be monitored using standard coagulation assays; however, the risk of an anamnestic increase in inhibitor titer exists. In general, FVIII products are no longer effective when the inhibitor titers are >5 BU. The use of plasma exchange or immunoabsorption to decrease the inhibitor titer requires highly specialized equipment and is used rarely in patients with hemophilia B where immune tolerance induction may not be possible. The activated prothrombin complex concentrate FEIBA (Factor VIII Inhibitor By-passing Activity, FEIBA®VH, Baxter® Healthcare Corp, CA, USA) and recombinant FVIIa (Novoseven®, Novo Nordisk A/S, Bagsvaerd, Denmark) are two bypassing agents currently available to treat bleeding in patients with inhibitors.

FEIBA is used for the treatment of acute bleeding episodes at a dose of 50–100 U/kg body weight administered every 8–12 hours, with a maximum of 200 U/kg/day. The mechanism of action, although not completely understood, may be mediated through prothrombin and FXa [29]. The efficacy has been shown to be ≥65% for treatment of acute joint bleeds [30]. The ProFEIBA Study showed that prophylaxis three times a week with 85 U/kg reduced the occurrence of joint hemorrhage by 61%, compared to on-demand treatment [31].

Recombinant factor VIIa (rFVIIa) works by directly activating platelet-bound FX and inducing a thrombin burst [9]. The major drawback is its short half-life. rFVIIa has been found to be efficacious at a dose of 90–120 μg/kg given every 2–3 hours. Kenet et al. showed that a single larger dose of 200–300 μg/kg was effective in children [32]. rFVIIa has also been used as prophylaxis for the prevention of joint bleeds [33,34].

The FENOC study compared both FEIBA and rFVIIa and found them to be equally efficacious in the treatment of joint bleeds in hemophilia patients with inhibitors [34]. Following infusion, both FEIBA and rFVIIa can only be monitored using newer global assays such as thrombin generation or thromboelastography [35]. Both agents have reportedly been associated with a slightly increased risk of thrombosis and therefore should be employed with caution especially when used concomitantly or sequentially in a life- or limb-threatening situation [36], or in patients with coronary heart disease. There is a risk of anamnestic increase in anti-FVIII inhibitor levels with the use of FEIBA, which contains trace amounts of FVIII antigen. This increase in inhibitor titer does not seem to decrease the clinical efficacy and the inhibitor levels have been noted to gradually decrease with continued use of the product.

In the 1990s, an alternative to bypassing agents was porcine FVIII, which was used both in patients with autoantibodies as well as alloanti-bodies to FVIII [37,38] since the cross-reactivity between anti-human FVIII antibodies and porcine FVIII is only 15%. However, the older porcine FVIII product was discontinued because of laboratory evidence of porcine parvovirus in batches of product [39], even though there was no evidence of transmission in human recipients. A recombinant B-domain-deleted porcine FVIII (OBI-1) has recently been studied in pre-licensure clinical trials, and the results are awaited. An analog of rFVIIa, NN1731 has been shown to have a longer half-life in ex vivo studies [40].

In patients with mild hemophilia A who develop inhibitors, desmo-pressin acetate should be considered as an alternative to treatment with FVIII products. Inhibitors in mild hemophilia A occur later in life and are associated with certain high-risk mutations. Immune tolerance induction has been less successful in eradicating these inhibitors and immunomodu-lation may increase the chances of successful tolerization. Again, clinical trials would be necessary but are difficult to perform in this rare disease.

Immune tolerance induction for the eradication of inhibitors

The ultimate goal in the management of a patient with inhibitors is to eradicate the inhibitor. Immune tolerance induction (ITI) is the only proven method to achieve tolerance to FVIII or FIX. This was first described by Brackmann and Goremsen in 1977, where patients were given repeated doses of FVIII concentrate (200–300 U/kg/day) along with prothrombin complex concentrates until the inhibitor disappeared and the half-life of the FVIII normalized. While several modifications of this protocol have been described, the basic principles remain the same, where frequent FVIII administration is used with the intention of achieving and maintaining tolerance. The International ITI study compared the use of high dose (200 U/kg daily) with low dose (50 U/kg, three times a week) and found no difference in efficacy (76%) but the high-dose group achieved tolerance earlier and had fewer bleeding episodes [41]. Low titer of inhibitor prior to start of ITI (<10 BU) and historical peak inhibitor titer of <200 BU were consistently associated with successful tolerization. The use of von Willebrand factor containing concentrate to induce tolerance is currently being investigated in the RESIST trial, both in patients who have already experienced and failed ITI with von Willebrand factor-free concentrates and as a first-line modality in newly diagnosed inhibitor patients (http://www.itistudy-resist.com/).

While the success of treating patients with hemophilia A with inhibitors is approximately 80%, the success rate in hemophilia B is dismally low at 15%, along with the occurrence of nephrotic syndrome while on ITI, as noted in the ISTH registry [42].

Immune modulation

Monoclonal antibodies such as rituximab, a humanized anti-CD-20 antibody, has been used with limited success in inhibitor patients with hemophilia A and B who have failed the standard ITI therapy. Randomized controlled trials are necessary but difficult to conduct in this small population of patients.

Conclusion

Inhibitor formation is currently the most important and difficult to manage complication in patients with hemophilia. Understanding the mechanisms involved in the development of inhibitors and preventing inhibitor development would be the ultimate goal of physicians treating these patients. Clinical trials, although difficult to perform, are crucial to a better understanding of this problem. Our understanding of the mechanisms of tolerance has come a long way and hopefully will progress rapidly to facilitate a successful outcome for inhibitor patients. Immune tolerance induction remains the sole known method of inhibitor eradication but is only successful in a small group of patients.

References

1. Key NS. Inhibitors in congenital coagulation disorders. *Br J Haematol* 2004; 127:379–91.
2. Sahud MA. Factor VIII inhibitors: laboratory diagnosis of inhibitors. *Semin Thromb Hemost* 2000;26:195–203.
3. Verbruggen B, Novakova I, Wessels H, et al. The Nijmegen modification of the Bethesda assay for factor VIII:C inhibitors: improved specificity and reliability. *Thromb Haemost* 1995;73:247–51.

4. Gitschier J, Wood WI, Goralka TM, et al. Characterization of the human factor VIII gene. *Nature* 1984;312(5992):326–30.

5. Jayandharan G, Shaji RV, Baidya S, et al. Identification of factor VIII gene mutations in 101 patients with haemophilia A: mutation analysis by inversion screening and multiplex PCR and CSGE and molecular modeling of 10 novel missense substitutions. *Haemophilia* 2005;11:481–91.

6. Lakich D, Kazazian HH Jr., Antonarakis SE, Gitschier J. Inversions disrupting the factor VIII gene are a common cause of severe haemophilia A. *Nat Genet* 1993;5:236–41.

7. Jacquemin M, De Maeyer M, D'Oiron R, et al. Molecular mechanisms of mild and moderate hemophilia A. *J Thromb Haemost* 2003;1(3):456–63.

8. Pratt KP, Thompson AR. B-cell and T-cell epitopes in anti-factor VIII immune responses. *Clin Rev Allergy Immunol* 2009;37(2):80–95.

9. Lee CA, Berntorp E, Hoots WK, editors. *Textbook of Hemophilia.* Second edition. Oxford: Blackwell Publishing Ltd, 2010.

10. Carroll RR, Panush RS, Kitchens CS. Spontaneous disappearance of an IgA anti-factor IX inhibitor in a child with Christmas disease. *Am J Hematol* 1984;17:321–5.

11. Sawamoto Y, Shima M, Yamamoto M, et al. Measurement of anti-factor IX IgG subclasses in haemophilia B patients who developed inhibitors with episodes of allergic reactions to factor IX concentrates. *Thromb Res* 1996;83:279–86.

12. Aledort LM, Dimichele DM. Inhibitors occur more frequently in African-American and Latino haemophiliacs. *Haemophilia* 1998;4:68.

13. Viel KR, Ameri A, Abshire TC, et al. Inhibitors of factor VIII in black patients with hemophilia. *N Engl J Med* 2009;360:1618–27.

14. Boekhorst J, Lari GR, D'Oiron R, et al. Factor VIII genotype and inhibitor development in patients with haemophilia A: highest risk in patients with splice site mutations. *Haemophilia* 2008;14:729–35.

15. DiMichele D. Inhibitor development in haemophilia B: an orphan disease in need of attention. *Br J Haematol* 2007;138:305–15.

16. Gill JC. The role of genetics in inhibitor formation. *Thromb Haemost* 1999;82:500–4.

17. Astermark J, Berntorp E, White GC, Kroner BL. The Malmo International Brother Study (MIBS): further support for genetic predisposition to inhibitor development in hemophilia patients. *Haemophilia* 2001;7:267–72.

18. Gouw SC, van der Bom JG, Marijke van den Berg H. Treatment-related risk factors of inhibitor development in previously untreated patients with hemophilia A: the CANAL cohort study. *Blood* 2007;109:4648–54.

19. Gouw SC, van der Bom JG, Auerswald G, et al. Recombinant versus plasma-derived factor VIII products and the development of inhibitors in previously untreated patients with severe hemophilia A: the CANAL cohort study. *Blood* 2007;109:4693–7.

20. Coppola A, Santoro C, Tagliaferri A, Franchini M, Dim G. Understanding inhibitor development in haemophilia A: towards clinical prediction and prevention strategies. *Haemophilia* 2010;16(suppl 1):13–19.

21. Lusher JM. First and second generation recombinant factor VIII concentrates in previously untreated patients: recovery, safety, efficacy, and inhibitor development. *Semin Thromb Hemost* 2002;28:273–6.

22. Oldenburg J, Goudemand J, Valentino L, et al. Postauthorization safety surveillance of ADVATE [antihaemophilic factor (recombinant), plasma/albumin-free method]

demonstrates efficacy, safety and low-risk for immunogenicity in routine clinical practice. *Haemophilia* 2010;16:866–77.

23. Lorenzo JI, Lopez A, Altisent C, Aznar JA. Incidence of factor VIII inhibitors in severe haemophilia: the importance of patient age. *Br J Haematol* 2001;113: 600–3.

24. van der Bom JG, Mauser-Bunschoten EP, Fischer K, van den Berg HM. Age at first treatment and immune tolerance to factor VIII in severe hemophilia. *Thromb Haemost* 2003;89:475–9.

25. Auerswald G, Bidlingmaier C, Kurnik K. Early prophylaxis/FVIII tolerization regimen that avoids immunological danger signals is still effective in minimizing FVIII inhibitor developments in previously untreated patients: long-term follow-up and continuing experience. *Haemophilia* 2012;18:e18–20.

26. Kurnik K, Bidlingmaier C, Engl W, et al. New early prophylaxis regimen that avoids immunological danger signals can reduce FVIII inhibitor development. *Haemophilia* 2010;16: 256–62.

27. Hay CR, Ludlam CA, Colvin BT, et al. Factor VIII inhibitors in mild and moderate-severity haemophilia A. UK Haemophilia Centre Directors Organization. *Thromb Haemost* 1998;79:762–6.

28. Warrier I, Ewenstein BM, Koerper MA, et al. Factor IX inhibitors and anaphylaxis in hemophilia B. *J Pediatr Hematol Oncol* 1997;19:23–7.

29. Turecek PL, Varadi K, Gritsch H, Schwarz HP. FEIBA: mode of action. *Haemophilia* 2004;10(suppl 2):3–9.

30. Barthels M. Clinical efficacy of prothrombin complex concentrates and recombinant factor VIIa in the treatment of bleeding episodes in patients with factor VII and IX inhibitors. *Thromb Res* 1999;95(4 suppl 1):S31–8.

31. Leissinger C, Gringeri A, Antmen B, et al. Anti-inhibitor coagulant complex prophylaxis in hemophilia with inhibitors. *N Engl J Med* 2011;365:1684–92.

32. Kenet G, Martinowitz U. Single-dose recombinant activated factor VII therapy in hemophilia patients with inhibitors. *Semin Hematol* 2008;45(2 suppl 1): S38–41.

33. Konkle BA, Ebbesen LS, Erhardtsen E, et al. Randomized, prospective clinical trial of recombinant factor VIIa for secondary prophylaxis in hemophilia patients with inhibitors. *J Thromb Haemost* 2007;5:1904–13.

34. Astermark J, Donfield SM, DiMichele DM, et al. A randomized comparison of bypassing agents in hemophilia complicated by an inhibitor: the FEIBA NovoSeven Comparative (FENOC) Study. *Blood* 2007;109:546–51.

35. Brophy DF, Martin EJ, Christian Barrett J, et al. Monitoring rFVIIa 90 mug kg(1) dosing in haemophiliacs: comparing laboratory response using various whole blood assays over 6 h. *Haemophilia* 2011;17:e949–57.

36. Schneiderman J, Rubin E, Nugent DJ, Young G. Sequential therapy with activated prothrombin complex concentrates and recombinant FVIIa in patients with severe haemophilia and inhibitors: update of our previous experience. *Haemophilia* 2007: 13:244–8.

37. Brettler DB, Forsberg AD, Levine PH, et al. The use of porcine factor VIII concentrate (Hyate:C) in the treatment of patients with inhibitor antibodies to factor VIII. A multicenter US experience. *Arch Intern Med* 1989;149:1381–5.

38. Morrison AE, Ludlam CA, Kessler C. Use of porcine factor VIII in the treatment of patients with acquired hemophilia. *Blood* 1993;81:1513–20.

39. Gringeri A, Santagostino E, Tradati F, et al. Adverse effects of treatment with porcine factor VIII. *Thromb Haemost* 1991;65:245–7.

40. Gray LD, Hussey MA, Larson BM, et al. Recombinant factor VIIa analog NN1731 (V158D/E296V/M298Q-FVIIa) enhances fibrin formation, structure and stability in lipidated hemophilic plasma. *Thromb Res* 2011;128:570–6.

41. DiMichele D. The North American Immune Tolerance Registry: contributions to the thirty-year experience with immune tolerance therapy. *Haemophilia* 2009;15: 320–8.

42. Chitlur M, Warrier I, Rajpurkar M, Lusher JM. Inhibitors in factor IX deficiency a report of the ISTH-SSC international FIX inhibitor registry (1997–2006). *Haemophilia* 2009;15:1027–31.

CHAPTER 8

Treatment Options for Acquired Hemophilia

Anjali Sharathkumar and David Green

Departments of Pediatrics and Medicine, Feinberg School of Medicine of Northwestern University, Chicago, IL, USA

Introduction

Acquired hemophilia (AH) is a rare but potentially life-threatening autoimmune disorder that is characterized by the abrupt onset of bleeding in patients with negative family and personal history of bleeding [1,2]. It is more frequently reported in the elderly and is caused by autoantibodies that are directed against functional epitopes of factor VIII (FVIII), causing its neutralization and/or accelerated clearance from the plasma [3,4]. Morbidity and mortality associated with AH are high, and successful management relies on a high index of suspicion, early diagnosis, and appropriate medical intervention.

In this chapter, we will briefly review the epidemiology, pathophysiology, and criteria for diagnosis, but the main focus will be on disease management. Methods for controlling hemorrhage will be described and steps to suppress or eliminate autoantibody formation will be discussed.

Epidemiology

Since the first description of AH in 1940 [5], much progress has been made in unfolding the epidemiology of this condition. The estimated annual incidence is between 0.2 and 1.48 cases per million [6,7], and the age distribution is biphasic, with a small peak at 20–30 years (mainly postpartum women) and a larger peak in patients aged 70–80 years. The annual incidence increases with age and is estimated to be 0.045 per million in children under 16 and 14.5 per million in people over 85 [6]. Women

Hemostasis and Thrombosis: Practical Guidelines in Clinical Management, First Edition.
Hussain I. Saba and Harold R. Roberts.
© 2014 John Wiley & Sons, Ltd. Published 2014 by John Wiley & Sons, Ltd.

predominate in the younger age group because of the association with
pregnancy, while there is male predominance in those over 60 [7].

Etiology

The decrease in FVIII is due to the presence of FVIII autoantibodies [8].
Most patients do not have concomitant illnesses, but in others antibodies
appear in conjunction with underlying medical conditions such as autoimmune diseases, solid tumors, lymphoproliferative malignancies, and pregnancy [6,7,9]. Pregnancy-related antibodies generally occur in primiparous
women within the first 3 months of delivery [6,7]. When the inhibitor
develops during pregnancy, there is a risk of transplacental transfer of
antibody to the fetus or newborn, causing "neonatal AH" [10].

Circulating FVIII is non-covalently bound to von Willebrand factor
(VWF). Upon initiation of coagulation, FVIII becomes activated and,
together with activated FIX, forms the intrinsic tenase complex. This
complex is a major participant in thrombin generation and amplifies the
coagulation cascade [11]. Autoantibodies bind to one or more of the
domains of FVIII and interfere with its various hemostatic properties
[12–16].

Depending on the domain specificity, antibodies might block the binding
of FVIIIa to FIXa, FX or phospholipid, or interfere with the proteolytic
activation of FVIII. Furthermore, antibodies that interfere with the
binding to VWF increase the clearance of FVIII [17]. The ultimate result
is that FVIII autoantibodies decrease thrombin generation and impair
hemostasis.

The autoantibodies are polyclonal [18–20], and the major antibody
subclass is IgG4 (less frequently, IgG1). Since IgG1 and IgG4 antibodies do
not bind complement, they do not cause immune-complex-mediated reactions. Interestingly, antibodies to FVIII have been demonstrated in 17%
of healthy people, implying that not all antibodies are pathogenic [21].
Those antibodies that are clinically important usually have type 2 inactivation kinetics [22]; they inactivate FVIII incompletely and display residual
FVIII activity [8,23]. This has implications for measurement of anti-FVIII
antibody titers and may play a role in the typical bleeding patterns
observed.

Why persons develop anti-FVIII autoantibodies is not fully understood. The association of AH with autoimmune disorders and older
age suggests immune dysregulation. Genetic polymorphisms that affect
T-cell regulatory factors have been described in patients with AH [24].
Also, polymorphisms within the *f8* gene may contribute to inhibitor
formation [25].

Clinical presentation

The clinical presentation of AH differs from that of congenital hemophilia [6,7]. Most patients with FVIII autoantibodies have hemorrhages into the skin, muscles, soft tissues, or mucous membranes (e.g., epistaxis, gastrointestinal and urological bleeding, retroperitoneal hematoma, and postpartum bleeding), but hemarthroses, a typical feature of congenital FVIII deficiency, are uncommon. Patients with AH may have overt hemorrhage or anemia due to occult bleeding. Life-threatening hemorrhage occurs in 9–22% [6,7], while 30% have mild bleeding requiring no treatment [26]. Occasionally, patients without clinical evidence of bleeding are diagnosed during routine blood tests.

Because of delays in diagnosis, patients with AH are at higher risk of bleeding-related death compared to congenital hemophilia patients with inhibitors. Delays of as long as 58 days between bleeding onset and diagnosis, and 69 days between the first abnormal activated partial thromboplastin time (aPTT) and diagnosis, have been reported [27]. Death may result from bleeding, from the underlying disease, or from the side effects of treatment. If the inhibitor is not eradicated, severe bleeding might occur at any time. Some patients bleed persistently until the inhibitor is eradicated, whereas others live normally for years with a detectable inhibitor. Treatment decisions are usually based on the clinical bleeding phenotype.

Infrequently, acquired hemophilia occurs in a child, as illustrated by the following Case:

Case: Acquired hemophilia in a child [95]

A 14-year-old girl with a recent history of bruising on her legs developed an acute abdomen. Abdominal ultrasound revealed a cystic, hemorrhagic lesion of the left ovary. In the emergency room she became hypotensive and received multiple fluid boluses, packed red cells, and fresh frozen plasma. Coagulation studies showed prolongation of aPTT and a normal PT; the addition of normal plasma to the patient's plasma failed to correct the aPTT. The FVIII level was 8% and Bethesda assay showed an inhibitor titer of 110 BU. These findings were consistent with a diagnosis of acquired hemophilia. Treatment with 90 μg/kg/dose of rFVIIa at 2-hourly intervals controlled her bleeding.

Laboratory diagnosis

Laboratory investigation for the evaluation of a patient with suspected AHA should include screening coagulation tests, mixing studies, specific factor assays, and Bethesda assay to quantify the inhibitor. Figure 8.1

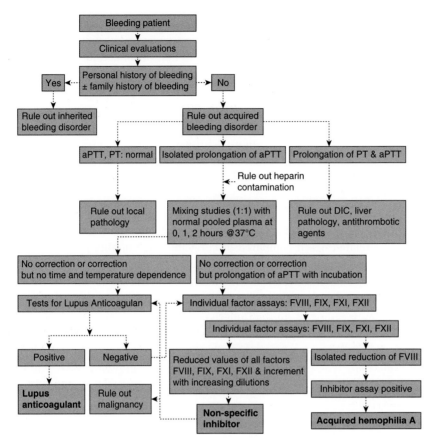

Figure 8.1 Algorithm for evaluating bleeding if FVIII autoantibody is suspected. Source: Adapted from Collins 2011 [55]. Reproduced with permission of John Wiley & Sons Ltd.

shows an algorithm for evaluating bleeding in a patient suspected of harboring a FVIII autoantibody [6]. Screening coagulation assays typically reveal a prolongation of activated partial thromboplastin time (aPTT) and a normal prothrombin time (PT). The next step is a mixing test, to determine if patient plasma prolongs the aPTT of normal plasma. Because many autoantibodies inactivate FVIII in a time- and temperature-dependent manner, the aPTT should be repeated after the mixture has been incubated for up to 2 hours at 37°C. On occasion, it is necessary to exclude the presence of a lupus anticoagulant [28], although such anticoagulants are infrequently associated with bleeding. If antiphospholipid antibodies interfere with the Bethesda assay, an enzyme-linked immunosorbent assay (ELISA) can be used to screen for FVIII inhibitors [29]. The presence of heparin is likely if the thrombin time is prolonged and the reptilase time is normal.

The Bethesda titer is defined as the dilution of patient plasma that produces a 50% decrease in the FVIII activity of normal plasma [30]. The original Bethesda assay has been modified to decrease spurious results [31,32], and an ELISA assay may be useful in complicated cases [33]. Inhibitors are classified as low titer if the Bethesda titer is <5 BU.

Treatment options for acquired hemophilia

The main principles of treatment for AH are:
- control of acute bleeding;
- avoid non-essential invasive procedures;
- resolve underlying disorders;
- eradicate the inhibitor; and
- educate patients about the importance of not exposing themselves to injury.

It is strongly recommended that physicians managing a patient with suspected or confirmed AH should not delay in consulting a hemophilia center with expertise in managing inhibitors [27]. It is important to underscore that the severity of bleeding correlates poorly with the FVIII activity level and Bethesda titer, and that even patients with measurable FVIII levels and low inhibitor titers can have life-threatening hemorrhages. Therefore, decisions about management need to rely on the clinical severity of bleeding.

Control of acute bleeding
Table 8.1 displays agents useful in controlling bleeding. Two approaches to achieve haemostasis are the use of bypassing agents and strategies to

Table 8.1 Agents used to control bleeding in patients with factor VIII autoantibodies.

Clotting factor concentrates	
FEIBA (Factor VIII Inhibitor Bypassing Agent)	50–100 U/kg every 8–12 hours, not to exceed 200 U/kg/day
rFVIIa (recombinant factor VIIa)	90–120 µg/kg every 2–3 hours until response
rFVIII (recombinant factor VIII)	Inhibitor <5 BU: 100 U/kg; repeat as necessary
Adjunctive agents	
DDAVP (desmopressin)	Inhibitor <5 BU: 0.3 µg/kg IV/SC
Tranexamic acid	10 mg/kg IV every 6 hours
ε-aminocaproic acid	Loading: 100 mg/kg IV; maintenance: 50 mg/kg every 6 hours

raise the level of circulating FVIII. Local measures such as topical fibrin glue for mucosal hemorrhages can be helpful. While the concurrent administration of antifibrinolytic agents (tranexamic acid, ε-aminocaproic acid) is occasionally beneficial, they increase the risk of thrombosis and should be used with caution in patients with hematuria. Besides focusing on achieving hemostatic control, close clinical and laboratory monitoring is necessary to prevent hemodynamic instability due to acute blood loss.

Recombinant factor VIIa

Recombinant factor VIIa (rFVIIa, NovoSeven®) was initially developed for use in patients with congenital hemophilia with inhibitors, but it has been approved for the treatment of AH [34]. By directly activating FX on the surface of activated platelets at the site of injury (thereby bypassing FVIII and FIX), rFVIIa can circumvent the actions of inhibitory antibodies [35].A retrospective analysis by Hay et al. [36] showed that bleeding was controlled in all of 38 patients when rFVIIa was used as a first-line treatment and a 75% response rate when it was used as salvage therapy. Sumner et al. [37] performed a meta-analysis of the published literature as well as the Hemophilia and Thrombosis Research Society Registry data and reported similar results. rFVIIa is initiated in doses of 90 μg/kg every 2–4 hours until bleeding is controlled, followed by further, less frequent dosing, to prevent recurrence [38]. Although doses of up to 270 μg/kg have been used in the management of congenital hemophilia with inhibitors [39], such doses should be used cautiously in patients with AH because of the risk of thromboembolic complications. Such events occur in 7% of patients [40]. If bleeding remains poorly controlled despite a trial of rFVIIa, it may be prudent to switch to activated prothrombin complex concentrate.

Activated prothrombin complex concentrate

Activated prothrombin complex concentrate (aPCC, FEIBA®) is a plasma-derived concentrate containing mainly non-activated factors II, IX, X, and activated FVII, as well as 1–6 units of FVIII antigen. A retrospective study of 34 patients with AH showed an overall complete response rate of 86% with a dosing regimen of FEIBA of 75 U/kg every 8–12 hours, with a median of 10 doses to control severe bleeding [41]. Thrombotic complications are relatively infrequent, and occur mainly when recommended doses (Table 8.1) are exceeded. The duration of treatment is dependent on clinical judgment.

Monitoring therapy with bypassing agents

The utility of thrombin generation assays (TGA) and modified thromboelastography in monitoring therapy with bypassing agents appears promising but these assays are not widely available for clinical use [38,42].

FVIII concentrates

If the level of the inhibitor is <5 BU and no bypassing agent is available, hemostasis may be achieved with high doses of FVIII (Table 8.1). The response to this treatment, however, is unpredictable and the use of FVIII should not delay the use of agents (rFVIIa or aPCC) more likely to control bleeding. FVIII is more efficacious when used as part of multimodal treatment regimens that include immunoadsorption to temporarily remove the inhibitor [43].

When porcine FVIII was available, it controlled 78% of bleeds in patients with AH [44–46]. However, it was withdrawn because of safety considerations, and a recombinant porcine FVIII is currently under development (see below).

Desmopressin

Desmopressin or DDAVP (1-deamino-8-D-arginine vasopressin) (Table 8.1) can occasionally be useful in managing minor bleeding episodes in patients with very low titer inhibitors (<5 BU). However, DDAVP should not replace the use of more effective agents [47]. The European Acquired Hemophilia (EACH2) Registry reported that bleeding control was similar between rFVIIa and aPCC, but was significantly higher with these bypassing agents than with FVIII/DDAVP (93.3% vs 68.3%; $P = 0.003$) [48].

Antifibrinolytic agents

Antifibrinolytics have equivocal benefits [49], but there are no guidelines or consensus on the dosing in patients with AH, and the doses given in Table 8.1 are representative of doses given for bleeding in other disorders.

Immunoadsorption/plasmapheresis

Factor VIII autoantibodies can be removed by plasmapheresis or immunoadsorption with staphylococcal protein A [50,51]. Implementation of these measures requires a skilled team, expensive equipment, and large-bore IV access. They are most useful in bleeding or presurgical patients with high-titer inhibitors who have failed to respond to bypassing agents. Following pheresis or immunoadsorption, FVIII concentrates are given to achieve hemostasis.

Immune tolerance induction

Immune tolerance induction (ITI) protocols, like those used for the treatment of alloantibody inhibitors against FVIII or fIX in patients with congenital hemophilia A or B, have been proposed for the management of autoantibodies. Evidence of effectiveness and safety has been demonstrated using the Budapest protocol (FVIII combined with cyclophosphamide and methylprednisolone) [52]. The protocol comprises 3 weeks of treatment with FVIII concentrate (30 U/kg/day for the first week, 20 U/kg/day for the second, and 15 U/kg/day for the third week) along with cyclophosphamide (200 mg/day to a total dose of 2–3 g) plus methylprednisolone (100 mg/day IV for 1 week and then tapering the dose gradually over 2 weeks). Eradication of the inhibitor occurred in 13 of 14 ITI patients vs. 4 of 6 patients in a control group treated with traditional immunosuppressive therapy. Similar results (complete response of 88%) have been reported with a modified Malmo protocol (immunoadsorption, high doses of FVIII, high-dose immunoglobulin, cyclophosphamide, and corticosteroids) [53].

Eradication of inhibitors

Table 8.2 shows the agents most commonly selected to eliminate autoantibodies. Corticosteroids have been used for more than 50 years and are effective in up to 70% of patients [54,55]. Patients with low inhibitor titers are more likely to respond, although even those with high titers occasionally will remit. Because of steroid-associated side effects, doses are usually reduced after 3 weeks, and the drug discontinued by 6 weeks. Because of response failures in patients with high titer inhibitors, and occasional relapses after discontinuation of steroids, most clinicians combine steroids with a cytotoxic agent such as cyclophosphamide [56–58]. An analysis of 331 patients that compared steroids alone to combined therapy found an odds ratio of 3.25 ($P < 0.001$) in favor of combined therapy [53]. Therefore, prednisone and cyclophosphamide should be the initial therapy for most patients with autoantibodies. This regimen can be modified based on patient characteristics; for example, cyclophosphamide might be avoided in persons of reproductive age, or steroids omitted in diabetic patients. Some clinicians favor other immunosuppressive agents such as azathioprine, vincristine, and cyclosporine, but there is no convincing evidence

Table 8.2 Agents used for the eradication of factor VIII autoantibodies.

Agent*	Dose
Corticosteroids	Prednisone, 1 mg/kg/day, for 3 weeks; then taper gradually over 1–2 weeks
Cyclophosphamide	Oral: 1–2 mg/kg/day; IV: 1.0–1.5 g/week; continue for up to 6 weeks
Cyclosporine	200–300 mg/kg/day
Rituximab (anti-CD20 antibody)	375 mg/m² IV each week for 4 weeks

*Immunoadsorption, plasmapheresis, and immune tolerance induction are alternatives (see text).

that they improve on the results with prednisone and cyclophosphamide [6]. While early, anecdotal reports suggested IV immunoglobulin might be beneficial, further studies did not confirm its effectiveness [59,60], and it is no longer recommended [53].

Rituximab

Rituximab has emerged as a promising new agent for the eradication of inhibitors in patients with acquired hemophilia [61–65]. The largest published study reported complete remissions in 8 of 10 patients [59]. The usual dose is $375\,mg/m^2$ each week for 4 weeks. Most responses are seen within the first 2 weeks of therapy, but the presence of high inhibitor titers ($>100\,BU/mL$) is a negative prognostic factor for responsiveness. The general consensus is that rituximab should be considered in patients who are resistant to first-line therapy or cannot tolerate standard immunosuppressive therapy. However, some groups propose that rituximab should be included as first-line therapy in combination with prednisolone for patients with an inhibitor titer above 5 but less than 30, and in addition to prednisone and cyclophosphamide for those patients with a titer above 30 [66].

Case continued (evaluating response to therapy)

After the acute bleeding subsided, prophylactic therapy with FEIBA, 50 U/kg/dose every other day, was started. To suppress the inhibitor, prednisone, 2 mg/kg/day, was given and the patient was discharged. With this regimen, she did not have serious bleeding for the next 2 weeks although she continued to have occasional bruises. Because the inhibitor titer failed to decline, the prednisone dose was gradually tapered over a 2-week period (Figure 8.2). After discontinuation of steroids, she experienced a spontaneous left shoulder soft tissue bleed. She was then given rituximab, 375 mg/kg/dose, weekly for 4 weeks. After commencement of rituximab, the inhibitor disappeared and she has remained in continuous remission without further bleeding. Since she had residual FVIII activity despite the presence of inhibitors, thrombin generation assays were performed to better evaluate her hemostasis. Thrombin generation correlated with the FVIII levels and inhibitor titers (Table 8.3).

Relapse

Relapses occur in 20% of patients at a median of 7.5 months (range 1 week to 14 months) [6]. An interim analysis of 176 evaluable patients in the EACH2 registry reported relapse in 19% of those treated only with steroids and 13% for the combination of steroids and cyclophosphamide. While no relapses were observed in those treated with front-line rituximab [67], the number of patients was small and follow-up short. Therefore,

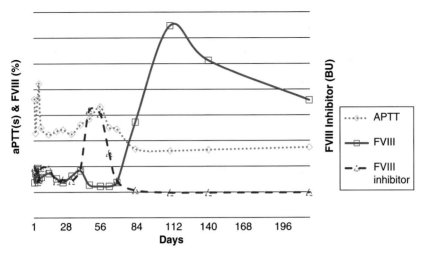

Figure 8.2 The clinical course and management of a pediatric patient with acquired hemophilia. Steroids were given from day 2 to day 30, and rituximab on days 69, 75, and 83.

Table 8.3 Case presentation: thrombin generation (peak thrombin activity), factor VIII activity, and inhibitor titers during immunosuppressive therapy modified from Batra et al [102], with permission (see also Figure 8.2).

Day	Peak thrombin (nM)	FVIII (U/mL)	Inhibitor (BU)
41	12	0.02	66
81	63	0.18	7.8
91	141	0.55	1.8
123	249	1.30	Undetectable

prolonged observation is required and patients should be advised to promptly report any bleeding.

New approaches to the management of factor VIII autoantibodies

Investigational agents

There are two approaches to augmenting hemostasis in patients with antibodies to FVIII. The first relies on providing a form of FVIII that is resistant to the inhibitory effects of the antibody. FVIII of porcine and bovine origin lacks binding sites favored by human FVIII antibodies, and therefore is less inhibited. OBI-1 is a recombinant, B-domain deleted porcine FVIII that is currently in clinical trials [68,69]. Advantages of this product are that the recombinant technology precludes contamination with porcine viruses, and that FVIII levels can be monitored, informing appropriate dose selection. A disadvantage is the potential for anti-porcine antibodies to develop, causing progressive waning of product effectiveness. An in vitro study of OBI-1 showed dose-dependent correction of thrombin generation and clot structure in plasma containing 2.7 BU of anti-porcine antibody, but little improvement if the titer was 19.1 BU [70].

The second approach is to secure hemostasis without the participation of FVIII. This can be done by enhancing the tissue factor–FVIIa coagulation pathway. Two strategies have been employed. First, relatively high concentrations of FVIIa or combinations of factors VIIa, IXa, Xa, and XIa can be infused. Second, the tissue factor pathway inhibitor (TFPI) can be blocked, resulting in uninhibited FVIIa/FXa activity.

Modifications of recombinant factor VIIa
GlycoPEGylated recombinant activated factor VII
Recombinant FVIIa has a half-life of only 2–4 hours. A pegylated form of rFVIIa is currently undergoing evaluation [71]. It has a mean half-life of 15 hours, and activity was measurable for up to 72 hours. A dose-dependent decrease in the prothrombin time was noted. No adverse effects, such as thrombotic events, were noted in the healthy persons studied. Trials in patients with bleeding disorders are anticipated.

NN1731
This is a rFVIIa analog that stabilizes the molecule in its active conformation, with functional activity similar to the FVIIa–tissue factor complex [72]. As compared with FVIIa, NN1731 binds to a greater number of sites on activated platelets [73]. An ex-vivo study of hemophilic plasma with and without inhibitors showed that the agent, at a concentration of 80 μg/kg, normalized clot stability [74]. A dose-escalation study in hemophilic patients with inhibitors and joint bleeds found that the analog was well-tolerated and appeared efficacious [75].

AAV8-FVIIa
AAV-mediated gene therapy provides another approach to compensate for the short half-life of FVIIa. Transduction of an AAV8-FVIIa construct into the hepatocytes of hemophilic mice and dogs led to sustained FVIIa expression and amelioration of bleeding episodes [76]. Further investigation using this novel approach continues.

Recombinant prothrombin complex concentrate

A concentrate of recombinant prothrombin and FXa provided hemostasis and lacked thrombogenicity in a rabbit model [77], but human studies have yet to be reported.

Inhibition of TFPI

BAX499 is an aptamer that binds to TFPI and blocks its inhibition of the tissue factor–FVIIa complex and FXa. In a monkey model of hemophilia, the aptamer corrected prolonged bleeding and clotting times [78]. When added to normal or hemophilic plasma, it dose-dependently improved tissue factor-induced coagulation by shortening lag times and increasing clot size [79]. Another product, a high-affinity humanized monoclonal antibody directed against TFPI, binds to the second Kunitz domain and blocks the interaction of TFPI and FXa [80]. When given to rabbits made hemophilic by infusion of a monoclonal anti-human FVIII antibody, a single dose of anti-TFPI was able to decrease cuticle bleeding for up to 7 days [81]. These TFPI antagonists control bleeding, but still unknown is whether they pose a risk for thrombosis.

Eliminating autoantibodies
Inducing tolerance to factor VIII

T-regulatory cells (Treg; CD4+Foxp3+) play a key role in modulating immune responses to self-antigens; in animal models, elimination of these cells results in the development of autoimmune disease. The immunosuppressive activity of Tregs is regulated by a number of cytokines including interleukin-2 (expands Tregs) [82] and interleukin-17 (inhibits Treg generation) [83]. Liu et al. [84] increased Tregs five- to sevenfold by injecting an IL-2/IL-2 antibody complex into hemophilic mice, and showed that these mice failed to develop antibodies after exposure to FVIII. IL-17 has been implicated in several disorders characterized by autoimmunity [85,86], as well as in immune responses to FVIII [87]. Monoclonal antibodies against IL-17 are currently in clinical trials for the treatment of a variety of autoimmune disorders [16], and could be considered for the management of autoimmune FVIII inhibitors.

Another approach is modulation of the immunological synapse between CD80/86 on dendritic cells and CTLA4 on T-cells [88]. In 2000, it was shown by Hoyer et al. [89,90] that the T-cell costimulatory molecule, B7, was required for inhibitor development in hemophilic mice. Blocking B7 with CTLA4-Ig prevented inhibitor formation. Subsequently, Hausl et al. [91] reported that blocking B7 inhibits the re-stimulation and differentiation of FVIII-specific memory B-cells in vitro and in vivo. They also observed that while low concentrations of FVIII (3–10 ng/mL) stimulated B-cells, higher levels (100–300 ng/mL) inhibited these cells [92]. Their experiments suggest that regimens that combine blocking of essential costimulating interactions (CD80/86-CD28, CD40-CD40L) with large doses of FVIII might restore tolerance to FVIII. A fusion protein composed of CTLA-4 and immunoglobulin (abatacept) is currently approved for the treatment of rheumatoid arthritis. It decreases the number but enhances the function of Tregs [93] and, if it were given in conjunction with FVIII, might decrease autoantibody formation.

In a murine model of hemophilia with inhibitor, it was shown that CD11c$^+$ dendritic cells facilitated the differentiation of FVIII-specific memory B-cells in the presence of FVIII and a toll-like receptor agonist [94]. However, it is possible to modify dendritic cells so that they express lower levels of costimulatory molecules and secrete high levels of IL-10 [95]. Modification of dendritic cells in patients with autoimmune disorders might result in tolerance to FVIII antigen.

Monoclonal antibodies

New CD20 monoclonal antibodies are under development that might have improved ability to delete B-cells. Type I antibodies bind to the amino-terminus of CD20 and redistribute it into lipid rafts, enhancing complement binding and cytotoxicity, whereas type II antibodies bind to the carboxy-terminus, triggering homotypic adhesion and lysosomal cell death [96]. Type I antibodies are bound by surface membrane Fc gamma receptor IIb, which promotes internalization and reduces efficacy [97]; type II antibodies do not engage with the Fc receptor and, therefore, might be more clinically effective.

Another approach might use a combination of a CD20 monoclonal antibody and alemtuzumab, an anti-CD52 antibody which has shown efficacy in the treatment of autoimmune diseases. In vitro, alemtuzumab interferes with the down-modulation of CD20 by phagocytic cells, and increases the susceptibility of CD52-negative cells to rituximab [98]. Using low doses of both drugs, Gomez-Almaguer et al. [99] reported responses in 21 patients with steroid-refractory autoimmune hemolytic anemia and immune thrombocytopenic purpura, and comparable results might occur in patients with acquired hemophilia.

A serious adverse effect of treatment with monoclonal antibodies is depletion of immunocytes, increasing patient vulnerability to infection. A more targeted strategy would focus on directly eliminating circulating FVIII autoantibodies. Gilles et al. [100,101] prepared high-affinity monoclonal anti-idiotypic antibodies against antibodies directed toward the A2, C1, or C2 domains of FVIII. In a mouse model, they showed that a combination of five of these anti-idiotypic antibodies neutralized almost all inhibitors and protected FVIII from inactivation. Clinical trials in acquired hemophilia are under consideration.

References

1. Franchini M. Acquired hemophilia A. *Hematology* 2006;11:119–25.
2. Collins PW, Percy CL. Advances in the understanding of acquired haemophilia A: implications for clinical practice. *Br J Haematol* 2010;148:183–94.
3. Ly B, Michaelsen TE, Dahl O, Froland SS. Characterization of an antibody to factor VIII in a patient with acquired hemophilia with circulating immune complexes. *Scand J Haematol* 1982;28:132–40.
4. Margolius A, Jackson D, Ratnoff O. Circulating anticoagulants: a study of 40 cases and a review of the literature. *Medicine* 1961;40:145–202.
5. Lozier E, Jolliffe L, Taylor F. Hemorrhagic diathesis with prolonged coagulation time associated with a circulating anticoagulant. *Am J Med Sci* 1940;318–27.
6. Collins PW, Hirsch S, Baglin TP, et al. Acquired hemophilia A in the United Kingdom: a 2-year national surveillance study by the United Kingdom Haemophilia Centre Doctors' Organisation. *Blood* 2007;109:1870–7.
7. Green D, Lechner K. A survey of 215 non-hemophilic patients with inhibitors to Factor VIII. *Thromb Haemost* 1981;45:200–3.
8. Biggs R, Bidwell E, Macfarlane RG. The mode of action and aetiology of antihaemophilic globulin inhibitors. *Sang* 1959;30:340–51.
9. Solymoss S. Postpartum acquired factor VIII inhibitors: results of a survey. *Am J Hematol* 1998;59:1–4.
10. Lulla RR, Allen GA, Zakarija A, Green D. Transplacental transfer of postpartum inhibitors to factor VIII. *Haemophilia* 2010;16:14–17.
11. Mann KG, Orfeo T, Butenas S, et al. Blood coagulation dynamics in haemostasis. *Hamostaseologie* 2009;29:7–16.
12. Lollar P, Parker ET, Curtis JE, et al. Inhibition of human factor VIIIa by anti-A2 subunit antibodies. *J Clin Invest* 1994;93:2497–504.
13. Scandella D, DeGraaf Mahoney S, Mattingly M, et al. Epitope mapping of human factor VIII inhibitor antibodies by deletion analysis of factor VIII fragments expressed in *Escherichia coli*.[Erratum appears in Proc Natl Acad Sci USA 1989;86:1387]. *Proc Natl Acad Sci USA* 1988;85:6152–6.
14. Scandella D, Kessler C, Esmon P, et al. Epitope specificity and functional characterization of factor VIII inhibitors. *Adv Exp Med Biol* 1995;386:47–63.
15. Scandella D, Mattingly M, de Graaf S, Fulcher CA. Localization of epitopes for human factor VIII inhibitor antibodies by immunoblotting and antibody neutralization. *Blood* 1989;74:1618–26.
16. Reding MT, Lei S, Lei H, et al. Distribution of Th1- and Th2-induced anti-factor VIII IgG subclasses in congenital and acquired hemophilia patients. *Thromb Haemost* 2002;88:568–75.
17. Wootla B, Dasgupta S, Dimitrov JD, et al. Factor VIII hydrolysis mediated by anti-factor VIII autoantibodies in acquired hemophilia. *J Immunol* 2008;180:7714–20.
18. Fulcher CA, Lechner K, de Graaf Mahoney S. Immunoblot analysis shows changes in factor VIII inhibitor chain specificity in factor VIII inhibitor patients over time. *Blood* 1988;72:1348–56.
19. Matsumoto T, Shima M, Fukuda K, et al. Immunological characterization of factor VIII autoantibodies in patients with acquired hemophilia A in the presence or absence of underlying disease. *Thromb Res* 2001;104:381–8.
20. Scandella DH, Nakai H, Felch M, et al. In hemophilia A and autoantibody inhibitor patients: the factor VIII A2 domain and light chain are most immunogenic. *Thromb Res* 2001;101:377–85.

21. Algiman M, Dietrich G, Nydegger UE, et al. Natural antibodies to factor VIII (anti-hemophilic factor) in healthy individuals. *Proc Natl Acad Sci USA* 1992;89:3795–9.

22. Leitner A, Bidwell E, Dike GW. An antihaemophilic globulin (factor VIII) inhibitor: purification, characterization and reaction kinetics. *Br J Haematol* 1963;9:245–58.

23. Bidwell E, Denson KW, Dike GW. Antibody nature of the inhibitor to antihaemophilic globulin (Factor 8). *Nature* 1966;210:746–7.

24. Pavlova A, Diaz-Lacava A, Zeitler H, et al. Increased frequency of the CTLA-4 49 A/G polymorphism in patients with acquired haemophilia A compared to healthy controls. *Haemophilia* 2008;14:355–60.

25. Tiede A, Eisert R, Czwalinna A, et al. Acquired haemophilia caused by non-haemophilic factor VIII gene variants. *Ann Hematol* 2010;89:607–12.

26. Lottenberg R, Kentro TB, Kitchens CS. Acquired hemophilia: a natural history study of 16 patients with factor VIII inhibitors receiving little or no therapy. *Arch Int Med* 1987;147:1077–81.

27. Knobl P, Marco P, Baudo F, et al. Demographic and clinical data in acquired haemophilia A: results from the European Acquired Haemophilia Registry (EACH2). *J Thromb Haemost* 2012;10:622–31.

28. Huth-Kuhne A, Baudo F, Collins P, et al. International recommendations on the diagnosis and treatment of patients with acquired hemophilia A. *Haematologica* 2009;94:566–75.

29. Kazmi MA, Pickering W, Smith MP, et al. Acquired haemophilia A: errors in the diagnosis. *Blood Coag Fibrinol* 1998;9:623–8.

30. Kasper CK, Aledort L, Aronson D, et al. Proceedings: a more uniform measurement of factor VIII inhibitors. *Thromb Diath Haemorrh* 1975;34:15.

31. Verbruggen B, Novakova I, Wessels H, et al. The Nijmegen modification of the Bethesda assay for factor VIII:C inhibitors: improved specificity and reliability. *Thromb Haemost* 1995;73:247–51.

32. Giles AR, Verbruggen B, Rivard GE, et al. A detailed comparison of the performance of the standard versus the Nijmegen modification of the Bethesda assay in detecting factor VIII:C inhibitors in the haemophilia A population of Canada. Association of Hemophilia Centre Directors of Canada. Factor VIII/IX Subcommittee of Scientific and Standardization Committee of International Society on Thrombosis and Haemostasis. *Thromb Haemost* 1998;79:872–5.

33. Sahud MA, Pratt KP, Zhukov O, et al. ELISA system for detection of immune responses to FVIII: a study of 246 samples and correlation with the Bethesda assay. *Haemophilia* 2007;13:317–22.

34. Lak M, Sharifian RA, Karimi K, Mansouritorghabeh H. Acquired hemophilia A: clinical features, surgery and treatment of 34 cases, and experience of using recombinant factor VIIa. *Clin Appl Thromb/Hemost* 2010;16:294–300.

35. Butenas S, Brummel KE, Bouchard BA, Mann KG. How factor VIIa works in hemophilia. *J Thromb Haemost* 2003;1:1158–60.

36. Hay CR, Negrier C, Ludlam CA. The treatment of bleeding in acquired haemophilia with recombinant factor VIIa: a multicentre study. *Thromb Haemost* 1997;78: 1463–7.

37. Sumner MJ, Geldziler BD, Pedersen M, Seremetis S. Treatment of acquired haemophilia with recombinant activated FVII: a critical appraisal. *Haemophilia* 2007; 13:451–61.

38. Franchini M, Capra F, Capelli C, et al. Clinical efficacy of recombinant activated factor VII (rFVIIa) during acute bleeding episode and surgery in a patient with acquired hemophilia A with high inhibitor titer. *Haematologica* 2001;86:E12.

39. Santagostino E, Mancuso ME, Rocino A, et al. A prospective randomized trial of high and standard dosages of recombinant factor VIIa for treatment of hemarthroses in hemophiliacs with inhibitors. *J Thromb Haemost* 2006;4:367–71.

40. Makris M, Van Veen JJ. Comparative thrombotic event incidence after infusion of recombinant factor VIIa versus factor VIII inhibitor bypass activity: a rebuttal. *J Thromb Haemost* 2005;3:818–19; author reply 819.

41. Sallah S, Aledort L. Treatment of patients with acquired inhibitors. *J Thromb Haemost* 2005;3:595–7.

42. Varadi K, Negrier C, Berntorp E, et al. Monitoring the bioavailability of FEIBA with a thrombin generation assay. *J Thromb Haemost* 2003;1:2374–80.

43. Pintado T, Taswell HF, Bowie EJ. Treatment of life-threatening hemorrhage due to acquired factor VIII inhibitor. *Blood* 1975;46:535–41.

44. Kessler CM, Ludlam CA. The treatment of acquired factor VIII inhibitors: worldwide experience with porcine factor VIII concentrate. International Acquired Hemophilia Study Group. *Sem Hem* 1993;30(2 Suppl 1):22–7.

45. Morrison AE, Ludlam CA, Kessler C. Use of porcine factor VIII in the treatment of patients with acquired hemophilia. *Blood* 1993;81:1513–20.

46. O'Gorman P, Dimichele DM, Kasper CK, et al. Continuous infusion of porcine factor VIII in patients with haemophilia A and high-responding inhibitors: stability and clinical experience. *Haemophilia* 2001;7:537–43.

47. Mannucci PM. Desmopressin: a nontransfusional form of treatment for congenital and acquired bleeding disorders. *Blood* 1988;72:1449–55.

48. Baudo F, Collins P, Huth-Kuehne A, et al. Management of bleeding in acquired hemophilia A: results from the Europena Acquired Hemophilia (EACH2) Registry. *Blood* 2012;120:39–46.

49. Sahu S, Raipancholia R, Pardiwalla FK, Pathare AV. Hemostasis in acquired hemophilia: role of intracavitary instillation of EACA. *J Postgrad Med* 1996;42:88–90.

50. Uehlinger J, Button GR, McCarthy J, et al. Immunoadsorption for coagulation factor inhibitors. *Transfusion* 1991;31:265–9.

51. Rivard GE, St Louis J, Lacroix S, et al. Immunoadsorption for coagulation factor inhibitors: a retrospective critical appraisal of 10 consecutive cases from a single institution. *Haemophilia* 2003;9:711–16.

52. Nemes L, Pitlik E. New protocol for immune tolerance induction in acquired hemophilia. *Haematologica* 2000;85(10 Suppl):64–8.

53. Zeitler H, Ulrich-Merzenich G, Hess L, et al. Treatment of acquired hemophilia by the Bonn-Malmo Protocol: documentation of an in vivo immunomodulating concept. *Blood* 2005;105:2287–93.

54. Green D, Rademaker AW, Briet E. A prospective, randomized trial of prednisone and cyclophosphamide in the treatment of patients with factor VIII autoantibodies. *Thromb Haemost* 1993;70:753–7.

55. Collins PW. Management of acquired haemophilia A. *J Thromb Haemost* 2011; 9:226–35.

56. Green D. Suppression of an antibody to factor VIII by a combination of factor VIII and cyclophosphamide. *Blood* 1971;37:381–7.

57. Green D. The management of factor VIII inhibitors in non-hemophilic patients. *Prog Clin Biol Res* 1984;150:337–352.

58. Green D. Oral immunosuppressive therapy for acquired hemophilia. *Ann Intern Med* 1998;128:325.

59. Schwartz RS, Gabriel DA, Aledort LM, et al. A prospective study of treatment of acquired (autoimmune) factor VIII inhibitors with high-dose intravenous gammaglobulin. *Blood* 1995;86:797–804.

60. Delgado J, Jimenez-Yuste V, Hernandez-Navarro F, Villar A. Acquired hemophilia: review and meta-analysis focused on therapy and prognostic factors. *Br J Haematol* 2003;121:21–35.

61. Stasi R, Brunetti M, Stipa E, Amadori S. Selective B-cell depletion with rituximab for the treatment of patients with acquired hemophilia. *Blood* 2004;103:4424–8.

62. Cretel E, Jean R, Chiche L, Durand JM. Successful treatment with rituximab in an elderly patient with acquired factor VIII inhibitor. *Geriatr Gerontol Int* 2009;9: 197–9.

63. Franchini M. Rituximab in the treatment of adult acquired hemophilia A: a systematic review. *Crit Rev Oncol Hematol* 2007;63:47–52.

64. Franchini M, Veneri D, Lippi G, Stenner R. The efficacy of rituximab in the treatment of inhibitor-associated hemostatic disorders. *Thromb Haemost* 2006;96: 119–25.

65. Stachnik JM. Rituximab in the treatment of acquired hemophilia. *Ann Pharmacotherapy* 2006;40:1151–7.

66. Aggarwal A, Grewal R, Green RJ, et al. Rituximab for autoimmune haemophilia: a proposed treatment algorithm. *Haemophilia* 2005;11:13–19.

67. Collins PW, Baudo F, Knobl P, et al. Immunosuppression for acquired hemophilia A: results from the European Acquired Haemophilia Registry (EACH2). *Blood* 2012;120:47–55.

68. Parker ET, Craddock HN, Barrow RT, Lollar P. Comparative immunogenicity of recombinant B domain-deleted porcine factor VIII and Hyate:C in hemophilia A mice presensitized to human factor VIII. *J Thromb Haemost* 2004;2:605–11.

69. Mahlangu J, Andreeva TA, Macfarlane D, et al. A phase II open-label study evaluating hemostatic activity, pharmacokinetics and safety of recombinant porcine factor VIII (OBI-1) in hemophilia A patients with alloantibody inhibitors directed against human FVIII. *Blood* 2007;110:241a.

70. Negrier C, Oldenburg J, Martinowitz U, et al. In vitro correction of thrombin generation and improvement of clot structure by recombinant porcine factor VIII in plasma containing anti-factor VIII inhibitory antibodies. Abstract ISTH;2011: P-TH-519.

71. Moss J, Rosholm A, Lauren A. Safety and pharmacokinetics of a glycoPEGylated recombinant activated factor VII derivative: a randomized first human dose trial in healthy subjects. *J Thromb Haemost* 2011;9:1368–74.

72. Tranholm M, Kristensen K, Kristensen AT, et al. Improved hemostasis with superactive analogs of factor VIIa in a mouse model of hemophilia A. *Blood* 2003;102:3615–20.

73. Hoffman M, Volovyk Z, Persson E, et al. Platelet binding and activity of a factor VIIa variant with enhanced tissue factor independent activity. *Thromb Haemost* 2011;9:759–66.

74. Rea CJ, Ezban M, Foley JH, Sorensen B. rFVIIa-analogue and rFVIIa enhance clot stability more than FVIII in haemophilia A. Abstract ISTH 2011: P-TU-503.

75. De Paula EV, Kavakli K, Mahlangu J, et al. Recombinant factor VIIa analog (vatreptacog alfa [activated])for treatment of joint bleeds in hemophilia patients with inhibitors: a randomized controlled trial. *J Thromb Haemost* 2012;10: 81–9.

76. High KA. Gene therapy for haemophilia: a long and winding road. *J Thromb Haemost* 2011;9(suppl 1):2–11.

77. Himmelspach M, Richter G, Muhr E, et al. A fully recombinant partial prothrombin complex effectively bypasses fVIII in vitro and in vivo. *Thromb Haemost* 2002;88: 1003–11.

78. Waters EK, Genga RM, Schwartz MC, et al. Aptamer ARC19499 mediates a pro-coagulant hemostatic effect by inhibiting tissue factor pathway inhibitor. *Blood* 2011;117:5514–22.

79. Parunov LA, Fadeeva OA, Balandina AN, et al. Improvement of spatial fibrin formation by the anti-TFPI aptamer BAX499: changing clot size by targeting extrinsic pathway initiation. *J Thromb Haemost* 2011;9:1825–34.

80. Breinholt J, Svensson LA, Hilden I, et al. The extensive epitope overlap of the humanized monoclonal antibody MAB2021 with the FXa binding site on K2 explains its neutralizing effect on TFPI. Abstract ISTH 2011; P-MO-111.

81. Hilden I, Lauritzen B, Sorensen BB, et al. Hemostatic effect of a monoclonal anti-antibody mAB2021blocking the interaction between FXa and TFPI in a rabbit hemophilia model. *Blood* 2012;119:5871–8.

82. Hoyer KK, Kuswanto WF, Gallo E, Abbas AK. Distinct roles of helper T-cell subsets in a systemic autoimmune disease. *Blood* 2009;113:389–95.

83. Mai J, Wang H, Yang XF. Th 17 cells interplay with Foxp3+ Tregs in regulation of inflammation and autoimmunity. *Front Biosci* 2010;15:986–1006.

84. Liu C-L, Ye P, Lin J, Miao CH. IL2/IL2 MAB complexes induce in vivo expansion of Treg cells and prevent anti-FVIII antibody production following FVIII protein replacement therapy in hemophilia A mice. Abstract ISTH 2011: O-TU-065.

85. Miossec P, Korn T, Kuchroo VK. Interleukin-17 and type 17 helper T cells. *N Engl J Med* 2009;361:888–98.

86. Peffault de Latour, Visconte V, Takaku T, et al. Th17 immune responses contribute to the pathophysiology of aplstic anemia. *Blood* 2010;116:4175–84.

87. Ettinger RA, James EA, Kwok WW, et al. Lineages of human T-cell clones, including T helper 17/T helper 1 cells, isolated at different stages of anti-factor VIII immune responses. *Blood* 2009;114:1423–8.

88. Shevach EM. Regulating suppression. *Science* 2008;322:202–3.

89. Hoyer LW, Qian J. Characterization of the immune response to factor VIII using hemophilia A mice. *Haematologica* 2000;85(suppl 10):100–2.

90. Qian J, Collins M, Sharpe AH, Hoyer LW. Prevention and treatment of factor VIII Inhibitors in murine hemophilia A. *Blood* 2000;95:1324–9.

91. Hausl C, Ahmad RU, Schwarz HP, et al. Preventing restimulation of memory B cells in hemophilia A: a potential new strategy for the treatment of antibody-dependent immune disorders. *Blood* 2004;104:115–22.

92. Hausl C, Ahmad RU, Sasgary MS, et al. High-dose factor VIII inhibits factor VIII-specific memory B cells in hemophilia A with factor VIII inhibitors. *Blood* 2005;106:3415–22.

93. Alvarez-Quiroga C, Abud-Mendoza C, Doniz-Padilla L, et al. CTLA-4-Ig therapy diminishes the frequency but enhances the function of Treg cells in patients with rheumatoid arthritis. *J Clin Immunol* 2011;31:588–95.

94. Pordes AG, Baumgartner CK, Allacher P, et al. T cell-independent restimulation of FVIII-specific murine memory B cells I facilitated by dendritic cells together with toll-like receptor 7 agonist. *Blood* 2011;118:3154–62.

95. Waller EK. Dendritic cells get VIP treatment. *Blood* 2006;107:3423–4.

96. Cragg MS. CD20 antibodies: doing the time warp. *Blood* 2011;118:219–20.

97. Lim SH, Vaughan AT, Ashton-Key M, et al. Fc gamma receptor IIb on target B cells promotes rituximab internalization and reduces clinical efficacy. *Blood* 2011;118:2530–40.

98. Nijmeijer BA, van Schie MLJ, Halkes CJM, et al. A mechanistic rationale for combining alemtuzumab and rituximab in the treatment of ALL. *Blood* 2010;116:5930–40.

99. Gomez-Almaguer D, Solano-Genesta M, Tarin-Arzaga L, et al. Low-dose rituximab and alemtuzumab combination therapy for patients with steroid-refractory autoimmune cytopenias. *Blood* 2010;116:4783–5.

100. Gilles JG. Role of anti-idiotypic antibodies in immune tolerance induction. *Haemophilia* 2010;16:80–3.

101. Gilles JG, Grailly SC, de Maeyer M, et al. In vivo neutralization of a C2 domain-specific human anti-factor VIII inhibitor by an anti-idiotypic Ab. *Blood* 2004;103:2617–23.

102. Batra S, Sharathkumar A, Glaubach T, et al. Autoimmune haemophilia in a teenager. *Haemophilia* 2013;19:e386–88.

CHAPTER 9

Factor XII Deficiency or Hageman Factor Deficiency

Evi X. Stavrou and Alvin H. Schmaier

Division of Hematology and Oncology, Department of Medicine, Case Western Reserve University, Cleveland, OH, USA

Introduction

In 1955, Ratnoff and Colopy demonstrated that there was an unrecognized clotting factor, which they initially named Hageman factor after the first patient, John Hageman, who presented with a prolonged Lee-White clotting time on preoperative screening [1]. In 1961, Ratnoff and Davie showed that the Hageman factor, which they named factor XII (FXII), has the ability to activate factor XI (FXI). Recognition of this pathway for FXI activation served as the basis for the development of the waterfall cascade hypothesis of the blood coagulation system [2]. FXII has the unique ability to autoactivate upon exposure to neutral or negatively charged surfaces to become the enzyme factor XIIa (α-FXIIa). The autoactivation mechanism of factor XII is called "contact activation." The mechanism(s) of FXII autoactivation is not known, but the protein changes shape as demonstrated by circular dichroism and sum frequency generation vibrational spectroscopy [3,4]. α-FXIIa then activates FXI to factor XIa, prekallikrein (PK) to plasma kallikrein, and C1 esterases (C1r, C1s), the first components of C1 and the classic complement cascade to active enzymes in enzyme–substrate interactions (Figure 9.1) [5]. All of these reactions are accelerated in vitro and in plasma by the cofactor protein, high-molecular-weight kininogen (HK). The initiation of contact activation by FXII autoactivation is amplified by activation of preakallikrein to plasma kallikrein. Plasma kallikrein reciprocally activates FXII. An initial cleavage causes (surface-bound) FXII to become α-FXIIa, the second cleavage causes dissociation of its light chain containing the protease domain [6,7]. Notably, this fragment of FXII, known as β-FXIIa (FXII fragment or Hageman factor fragment) activates prekallikrein in solution, but has no α-FXIIa surface

---

Hemostasis and Thrombosis: Practical Guidelines in Clinical Management, First Edition.
Hussain I. Saba and Harold R. Roberts.

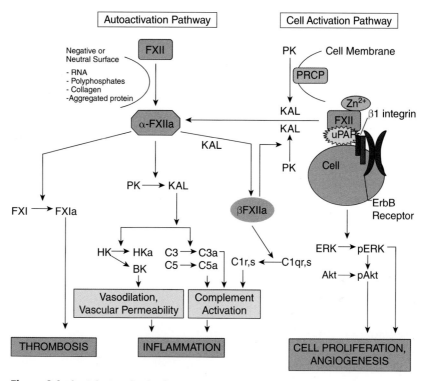

Figure 9.1 Physiologic roles for factor XII. FXII is involved in three physiologic pathways: thrombosis, inflammation, and angiogenesis. There are two activation pathways for FXII: autoactivation and cell-based. Zymogen FXII associates with neutral or negatively charged surfaces to autoactivate into enzyme. Biologic substances that can support FXII autoactivation include RNA, long-chain polyphosphates, collagen, and aggregated proteins. Formed FXIIa (α-FXIIa) activates factor XI (FXI) into factor XIa (FXIa) and prekallikrein (PK) to plasma kallikrein (KAL). Activated FXI contributes to thrombin formation, hemostasis, and thrombosis. When factor XI is activated by FXIIa, this mechanism mostly influences thrombosis. Formed plasma kallikrein proteolyzes high-molecular-weight kininogen (HK) into an activated form of cleaved HK (HKa), liberating bradykinin (BK) in the process. α-FXIIa also has the ability to cleave HK and liberate BK (not shown). Formed plasma kallikrein activates C3 to C3a and C5 to C5a, and C3a also leads to C5 activation. BK formation leads to vasodilation and vascular permeability which, along with complement activation, contribute to the inflammatory response. Plasma kallikrein also proteolyzes α-FXIIa to make β-FXIIa, a fluid phase prekallikrein activator and an activator of C1r and C1s in a macromolecular complex with C1q. These pathways influence inflammation. Plasma prekallikrein also can be activated on endothelial cells by a serine protease, prolylcarboxypeptidase (PRCP), independent of activated forms of FXII. Independent of autoactivation of FXII or activated forms of FXII, zymogen FXII binds cells through uPAR, initiating a signaling cascade through beta-1 integrins, ErbB receptors leading to phosphorylation of ERK1/2 and Akt[S473] that is associated with cell growth and in vivo angiogenesis [21].

activation or coagulation initiation ability (Figure 9.1) [8]. Activation of prekallikrein by α-FXIIa or β-FXIIa is potentiated by HK, leading to generation of the potent vasoactive peptide, bradykinin (BK). BK mediates inflammation, such as vasodilation, increased capillary permeability, and leukocyte migration leading to local edema and, if sufficiently high, systemic changes in arterial blood pressure. Two distinct enzymatic systems are triggered by autoactivated FXII: one leading to hemostasis and the other to inflammation (Figure 9.1). Thus, the in vivo physiologic activities of FXII are now recognized to modulate thrombosis risk, angiogenesis, and the inflammatory response.

Factor XII structure

Factor XII (FXII) is the zymogen of a serine protease, factor XIIa (FXIIa). It is produced and secreted by the liver and is the product of a 12 kb gene consisting of 13 introns and 14 exons [9,10]. The protein consists of a heavy chain of 353 residues and a light chain of 243 amino acids, held together by a disulfide bond. FXII is comprised of several structural domains. These domains are homologous to those found in other serine proteases, except for the proline-rich region that is unique to FXII. Starting from the N-terminus, the domains are a leader peptide, a fibronectin domain type II, an epidermal-growth-factor-like (EGF-like) domain, a fibronectin domain type I, a second EGF-like domain, a kringle domain, a proline-rich region, and the catalytic domain. Each of these regions will be discussed in detail in the following section.

Fibronectin domain, type II homology

The amino-terminal region of FXII shares sequence homology with the type II homology regions of fibronectin [11]. Structure function analysis of human FXII using recombinant deletion mutants confirms that the N-terminus of FXII contains a binding site for negatively charged activating surfaces (amino acids 1–28) [12–14]. Another putative binding site for negatively charged surfaces that consists of residues 134–153 has been mapped in the fibronectin type I domain [15].

The FXII fibronectin type II region contains a binding site for FXI that spans amino acids 3–19 in the area where it binds artificial surfaces [16]. The FXII binding site on FXI is two-fold: a region on apple domain 4 (A4) and a substrate recognition site at the FXI cleavage site (Arg369-Ile370) [17].

In addition to protein–protein interactions in solution, FXII has been demonstrated to bind to endothelial cells, platelets, and neutrophils [18–20]. Amino acid sequence 39–47 of FXII has been shown to interact with endothelial cells [18]. Factor XII interacts through urokinase plasminogen activator receptor (uPAR), gC1qR, and cytokeratin 1, the same receptors that have been demonstrated to be HK binding sites [18]. On uPAR, HK, single chain urokinase, and vitronectin compete for a similar binding region on uPAR's domain 2. HK competes with FXII binding to endothelial cells better than FXII competes with HK [18]. Our investigations have recently demonstrated that FXII stimulates ERK1/2 and AktS^{473} phosphorylation through uPAR, β1 integrin, and a member(s) of the ErbB receptor family to induce human umbilical vein endothelial cell proliferation, growth, and angiogenesis [21] (Figure 9.1). FXII's interaction with human umbilical vein endothelial cells requires the free zinc ion concentration to be 30 times the constitutive level in plasma (0.2 mM) [18]. This fact serves as a regulatory mechanism to constitutively prevent its interaction with endothelium until such time as there is sufficient zinc ion loss from local cells that allows for its binding and subsequent cell activation [18,21]. There are two recognized zinc binding sites in the fibronectin type II region, residues 40–44 and 78–82 [22]. Two other zinc ion binding sites are also postulated for residues 94–131 in the first EGF-like domain and residues 174–176 in the second EGF-like domain [22]. In vivo, collagen-activated platelets release sufficient Zn^{2+} to support FXII binding [18]. On platelets, FXII additionally binds to the GPIbα–IX–V complex [20].

The fibronectin type II region also contains a collagen binding site for FXII. Collagen contributes to thrombin generation in at least two ways. First, collagen provides a surface for FXII autoactivation. α-FXIIa, after contact activation on collagen, activates FXI to initiate blood coagulation [23]. Second, in high-flow, shear-generating arterial vessels, platelets become activated on exposed collagen after vascular damage. The major collagen receptor on platelets is an adapted immunoglobulin receptor, glycoprotein VI (GPVI) [23]. Platelet activation leads to platelet procoagulant activity by the surface exposure of phosphatidylserine and the assembly of coagulation proteins leading to prothrombinase [23].

In addition to platelets and endothelium, all the essential components of the contact-phase system assemble on the surface of neutrophils. Data suggest that HK and FXII bind to similar sites exposed on the external face of the neutrophil membrane, whereas PK is secured to the cell surface indirectly through its docking protein, HK [19]. The array of contact proteins assembled on the surface of neutrophils provides a unique circulating platform (solid phase) for activation of these proteins leading to bradykinin formation. Formation of BK from this assembly of proteins contributes to transudation of plasma and passage of circulating neutrophils into the interstitial space surrounding the site of injury or inflammation. Additionally, in vitro studies show that purified FXIIa corrects neutrophil aggregation and degranulation defects evident in FXII-deficient plasma [24]. FXII has been recognized to regulate the expression of monocyte FcγII receptor and it stimulates monocytes and macrophages to release interleukin (IL)-1 and IL-6 [25,26]. Last, factor XII-deficient human patients have reduced leukocyte migration into forearm skin windows [27]. The sum of these in vitro and in vivo studies indicates that FXII has a role in inflammation.

EGF-like domains

Two regions of FXII are homologous to an epidermal-growth-factor-like sequence that has been found in many proteins including transforming growth factor type 1, tissue plasminogen activator (tPA), single-chain urokinase plasminogen activator, hepatocyte growth factor, and several clotting factors. It is of interest that all of these proteins have been shown to have both proteolytic and non-proteolytic activities. In each of these proteins, there is a highly conserved region of 50 amino acids with nine invariant cysteine and glycine residues [28]. The carboxyl-terminal growth factor domain also contains the invariant glycine residues; in the amino-terminal domain, however, one invariant glycine residue has been replaced with a histidine. Epidermal growth factor (EGF) is a known mitogen for a variety of cells and stimulates a pleiotropic response in target cells, including increased DNA and protein synthesis [29]. The mechanism of EGF action is characterized by EGF receptor binding and autophosphorylation followed by phosphorylation of tyrosine residues in intracellular proteins like the mitogen-activated/extracellular signal-regulated protein kinase (MAPK/ERK) pathways. FXIIa has been recognized to regulate the expression of the monocyte FcγII receptor [25]. FXII and α-FXIIa have also been shown to enhance cell proliferation, [³H] thymidine incorporation, and [³H] leucine incorporation in HepG2 cells. Furthermore, FXII induces MAP kinase in Hep G2 cells, smooth muscle fibroblasts, and endothelial cells [21,23,30,31]. FXII also increases cell proliferation and 5-bromo-2′-deoxyuridine (BrdU) incorporation in endothelial cells leading to angiogenesis (Figure 9.1) [21]. However, it is not currently known if FXII's EGF-like domains mediate these activities.

Fibronectin type I region

Separating the two growth factor-like regions of FXII is a 43 amino acid peptide that shares limited sequence homology with the type I regions of fibronectin, each of which are characterized by two disulfide bonds giving a two-loop structure that has been named a "finger" domain [11]. Its precise function is not known, but it has been characterized to participate in artificial surface binding by Citarella et al. [32].

Kringle domain

Another type of homology found in FXII is the kringle domain. Kringle domains are typically 80 amino acids in length and form three characteristic disulfide bonds. The kringle domains in FXII and tPA share approximately 41% sequence homology. Its function in FXII is not known, but it has been proposed as a putative artificial surface binding site [12].

Proline-rich region

The kringle structure is followed by a region in which 33% of the residues are proline residues. This region does not share any sequence homology with other proline-rich proteins. The significance of this region in FXII remains undetermined.

Catalytic domain

The catalytic domain of FXII remains the single largest and best described region of the protein. The active site of FXIIa consists of three amino acids, H394, D442, and S544, indicating that, in vivo, the catalytic domain is globular, bringing these three residues in close apposition. Proteolytic cleavage of its R353-V354 site converts single-chain zymogen FXII (80 kDa) to two-chain α-FXIIa. This cleaved protein circulates as a two-chain protein consisting of a heavy chain of ~50 kDa (353 residues) and a ~30 kDa light chain (243 residues), held together by a disulfide bond between two cysteines. Reduction of this disulfide bond liberates the light chain as β-FXIIa (Hageman factor fragment, HFf).

Although a number of biologic substances had been shown to support FXII activation, it has always been questioned whether FXII autoactivation occurs during endogenous physiologic or after pathophysiologic activities. FXII is activated through proteolytic cleavage by plasma proteases, such as plasma kallikrein and plasmin (fluid-phase activation). We have shown that, on cultured endothelial cells, the serine protease prolylcarboxypeptidase activates prekallikrein ($K_m = 9\,\mathrm{nM}$) and its formed plasma kallikrein leads to kinetically favorable FXII activation ($K_m = 11\,\mu\mathrm{M}$) [33,34]. This mechanism has not yet been demonstrated in vivo. In addition, upon contact with negatively charged surfaces FXII autoactivates (solid-phase activation) into α-FXIIa. Negatively charged surfaces such as glass, kaolin, ellagic acid, sulfatide micelles, high-molecular-weight dextran sulfate, bismuth subgallate, dacron, polyethylene, silicone rubber, and various polymers support FXII autoactivation in vitro. Biologic substances that support FXII autoactivation include articular cartilage, skin, fatty acids, endotoxin, sodium urate crystals, calcium pyrophosphate, L-homocysteine, hematin, protoporphyrins, heparins, chondroitin sulfate, and phosphatidylserine, phosphatidylglycerol, phosphatidic acid, and phosphatidylinositol. FXII autoactivation alone is a slow process that occurs over 90–120 min.

In plasma, FXII autoactivation is much faster (2–5 min) due to the presence of prekallikrein and HK [33]. The molecular basis for FXII autoactivation is not known since the FXII–FXIIa crystal structures are not yet available.

There has been renewed interest in FXII autoactivation in vivo by the recognition that, although dispensable for physiologic hemostasis, FXII contributes to the propagation of the developing thrombus. This observation will be discussed below in the section on thrombosis. Recently, several biologic substances have been shown to support FXII autoactivation. These substances include extracellular DNA and RNA [35], polyphosphate with chain lengths longer than 75 subunits [36], aggregated proteins [37], and collagen exposed in arterial tissue [23]. Last, FXII autoactivation also occurs under conditions of sepsis, by the negatively charged surface provided by bacteria. Adsorption and activation of FXII on bacterial surfaces may contribute to the host's defense system, mobilizing leukocytes and through fibrin formation, limiting the extent of bacterial dissemination [38,39].

The major plasma protease inhibitor of α-FXIIa and β-FXIIa is C1 esterase inhibitor (C1 inhibitor, C1INH), accounting for more than 90% of the inhibition of these proteases in plasma [40]. C1 inhibitor binds both of these enzymes and irreversibly inactivates them. When associated with a kaolin surface, FXIIa is protected from C1 inhibitor inactivation [41]. HK also protects FXIIa from C1 inhibitor. Antithrombin (AT) also inhibits FXIIa [42]. Heparin, even at therapeutic levels, does not, however, significantly enhance the ability of AT to inhibit FXIIa [42]. A deficiency (type I) or defect (type II) in C1 esterase inhibitor results in the inflammatory condition called hereditary angioedema (HAE), a disorder associated with tissue swelling due to locally increased bradykinin formation [43]. Type III HAE is caused by one of two known rare mutations in FXII that lead to increased (gain-of-function) FXII activity [44]. This form of acquired C1 inhibitor deficiency is the first disease directly associated with a specific abnormality in factor XII.

Regulation of factor XII expression

Little is known about FXII expression. The FXII gene has a consensus estrogen-response element and estrogen therapy is known to increase liver production of FXII [45]. The hepatocyte nuclear factor-4 (HNF-4) transcription factor inhibits estrogen induction of the FXII promoter in fibroblasts but not in HepG2 cells where it potentiates estrogen-induced FXII expression [46]. HNF-4 null mice show reduced FXII expression [47]. This latter mechanism is important to understand the mechanism(s) for deficiency seen in patients with apparent FXII decrease. FXII stimulates

ERK1/2 in vascular endothelial and smooth muscle cells (VSMC) [21,48]. TGF-β1 has been recognized to upregulate transcriptionally FXII expression in fibroblasts and has been linked to conditions such as pulmonary fibrosis [49]. FXII immunochemical expression is increased in human atherosclerotic vessels [50].

Role of factor XII in hemostasis and thrombosis

Role in hemostasis

There is a dichotomy between abnormal laboratory assay findings due to FXII deficiency and clinical hemostasis. The contact activation phenomenon of FXII serves as the basis for all surface-activated blood coagulation tests such as the activated partial thromboplastin time (aPTT) assay and activated clotting times performed in millions of people annually. However, FXII does not contribute to physiologic hemostasis, since its deficiency is not associated with bleeding. Spronk et al. demonstrated that tissue factor (TF) is the physiologic initiator of blood coagulation leading to hemostasis. Mice with total deficiency of FXII and low TF are viable and phenotypically similar to low-TF mice with normal FXII expression.

Role in thrombosis

The observation in 1991 that thrombin directly activates factor XI (FXI) provided an alternative route for FXI activation independent of FXIIa, further diminishing interest in FXII in hemostasis [51]. The discovery that the first FXII knockout (KO) ($F12^{-/-}$) mouse is protected from contact activation-induced and ferric chloride-induced small vessel thrombosis without an associated bleeding diathesis has sparked new interest in FXII [36,52]. It suggests a role for FXII in thrombus formation in stroke and venous thrombosis [53,83]. In 1968, collagen was suggested as a FXII activating surface, but this observation was questioned. Recently, this observation was re-examined and collagen and several other biologic substances have been shown to support FXII autoactivation. As already mentioned above, these substances include extracellular RNA, aggregated proteins, collagen exposed in arterial tissue, and long-chain polyphosphate (mean polymer size 75 phosphate units) released from damaged cells [23,35–37]. A recombinant tick inhibitor for FXIIa abolishes thrombin formation in mice and was highly protective in a murine model of ischemic stroke without altering hemostasis [54]. The sum of these studies indicates novel in vivo functions of FXII, not previously appreciated, suggesting a new approach for selective thrombo-protection. However, caution should be given to the simple interpretation that FXII regulates thrombosis without influences on hemostasis. Recent published thrombosis studies were performed with only murine contact activation and small vessels thrombosis models. It is possible that other thrombosis models may give different results.

Factor XII in thromboembolic disease: human epidemiologic data

In contrast to murine data, human epidemiologic studies do not all agree that FXII deficiency protects from thrombosis. As part of an all-cause mortality study, an inverse correlation was found between levels of FXII and the risk of cardiovascular disease [55]. Similarly, lower FXII levels were found in patients with coronary heart disease. The concentration of plasma FXII antigen is regulated by cellular expression and secretion. A common genetic polymorphism, C46T, located in the promoter region of the F12 gene on chromosome 5, disturbs the consensus sequence [56]. The C46T polymorphism creates a new ATG codon that reduces the translation efficiency and leads to low levels of FXII antigen [57,58]. A higher percentage of T46 was also observed in patients with a myocardial infarction than in the control group, whether patients were hypercholesterolemic or not [59]. However, the odds ratio was higher in the hypercholesterolemic cohort than in the control group [59]. The high incidence of homozygous T46, which leads to reduced FXII activity, was further discovered to be a risk factor for ischemic stroke among Europeans [60], but not Japanese [61]. More recently, Sabeter-Lleal et al. described two new mutations, a C/G substitution at position 8 and a C/T substitution at position 17 of the FXII gene [62]. Both mutations are located in the promoter region of the FXII gene in a putative binding site for the hepatocyte nuclear factor 4-α transcription factor (HNF4α). HNF4-α is a liver-enriched transcription factor that influences expression of FXII. Each of these promoter region mutations summates with the 46C/T polymorphism to lower plasma FXII levels [62]. Thus, unlike the murine data, human clinical data suggest that lowered, but not totally deficient, levels of FXII are associated with deleterious cardiovascular outcomes. The actual meaning of these findings is not completely known, but suggests a dichotomy in the role of FXII in thrombosis risk.

Role in inflammation

There are many disorders that are believed to be influenced by FXII and its contact activation such as chronic renal disease [63], proliferative diabetic retinopathy [64], Alzheimer's disease [65], arthritis [66,67], vasculitis, bowel disease [66], sepsis [38], allergy [68, 69], preeclampsia [70], and malignancy [71]. However, the role of FXII in these conditions may not be related to its activity in thrombosis. Activation of FXII results not only in the activation of the coagulation system via FXI, but also activation of prekallikrein and direct or indirect release of bradykinin [37,72]. Factor XII-deficient mice have reduced constitutive plasma bradykinin levels [73]. Kallikrein and bradykinin have numerous roles. First, bradykinin leads to inflammation by causing classic symptoms such as redness, fever, swelling, and blood pressure changes. The peptide acts through two G-protein-coupled receptors, B1 and B2, present on a large number of cell types, but most notably endothelial cells. Unlike the B2 receptor (B2R) that is constitutively active, the B1R arises only after inflammation. Activation of these receptors leads to leukocyte recruitment and also the secretion of a number of proinflammatory and chemotactic cytokines [74]. The ability of excess negatively charged material in vivo to produce disease was driven home by the clinical outcomes of patients who received certain lots of porcine heparin sulfate adulterated with chondroitin sulfate [75]. Patients who received the chondroitin sulfate-adulterated heparin had allergic reactions and hypotension secondary to FXII contact activation with secondary formation of plasma kallikrein leading to bradykinin formation and C5 activation [75]. Second, tissue-type plasminogen activator (tPA) is released by bradykinin-stimulated endothelial cells [76–78]. Third, activated FXII is able to activate the complement system directly through activation of C1r and C1s, and indirectly through plasma prekallikrein activation and plasma kallikrein activation of C3 and C5 [5,79,80]. As already mentioned, a gain-of-function mutation of FXII results in acquired type III C1 inhibitor deficiency, an inflammatory disorder [44].

Finally, there may be some fundamental, but as yet not fully appreciated, role for FXII in neutrophil and macrophage function. As already mentioned, FXII-deficient persons have reduced leukocyte migration into skin windows [27]. Purified FXIIa aggregates neutrophils and FXII stimulates monocyte expression of receptors [24,25]. Our own ongoing studies show defective murine leukocyte migration in two inflammation models and bone marrow of wild type mice corrects the leukocyte migration defect in the $F12^{-/-}$ mice [81]. The reduced inflammatory response seen in stroke and venous thrombosis in FXII-deficient mice has suggested to others that this injury, and perhaps the other illnesses associated with FXII deficiency, may be mainly due to less inflammation [52,82,83]. Additional studies are needed to elucidate the role of FXII in inflammation.

Summary

In summary, our knowledge of FXII is starting to grow after a long hiatus in support for research in this area. The finding that $F12^{-/-}$ mice are protected from thrombosis has stirred new interest in this protein. FXII influences thrombosis risk without changing hemostasis. It also has a role in inflammation and leukocyte function. Finally, its zymogen is a growth factor that can stimulate cell growth and postnatal angiogenesis. FXII-deleted mice constitutively have reduced vessel number in skin biopsies. FXII/FXIIa is unique in that its proteolytic activity has precise roles in coagulation amplification through activation of FXI and inflammation. FXII, the zymogen, is a growth factor promoting vascular wellbeing and angiogenesis. These activities are important physiologic functions that with better understanding will make FXII a novel target for specific disease states independent of hemostasis.

References

1. Ratnoff OD, Colopy JE. A familial hemorrhagic trait associated with a deficiency of a clot-promoting fraction of plasma. *J Clin Invest* 1955;34:602–13.
2. Davie EW, Ratnoff OD. Waterfall sequence for intrinsic blood clotting. *Science* 1964;145:1310–12.
3. Samuel M, Pixley RA, Villanueva MA, et al. Human factor XII (Hageman factor) autoactivation by dextran sulfate. Circular dichroism, fluorescence, and ultraviolet difference spectroscopic studies. *J Biol Chem* 1992;25:19691–7.
4. Chen X, Wang J, Paszti Z, et al. Ordered adsorption of coagulation factor XII on negatively charged polymer surfaces probed by sum frequency generation vibrational spectroscopy. *Anal Bioanal Chem* 2007;388:65–72.
5. Ghebrehiwet B, Silverberg M, Kaplan AP. Activation of the classical pathway of complement by Hageman factor fragment. *J Exp Med* 1981;153:665–76.
6. Revak SD, Cochrane CG, Griffin JH. The binding and cleavage characteristics of human Hageman factor during contact activation. A comparison of normal plasma with plasmas deficient in factor XI, prekallikrein, or high molecular weight kininogen. *J Clin Invest* 1977;59:1167–75.
7. Fujikawa K, McMullen BA. Amino acid sequence of human beta-factor XIIa. *J Biol Chem* 1983;258:10924–33.
8. Dunn JT, Silverberg M, Kaplan AP. The cleavage and formation of activated human Hageman factor by autodigestion and by kallikrein. *J Biol Chem* 1982;257: 1779–84.
9. Cool DE, MacGillivray RT. Characterization of the human blood coagulation factor XII gene. Intron/exon gene organization and analysis of the 5′-flanking region. *J Biol Chem* 1987;262:13662–73.
10. Citarella F, Tripodi M, Fantoni A, et al. Assignment of human coagulation factor XII (fXII) to chromosome 5 by cDNA hybridization to DNA from somatic cell hybrids. *Hum Genet* 1988;80:397–8.
11. Petersen TE, Thogersen HC, Skorstengaard K, et al. Partial primary structure of bovine plasma fibronectin: three types of internal homology. *Proc Natl Acad Sci USA* 1983;80:137–41.
12. Citarella F, Ravon DM, Pascucci B, Fet al. Structure/function analysis of human factor XII using recombinant deletion mutants: evidence for an additional region

involved in the binding to negatively charged surfaces. *Eur J Biochem* 1996; 238:240–9.

13. Clarke BJ, Cote HC, Cool DE, et al. Mapping of a putative surface-binding site of human coagulation factor XII. *J Biol Chem* 1989;264:11497–502.

14. Samuel M, Samuel E, Villanueva GB. Histidine residues are essential for the surface binding and autoactivation of human coagulation factor XII. *Biochem Biophys Res Commun* 1993;191:110–17.

15. Pixley RA, Stumpo LG, Birkmeyer K, et al. A monoclonal antibody recognizing an icosapeptide sequence in the heavy chain of human factor XII inhibits surface-catalyzed activation. *J Biol Chem* 1987;262:10140–5.

16. Citarella F, Fedele G, Roem D, et al. The second exon-encoded factor XII region is involved in the interaction of factor XII with factor XI and does not contribute to the binding site for negatively charged surfaces. *Blood* 1998;92:4198–206.

17. Baglia FA, Jameson BA, Walsh PN. Identification and characterization of a binding site for factor XIIa in the Apple 4 domain of coagulation factor XI. *J Biol Chem* 1993;268:3838–44.

18. Mahdi F, Madar ZS, Figueroa CD, Schmaier AH. Factor XII interacts with the multiprotein assembly of urokinase plasminogen activator receptor, gC1qR, and cytokeratin 1 on endothelial cell membranes. *Blood* 2002;99:3585–96.

19. Henderson LM, Figueroa CD, Muller-Esterl W, Bhoola KD. Assembly of contact-phase factors on the surface of the human neutrophil membrane. *Blood* 1994; 84:474–82.

20. Bradford HN, Pixley RA, Colman RW. Human factor XII binding to the glycoprotein Ib-IX-V complex inhibits thrombin-induced platelet aggregation. *J Biol Chem* 2000;275:22756–63.

21. LaRusch GA, Mahdi F, Shariat-Madar Z, et al. Factor XII stimulates ERK1/2 and Akt through uPAR, integrins, and the EGFR to initiate angiogenesis. *Blood* 2010;115: 5111–20.

22. Rojkaer R, Schousboe I. Partial identification of the Zn2+-binding sites in factor XII and its activation derivatives. *Eur J Biochem* 1997;247:491–6.

23. van der Meijden PE, Munnix IC, Auger JM, et al. Dual role of collagen in factor XII-dependent thrombus formation. *Blood* 2009;114:881–90.

24. Wachtfogel YT, Pixley RA, Kucich U, et al. Purified plasma factor XIIa aggregates human neutrophils and causes degranulation. *Blood* 1986;67:1731–7.

25. Chien P, Pixley RA, Stumpo LG, et al. Modulation of the human monocyte binding site for monomeric immunoglobulin G by activated Hageman factor. *J Clin Invest* 1988;82:1554–9.

26. Toossi Z, Sedor JR, Mettler MA, et al. Induction of expression of monocyte interleukin 1 by Hageman factor (factor XII). *Proc Natl Acad Sci USA* 1992; 89:11969–72.

27. Rebuck JW. The skin window as a monitor of leukocytic functions in contact activation deficiencies in man. *Am J Pathol* 1983;79:405–13.

28. Cool DE, Edgell CJ, Louie GV, et al. Characterization of human blood coagulation factor XII cDNA. Prediction of the primary structure of factor XII and the tertiary structure of beta-factor XIIa. *J Biol Chem* 1985;260:13666–76.

29. Cohen S. Epidermal growth factor. *In Vitro Cell Dev Biol* 1987;23:239–46.

30. Gordon EM, Venkatesan N, Salazar R, et al. Factor XII-induced mitogenesis is mediated via a distinct signal transduction pathway that activates a mitogen-activated protein kinase. *Proc Natl Acad Sci USA* 1996;93:2174–9.

31. Schmeidler-Sapiro KT, Ratnoff OD, Gordon EM. Mitogenic effects of coagulation factor XII and factor XIIa on HepG2 cells. *Proc Natl Acad Sci USA* 1991;88:4382–5.

32. Citarella F, te Velthuis H, Helmer-Citterich M, Hack CE. Identification of a putative binding site for negatively charged surfaces in the fibronectin type II domain of human factor XII: an immunochemical and homology modeling approach. *Thromb Haemost* 2000;84:1057–65.

33. Rojkjaer R, Hasan AA, Motta G, et al. Factor XII does not initiate prekallikrein activation on endothelial cells. *Thromb Haemost* 1998;80:74–81.

34. Shariat-Madar Z, Mahdi F, Schmaier AH. Identification and characterization of prolylcarboxypeptidase as an endothelial cell prekallikrein activator. *J Biol Chem* 2002;277:17962–9.

35. Kannemeier C, Shibamiya A, Nakazawa F, et al. Extracellular RNA constitutes a natural procoagulant cofactor in blood coagulation. *Proc Natl Acad Sci USA* 2007;104:6388–93.

36. Muller F, Mutch NJ, Schenk WA, et al. Platelet polyphosphates are proinflammatory and procoagulant mediators in vivo. *Cell* 2009;139:1143–56.

37. Maas C, Govers-Riemslag JW, Bouma B, et al. Misfolded proteins activate factor XII in humans, leading to kallikrein formation without initiating coagulation. *J Clin Invest* 2008;118:3208–18.

38. Frick IM, Bjorck L, Herwald H. The dual role of the contact system in bacterial infectious disease. *Thromb Haemost* 2007;98:497–502.

39. Colman RW. Biologic activities of the contact factors in vivo: potentiation of hypotension, inflammation, and fibrinolysis, and inhibition of cell adhesion, angiogenesis and thrombosis. *Thromb Haemost* 1999;82:1568–77.

40. Forbes CD, Pensky J, Ratnoff OD. Inhibition of activated Hageman factor and activated plasma thromboplastin antecedent by purified serum C1 inactivator. *J Lab Clin Med* 1970;76:809–15.

41. Pixley RA, Schmaier A, Colman RW. Effect of negatively charged activating compounds on inactivation of factor XIIa by C1 inhibitor. *Arch Biochem Biophys* 1987;256:490–8.

42. Stead N, Kaplan AP, Rosenberg RD. Inhibition of activated factor XII by antithrombin-heparin cofactor. *J Biol Chem* 1976;251:6481–8.

43. Han ED, MacFarlane RC, Mulligan AN, et al. Increased vascular permeability in C1 inhibitor-deficient mice mediated by the bradykinin type 2 receptor. *J Clin Invest* 2002;109:1057–63.

44. Cichon S, Martin L, Hennies HC, et al. Increased activity of coagulation factor XII (Hageman factor) causes hereditary angioedema type III. *Am J Hum Genet* 2006;79:1098–104.

45. Farsetti A, Misiti S, Citarella F, et al. Molecular basis of estrogen regulation of Hageman factor XII gene expression. *Endocrinology* 1995;136:5076–83.

46. Farsetti A, Moretti F, Narducci M, et al. Orphan receptor hepatocyte nuclear factor-4 antagonizes estrogen receptor alpha-mediated induction of human coagulation factor XII gene. *Endocrinology* 1998;139:4581–9.

47. Inoue Y, Peters LL, Yim SH, et al. Role of hepatocyte nuclear factor 4alpha in control of blood coagulation factor gene expression. *J Mol Med (Berl)* 2006;84:334–44.

48. Fernando AN, Fernando LP, Fukuda Y, Kaplan AP. Assembly, activation, and signaling by kinin-forming proteins on human vascular smooth muscle cells. *Am J Physiol Heart Circ Physiol* 2005;289:H251–7.

49. Jablonska E, Markart P, Zakrzewicz D, et al. Transforming growth factor-beta1 induces expression of human coagulation factor XII via Smad3 and JNK signaling pathways in human lung fibroblasts. *J Biol Chem* 2010;285:11638–51.

50. Borissoff JI, Heeneman S, Kilinc E, et al. Early atherosclerosis exhibits an enhanced procoagulant state. *Circulation* 2010;122:821–30.

51. Gailani D, Broze GJ, Jr. Factor XI activation in a revised model of blood coagulation. *Science* 1991;253:909–12.
52. Renne T, Pozgajova M, Gruner S, et al. Defective thrombus formation in mice lacking coagulation factor XII. *J Exp Med* 2005;202:271–81.
53. Kleinschnitz C, Stoll G, Bendszuz M, et al. Targeting coagulation factor XII provides protection from pathological thrombosis in cerebral uschemia without interfering with hemostasis. *J Exp Med* 2006;203:513–18.
54. Hagedorn I, Schmidbauer S, Pleines I, et al. Factor XIIa inhibitor recombinant human albumin Infestin-4 abolishes occlusive arterial thrombus formation without affecting bleeding. *Circulation* 2010;121:1510–17.
55. Endler G, Marsik C, Jilma B, et al. Evidence of a U-shaped association between factor XII activity and overall survival. *J Thromb Haemost* 2007;5:1143–8.
56. Kozak M. Point mutations define a sequence flanking the AUG initiator codon that modulates translation by eukaryotic ribosomes. *Cell* 1986;44:283–92.
57. Kanaji T, Okamura T, Osaki K, et al. A common genetic polymorphism (46 C to T substitution) in the 5'-untranslated region of the coagulation factor XII gene is associated with low translation efficiency and decrease in plasma factor XII level. *Blood* 1998;91:2010–14.
58. Soria JM, Almasy L, Souto JC, et al. A quantitative-trait locus in the human factor XII gene influences both plasma factor XII levels and susceptibility to thrombotic disease. *Am J Hum Genet* 2002;70:567–74.
59. Roldan V, Corral J, Marin F, et al. Synergistic association between hypercholestero-lemia and the C46T factor XII polymorphism for developing premature myocardial infarction. *Thromb Haemost* 2005;94:1294–9.
60. Santamaria A, Mateo J, Tirado I, et al. Homozygosity of the T allele of the 46 C->T polymorphism in the F12 gene is a risk factor for ischemic stroke in the Spanish population. *Stroke* 2004;35:1795–9.
61. Oguchi S, Ito D, Murata M, et al. Genotype distribution of the 46C/T polymorphism of coagulation factor XII in the Japanese population: absence of its association with ischemic cerebrovascular disease. *Thromb Haemost* 2000;83:178–9.
62. Sabater-Lleal M, Chillon M, Mordillo C, et al. Combined cis-regulator elements as important mechanism affecting FXII plasma levels. *Thromb Res* 2010;125: e55–60.
63. Jozwiak L, Drop A, Buraczynska K, et al. Association of the human bradykinin B2 receptor gene with chronic renal failure. *Mol Diagn* 2004;8:157–61.
64. Gao BB, Chen X, Timothy N, et al. Characterization of the vitreous proteome in diabetes without diabetic retinopathy and diabetes with proliferative diabetic retin-opathy. *J Proteome Res* 2008;7:2516–25.
65. Bergamaschini L, Donarini C, Gobbo G, et al. Activation of complement and contact system in Alzheimer's disease. *Mech Aging Dev* 2001;122:1971–83.
66. Colman RW. Plasma and tissue kallikrein in arthritis and inflammatory bowel disease. *Immunopharmacology* 1999;43:103–8.
67. McLaren M, Alkaabi J, Connacher M, et al. Activated factor XII in rheumatoid arthritis. *Rheumatol Int* 2002;22:182–4.
68. Dotsenko VL, Nenasheva NM, Neshkova EA, et al. Mechanism of activation of the kallikrein-kinin system in plasma of patients with atopic allergic diseases. *Adv Exp Med Biol* 1989;247B:515–21.
69. Atkins PC, Miragliotta G, Talbot SF, et al. Activation of plasma Hageman factor and kallikrein in ongoing allergic reactions in the skin. *J Immunol* 1987;139:2744–8.
70. Vaziri ND, Toohey J, Powers D, et al. Activation of intrinsic coagulation pathway in pre-eclampsia. *Am J Med* 1986;80:103–7.

71. Maeda H, Wu J, Okamoto T, et al. Kallikrein-kinin in infection and cancer. *Immunopharmacology* 1999;43:115–28.
72. Schmaier AH. The elusive physiologic role of factor XII. *J Clin Invest* 2008; 118:3006–9.
73. Iwaki T, Castellino FJ. Plasma levels of bradykinin are suppressed in factor XII-deficient mice. *Thromb Haemost* 2006;95:1003–10.
74. Koyama S, Sato E, Nomura H, et al. Bradykinin stimulates type II alveolar cells to release neutrophil and monocyte chemotactic activity and inflammatory cytokines. *Am J Pathol* 1998;153:1885–93.
75. Kishimoto TK, Viswanathan K, Ganguly T, et al. Contaminated heparin associated with adverse clinical events and activation of the contact system. *N Engl J Med* 2008;358:2457–67.
76. Brown NJ, Nadeau JH, Vaughan DE. Selective stimulation of tissue-type plasminogen activator (t-PA) in vivo by infusion of bradykinin. *Thromb Haemost* 1997;77:522–5.
77. Brown NJ, Gainer JV, Stein CM, Vaughan DE. Bradykinin stimulates tissue plasminogen activator release in human vasculature. *Hypertension* 1999;33:1431–5.
78. Brown NJ, Gainer JV, Murphey LJ, Vaughan DE. Bradykinin stimulates tissue plasminogen activator release from human forearm vasculature through B(2) receptor-dependent, NO synthase-independent, and cyclooxygenase-independent pathway. *Circulation* 2000;102:2190–6.
79. DiScipio RG. The activation of the alternative pathway C3 convertase by human plasma kallikrein. *Immunology* 1982;45:587–95.
80. Wiggins RC, Giclas PC, Henson PM. Chemotactic activity generated from the fifth component of complement by plasma kallikrein of the rabbit. *J Exp Med* 1981;153:1391–404.
81. Stavrou E, LaRusch GA, Fullana MJ, et al. *Factor XII promotes leukocyte inflammation and its deficiency results in faster wound healing*. Abstract 368, American Society of Hematology, 2011. http://ash.confex.com/ash/2011/webprogram/Paper41208.html.
82. Nieswandt B, Kleinschnitz C, Stoll G. Ischaemic stroke: a thrombo-inflammatory disease? *J Physiol* 2011;589:4115–23.
83. von Bruhl M-L, Strak S, Steinhart A, et al. Monocytes, neutrophils, and platelets cooperate to initiate and propagate venous thrombosis in mice in vivo. *J Exp Med* 2012;209:819–35.

CHAPTER 10

Inherited Combined Factor Deficiency States

Asma Latif and Louis Aledort

Division of Hematology and Medical Oncology, Tisch Cancer Institute, Mount Sinai School of Medicine, New York, NY, USA

Introduction

Rare inherited bleeding disorders often present difficulties in diagnosis and management. Among the rarest of these coagulation disorders are the inherited combined factor deficiency states, which include combined inherited factor V and factor VIII deficiency (F5F8D), vitamin K-dependent clotting factor deficiency (VKCFD), and chance inheritance of multiple factor deficiencies. F5F8D results in the simultaneous decrease in both factor V (FV) and factor VIII (FVIII) activity levels. Defects in the *LMAN1* and *MCFD2* genes have been identified as the cause of F5F8D and lead to inhibition of the intracellular trafficking of both coagulation factors. Affected patients typically experience mild to moderate bleeding symptoms and laboratory data reveal prolonged prothrombin (PT) and partial thromboplastin times (PTT) [1]. VKCFD and chance inheritance of multiple factor deficiencies also present with bleeding symptoms and specific genetic mutations have been identified. All require prompt diagnosis and acute management of bleeding by treating providers.

Combined inherited factor V and factor VIII deficiency

F5F8D was first described in 1954 by Oeri et al. [2] as an autosomal recessive disorder distinct from the simultaneous chance inheritance of both FV deficiency and FVIII deficiency [1]. Affected patients typically experience mild to moderate bleeding symptoms which must be managed acutely [3]. Amongst affected patients 70% have been found to have mutations

Hemostasis and Thrombosis: Practical Guidelines in Clinical Management, First Edition.
Hussain I. Saba and Harold R. Roberts.
© 2014 John Wiley & Sons, Ltd. Published 2014 by John Wiley & Sons, Ltd.

in the *LMAN1* (lectin mannose binding protein) gene, formerly known as *ERGIC-53*, which encodes a chaperone protein in the endoplasmic reticulum (ER) [4,5]. An additional 15% of patients have mutations in the *MCFD2* (multiple coagulation factor deficiency 2) gene, which encodes a cofactor for LMAN1 [6]. F5F8D is characterized by defects in these genes, which lead to ineffective intracellular transport of FV and FVIII [6].

Epidemiology

F5F8D affects between 1:500,000 and 1:2,000,000 people in the general population [7], with males and females affected in equal numbers. Although rare, it is the most common combined hereditary coagulation factor deficiency and has a higher prevalence among Middle Eastern Jewish and non-Jewish Iranian populations, for whom incidence rates are as high as 1:100,000 [8,9]. The increased incidence rate among these groups, as compared to the general population, is postulated to be related to higher rates of consanguineous marriages. The highest rates of F5F8D are found in the Middle Eastern countries and India and lowest in North America [3], although the actual prevalence of F5F8D worldwide is difficult to determine due to ascertainment and publication bias, underdiagnosis due to mild symptomatology and misdiagnosis as a single factor deficiency in areas with limited hematologic resources.

Pathophysiology

FV and FVIII serve as essential cofactors for the proteolytic activation of prothrombin and factor X, respectively [10]. The combined deficiency is caused by a mutation in either the *LMAN1* or *MCFD2* gene which results in the defective intracellular transport of FV and FVIII. The first gene mutation involves the LMAN1 protein which normally functions as a chaperone for the intracellular trafficking of FV and FVIII in the endoplasmic reticulum Golgi intermediate compartment [3,11]. The second gene mutation involves the MCFD2 protein which normally forms a complex with LMAN1 and functions as a cargo receptor for ER to Golgi transport of FV and FVIII [12,13]. These mutations result in defective LMAN1 or MCFD2 proteins, unsuccessful intracellular transport of FV and FVIII, and concomitant decreased levels of both factors, generally in the range 5–20% [3].

Genetics and molecular basis

Congenital F5F8D has an autosomal recessive inheritance pattern and is found in highest concentration in regions where consanguineous marriage is common. Two distinct genes have been implicated in the etiology of F5F8D: *LMAN1* and *MCFD2*. *LMAN1* is located on chromosome 18q21 and since 1998 there have been over 30 mutations described in all 13 exons of the gene, the majority of which predict null alleles [5,13,14]. There are patients who are deficient in LMAN1 but have no mutations yet identified in the exons or exon-intron junctions, possibly suffering from mutations in the regulatory regions of the gene [5,13–16]. Interestingly, just two mutations in *LMAN1* have been linked to all Jewish cases of F5F8D [1].

Some affected families had two normal *LMAN1* alleles and in 2003 a second mutation in *MCFD2* was identified. *MCFD2* is located on chromosome 2p21 [6], and thus far over 15 mutations in the gene have been reported. One of the most commonly identified mutations is c.149 + 5G>A which has been observed in at least 13 unrelated families from around the world, including India, Italy, the United States, Serbia, and Germany [6,12,14,17,18]. While *LMAN1* and *MCFD2* have been linked to the majority of cases of F5F8D, there are affected families who do not have mutations in either of these genes, suggesting additional genetic mutations yet to be identified.

Phenotypic differences between *LMAN1* mutations and *MCFD2* mutations

While thought to be clinically indistinguishable, the phenotypes of F5F8D due to either *LMAN1* or *MCFD2* mutations reflect a small but statistically significant difference in factor levels. Patients with *MCFD2* mutations generally have lower mean FV and FVIII levels than those with *LMAN1* mutations, although considerable overlap in levels is present between the two populations [19]. Circulating FV exists in the plasma and in alpha granules of platelets, and the platelet source of FV is derived from the endocytosis of plasma FV. Both the *LMAN1* and *MCFD2* mutations similarly affect the steady-state levels of FV in both platelets and plasma [1].

Clinical manifestations

While in single coagulation factor deficiencies it is often possible to predict severity of disease based on the factor level, there is wide variation in clinical manifestations in patients with F5F8D [9]. Despite the presence of two coagulation defects, the hemorrhagic tendency in F5F8D is not enhanced beyond that typically seen with each defect separately [9], and the combined deficiency is most often associated with mild to moderate bleeding symptoms including easy bruising, epistaxis, and gingival bleeding [7]. Additionally, bleeding can be seen after surgical procedures, dental extractions, or with physical trauma and, for women, menorrhagia and postpartum hemorrhage are not uncommon [8]. Generally the levels of FV and FVIII are adequate in preventing severe bleeding symptoms but significant bleeding including hemarthroses and umbilical cord bleeding are commonly reported. Although rare, soft tissue hematomas, gastrointestinal and central nervous system bleeding, and persistent bleeding after

Table 10.1 Mean factor V and factor VIII concentrations among patients with F5F8D.

Reference	n	FV: mean % concentration (range)	FVIII: mean % concentration (range)
Seligsohn et al. 1982 [8]	13	17	19
Peyvandi et al. 1998 [20]	27	11.2 (2–21)	11.4 (2–22)
Shetty et al. 2000 [36]	9	6.7 (3–9)	1.5 (<1–3.8)
Mansouritorgabeh et al. 2004 [9]	19	9.3 (4–15)	12.6 (5–30)
Viswabandya et al. 2010 [37]	37	12.5 (5–31)	8.8 (1–27)

circumcision have also been noted [10,20]. Aside from bleeding tendency, there are no other consistent clinical manifestations of F5F8D and, unlike in isolated FV deficiency, F5F8D has not been reported in the literature to be associated with thrombotic events [21].

FV and FVIII levels vary in affected patients (Table 10.1), contributing to the variation in clinical bleeding symptoms. Patients who are obligatory carriers of the mutation generally have normal plasma factor levels without evidence of increased bleeding risk [1], although there have been reports suggesting that the heterozygous state may confer slightly lower levels of FV and FVIII concentrations associated with mild bleeding symptoms when compared with healthy subjects [8].

Diagnosis

The diagnosis for F5F8D is characterized by prolonged PT and PTT but normal platelet counts and bleeding times. When factor deficiency is suspected by mixing studies, specific assays for FV and FVIII coagulant activity should be performed to make the diagnosis and guide treatment [7]. Factor antigen assays are not necessary for either diagnosis or management of patients. Historically, F5F8D has been underdiagnosed due to its common assessment as a single factor deficiency (if only FV or FVIII levels are assessed) and thus it remains important to consider a combined deficiency in patients with prolonged PT and PTT [19]. Genotyping for specific mutation identification is possible in specific research laboratories and can be considered by treating providers.

Prenatal diagnosis of FVF8D is not generally recommended or performed due to the mild to moderate bleeding risk of the disease. In order to evaluate for the disease through prenatal diagnostic testing, a couple's carrier status must be known by already having one affected child, and chorionic villus sampling would need to be done at 10–12 gestational weeks in order to assess the fetal DNA for known genetic mutations found in both parents [3].

Disease management

The management of patients with F5F8D depends on the severity of bleeding and associated factor levels. Generally bleeding episodes are treated acutely and prophylaxis is not required, although it may be recommended in cases of severe recurrent bleeding. Guidelines focus on replacement therapy with FV and FVIII sources. As there are no FV concentrates currently available, fresh frozen plasma (FFP) is the only replacement option for FV, and although virus-inactivated plasma is preferred it is not available in many countries [22]. There are many products currently available for FVIII replacement, including FFP, desmopressin, plasma-derived concentrate, and recombinant FVIII (rFVIII).

For minor bleeding the goal is to raise the FV level to at least 25 IU/dL through replacement with FFP at a dose of approximately 15–20 mL/kg and FVIII levels should be raised to 30–50 IU/dL through the use of plasma-derived concentrate or rFVIII. Additionally, desmopressin (260 µg intranasal or 0.3 µg/kg intravenous) can be considered in the setting of minor bleeds as this synthetic hormone can raise the levels of both von Willebrand factor and FVIII, although its efficacy in individual patients must be verified and sodium parameters should be monitored [7]. While desmopressin has been described with successful effect during surgical intervention, there are no established guidelines for its optimal use [23].

For severe bleeding, FV levels should be maintained at ≥25 IU/dL with an initial dose of FFP of approximately 15–20 mL/kg followed by smaller doses every 12 hours based on the FV levels preferably, or PT and PTT. If bleeding remains uncontrolled, platelet transfusions can be considered although they have not been clearly shown to be effective. This recommendation is based on the premise that upon platelet activation and localized alpha granule release of FV at the bleeding site, FV will bind immediately to surface receptors and therefore optimize the prothrombinase complex activity. FVIII levels should be raised to at least 50–70 IU/dL in the setting of severe bleeding, and the relatively shorter half-life of FVIII (10–14 hours) as compared to FV (36 hours) should guide dosing frequency and monitoring [24].

In anticipation of surgical procedures, FFP and FVIII should be infused 30 minutes prior to and every 12 hours after the procedure, maintaining FV levels of ≥25 IU/dL and FVIII levels of ≥50 IU/dL until wound healing is demonstrated. Excessive menstrual bleeding in female patients may be managed with hormonal contraceptives or antifibrinolytic drugs [19]. Neonates can be diagnosed with F5F8D using peripheral or cord blood samples and should receive oral vitamin K replacement instead of intramuscular. Subcutaneous vaccinations can be continued and these patients can be managed expectantly [24].

There are no clear treatment guidelines for pregnant patients with F5F8D. These women should receive care in an obstetric unit with close consultation with a hemophilia center or coagulation program. FVIII levels are known to increase during normal pregnancy while FV levels may increase slightly or remain unchanged; therefore monitoring near term is prudent and FV and FVIII levels should be assessed in the patient's third trimester in order to plan any necessary hematologic interventions. Any bleeding during labor or the postpartum period is thought to be related to the FV deficiency, as the FVIII levels are known to rise during pregnancy [25]. During labor, FFP should be dosed to keep FV levels >15 IU/dL and FVIII levels should be maintained at >50 IU/dL. If a Caesarean section is necessary, FV replacement should be continued in patients with FV levels <15 IU/dL with close attention to maintaining a PT and PTT in the normal range until wound healing is complete. Epidurals may be safely performed if FV level is >15 IU/dL, FVIII level is >50 IU/dL and coagulation parameters are within the normal range.

Antibodies to FV have been demonstrated as a complication of FFP therapy in cases of FV deficiency. In F5F8D, there may be low levels of inhibitor to FV which require neutralization with large volumes of FFP and potential eradiation therapies. There is currently little literature as to whether IVIG, plasmapharesis, immunoadsorption, immunosuppressive regimens, or rituximab therapy is effective in the eradication of FV antibodies related to the treatment of the combined deficiency [19]. If large doses of FFP replacement are needed, diuretics can be used to manage volume status in the event that it is necessary. Lastly, upon diagnosis of F5F8D all patients should be considered for hepatitis B vaccinations due to projected blood product exposures over the lifetime.

Summary

F5F8D is a rare disease and the pathophysiology of the disorder involves complex genetic mutations. The resulting bleeding symptoms are often mild although there is marked variation in phenotypes which do not necessarily correlate with factor levels, more similar to FXI deficiency than to classic hemophilia. FVIII replacement is relatively simple with FVIII concentrate, while FV replacement is more complicated as there is no concentrate product or virally inactivated FFP currently available in the United States. While F5F8D remains one of the rarest bleeding disorders, hematologists must be alert to add this disease to the differential of prolonged PT and PTT in efforts to promptly diagnose and manage patients in the acute setting.

Vitamin K-dependent clotting factor deficiency

Vitamin K-dependent clotting factor deficiency is a very rare inherited disorder leading to deficiencies in factor II, VII, IX, and X. It results from defective γ-glutamyl carboxylation, which is necessary for the post-translational modification of vitamin K-dependent proteins. VKCFD is an autosomal recessive disorder with two variants, VKCFD1, which results from point mutations in the γ-glutamyl carboxylase gene (*GGCX*), and VKCFD2, which is associated with point mutations in the vitamin K epoxide reductase gene (*VKOR*) [26]. First described in 1966, fewer than 30 cases have been reported since, and most are associated with consanguinity [27,28]. Affected patients have factor levels in the range 1–30% and often present with early-life, mild to severe bleeding symptoms including umbilical cord and central nervous system bleeding. Infections and use of antibiotics will often further exacerbate symptoms [29]. Additionally, in affected patients proteins C, S, and Z have shown defective γ-glutamyl carboxylation which may portend a mild propensity for thrombosis [30]. Skeletal defects have also been reported [31].

Diagnosis is suspected with prolonged PT and PTT and factor II, VII, IX, and X levels are low. Warfarin use, malabsorption, and liver disease must be excluded and genotyping suspected patients should be considered. Current recommended management is prophylaxis treatment with high doses of daily oral vitamin K, which may partially increase factor levels in severely affected patients [32]. For the management of acute bleeding symptoms and surgical interventions, FFP is recommended [29] although prothrombin complex concentrates (PCCs) can also be used and may offer an alternative option with lower volume load. If parents are known to be carriers, prenatal diagnosis of VKCFD is possible and may allow early intervention and treatment [32].

Inheritance of multiple single-factor deficiencies

The inheritance of multiple single-factor deficiencies is rare but reported in the literature. Cases involving either factor II, VII, VIII, or XII deficiency with a factor X deficiency have been reported, both as chance inheritance of multiple mutations, and as autosomal dominant inheritance due to abnormalities in chromosome 13 (involving factor VII and X genes) [33]. Additionally, factor VII deficiency has been described with factor V, VIII, IX, and XI defects. The concurrent presence of von Willebrand disease and hemophilia A among families has also been identified, attesting to the broad range of inheritance possibilities [34]. Many patients with multiple inherited factor deficiencies display other clinical manifestations including

carotid body tumors, valvular and cardiac septal defects, mental retardation, metabolic disorders, and skeletal malformations [35]. Multiple factor
deficiencies can pose diagnostic dilemmas as diagnosis can be missed if the
prolonged PT and PTT can be explained by a single factor deficiency.
Therefore it is prudent to do a careful evaluation and check specific assays
for potential factor defects, especially in light of organ or skeletal malformations. The specific factor deficiencies will guide therapy with desmopressin, factor replacement concentrates, recombinant factor VIIa, PCCs,
and FFP.

References

1. Zhang B. Recent developments in the understanding of the combined deficiency of
   FV and FVIII. *Br J Haematol* 2009;145:15–23.
2. Oeri J, Matter M, Isenschmid H, et al. Congenital factor V deficiency (parahemo-
   philia) with true hemophilia in two brothers. *Bibl Paediatr* 1954;58:575–88.
3. Spreafico M, Peyvandi F. Combined FV and FVIII deficiency. *Haemophilia*
   2008;14:1201–8.
4. Nichols WC, Seligsohn U, Zivelin A, et al. Linkage of combined factors V and VIII
   deficiency to chromosome 18q by homozygosity mapping. *J Clin Invest* 1997;99:
   596–601.
5. Nichols WC, Seligsohn U, Zivelin A, et al. Mutations in the ER-Golgi intermediate
   compartment protein ERGIC-53 cause combined deficiency of coagulation factors
   V and VIII. *Cell* 1998;93:61–70.
6. Zhang B, Cunningham MA, Nichols WC, et al. Bleeding due to disruption of a
   cargo-specific ER-to-Golgi transport complex. *Nat Genet* 2003;34:220–5.
7. Mannucci PM, Duga S, Peyvandi F. Recessively inherited coagulation disorders.
   Blood 2004;104:1243–52.
8. Seligsohn U, Zivelin A, Zwang E. Combined factor V and factor VIII deficiency
   among non-Ashkenazi Jews. *N Engl J Med* 1982;307:1191–5.
9. Mansouritorgabeh H, Rezaieyazdi Z, Pourfathollah AA, et al. Haemorrhagic symptoms in patients with combined factors V and VIII deficiency in north-eastern Iran.
   Haemophilia 2004;10:271–5.
10. Cunningham MA, Pipe SW, Zhang B, et al. LMAN1 is a molecular chaperone for
    the secretion of coagulation factor VIII. *J Thromb Haemost* 2003;1:2360–2367.
11. Nishio M, Kamiya Y, Mizushima T, et al. Structural basis for the cooperative inter-
    play between the two causative gene products of combined factor V and factor VIII
    deficiency. *Proc Natl Acad Sci USA* 2010;107:4034–9.
12. Zhang B, McGee B, Yamaoka JS, et al. Combined deficiency of factor V and
    factor VIII is due to mutations in either LMAN1 or MCFD2. *Blood* 2006;107:
    1903–7.
13. Segal A, Zivelin A, Rosenberg N, et al. A mutation in LMAN1 (ERGIC-53) causing
    combined factor V and factor VIII deficiency is prevalent in Jews originating from
    the island of Djerba in Tunisia. *Blood Coagul Fibrinolysis* 2004;15:99–102.
14. Zhang B, Spreafico M, Zheng C, et al. Genotype-phenotype correlation in combined
    deficiency of factor V and factor VIII. *Blood* 2008;111:5592–600.

15. Neerman-Arbez M, Johnson KM, Morris MA, et al. Molecular analysis of the ERGIC-53 gene in 35 families with combined factor V-factor VIII deficiency. *Blood* 1999;93:2253–60.

16. Nichols WC, Terry VH, Wheatley MA, et al. ERGIC-53 gene structure and mutation analysis in 19 combined factors V and VIII deficiency families. *Blood* 1999; 93:2261–6.

17. Mohanty D, Ghosh K, Shetty S, et al. Mutations in the MCFD2 gene and a novel mutation in the LMAN1 gene in Indian families with combined deficiency of factor V and VIII. *Am J Hematol* 2005;79:262–6.

18. Jayandharan G, Spreafico M, Viswabandya A, et al. Mutations in the MCFD2 gene are predominant among patients with hereditary combined FV and FVIII deficiency (F5F8D) in India. *Haemophilia* 2007;13:413–19.

19. Lippi G, Favaloro EJ, Montagnana M, et al. Inherited and acquired factor V deficiency. *Blood Coagul Fibrinolysis* 2011;22:160–6.

20. Peyvandi F, Tuddenham EG, Akhtari AM, et al. Bleeding symptoms in 27 Iranian patients with the combined deficiency of factor V and factor VIII. *Br J Haematol* 1998;100:773–6.

21. Girolami A, Ruzzon E, Tezza F, et al. Arterial and venous thrombosis in rare congenital bleeding disorders: a critical review. *Haemophilia* 2006;12:345–51.

22. Di Paola J, Nugent D, Young G. Current therapy for rare factor deficiencies. *Haemophilia* 2001;7(suppl 1):16–22.

23. Bauduer F, Guichandut JP, Ducout L. Successful use of fresh frozen plasma and desmopressin for transurethral prostatectomy in a French Basque with combined factors V + VIII deficiency. *J Thromb Haemost* 2004;2:675.

24. Bolton-Maggs PH, Perry DJ, Chalmers EA, et al. The rare coagulation disorders–review with guidelines for management from the United Kingdom Haemophilia Centre Doctors' Organisation. *Haemophilia* 2004;10:593–628.

25. Kadir R, Chi C, Bolton-Maggs P. Pregnancy and rare bleeding disorders. *Haemophilia* 2009;15:990–1005.

26. Rost S, Fregin A, Ivaskevicius V, et al. Mutations in VKORC1 cause warfarin resistance and multiple coagulation factor deficiency type 2. *Nature* 2004;427: 537–41.

27. Brenner B. Hereditary deficiency of vitamin K-dependent coagulation factors. *Thromb Haemost* 2000;84:935–6.

28. McMillan CW, Roberts HR. Congenital combined deficiency of coagulation factors II, VII, IX and X. Report of a case. *N Engl J Med* 1966;274: 1313–15.

29. Brenner B, Tavori S, Zivelin A, et al. Hereditary deficiency of all vitamin K-dependent procoagulants and anticoagulants. *Br J Haematol* 1990;75: 537–42.

30. Bhattacharyya J, Dutta P, Mishra P, et al. Congenital vitamin K-dependent coagulation factor deficiency: a case report. *Blood Coagul Fibrinolysis* 2005;16:525–7.

31. Boneh A, Bar-Ziv J. Hereditary deficiency of vitamin K-dependent coagulation factors with skeletal abnormalities. *Am J Med Genet* 1996;65:241–3.

32. Weston BW, Monahan PE. Familial deficiency of vitamin K-dependent clotting factors. *Haemophilia* 2008;14:1209–13.

33. Girolami A, Ruzzon E, Tezza F, et al. Congenital FX deficiency combined with other clotting defects or with other abnormalities: a critical evaluation of the literature. *Haemophilia* 2008;14:323–8.

34. Miller CH, Hilgartner MW, Harris MB, et al. Concurrence of von Willebrand's disease and hemophilia A: implications for carrier detection and prevalence. *Am J Med Genet* 1986;24:83–94.

35. Girolami A, Ruzzon E, Tezza F, et al. Congenital combined defects of factor VII: a critical review. *Acta Haematol* 2007;117:51–6.
36. Shetty S, Madkaikar M, Nair S, et al. Combined factor V and VIII deficiency in Indian population. *Haemophilia* 2000;6:504–7.
37. Viswabandya A, Baidya S, Nair SC, et al. Clinical manifestations of combined factor V and VIII deficiency: a series of 37 cases from a single center in India. *Am J Hematol* 2010;85:538–9.

CHAPTER 11

Acute and Chronic Immune Thrombocytopenia: Biology, Diagnosis, and Management

Samir Dalia and Benjamin Djulbegovic
H. Lee Moffitt Cancer & Research Center, University of South Florida, Tampa, FL, USA

Introduction

Immune thrombocytopenia (ITP) is a common acquired autoimmune disorder characterized by isolated thrombocytopenia secondary to increased platelet destruction or antibody-induced decreased thrombopoiesis. ITP has also been called immune thrombocytopenic purpura and idiopathic thrombocytopenia purpura, but recently consensus groups renamed it immune thrombocytopenia due to immunologic pathophysiology [1–3]. ITP has been categorized into three categories: 1) newly diagnosed ITP, or acute ITP, is defined as those cases just diagnosed; 2) persistent ITP is defined by a period of 3–12 months from diagnosis. Included in this group are patients not achieving spontaneous remission or not maintaining their response after stopping treatment 3–12 months from diagnosis; 3) chronic ITP is reserved for those patients with ITP lasting more than 12 months [4].

The reported annual incidence of adult ITP is 5.5 per 100,000 persons when defined by a platelet count of less than 100×10^9/L. Adult ITP is more prevalent in females and the age-related incidence is twofold higher in populations older than age 60 than in those younger than 60 [5,6]. Children with ITP usually present between the ages of 2 and 10, with a peak incidence between 2 and 5 years of age [7,8]. ITP can occur as either an isolated primary disorder or a secondary consequence of other diseases. Secondary ITP has been identified by autoimmune diseases including systemic lupus erythematosus, chronic lymphocytic leukemia, Hodgkin lymphoma, human immunodeficiency virus, hepatitis C, *Helicobacter pylori*, myelodysplastic syndrome, immunoglobulin deficiencies, and

Hemostasis and Thrombosis: Practical Guidelines in Clinical Management, First Edition.
Hussain I. Saba and Harold R. Roberts.
© 2014 John Wiley & Sons, Ltd. Published 2014 by John Wiley & Sons, Ltd.

drug-induced ITP. Drug-induced causes include quinidine, gold, heparin, penicillin, procainamide, alpha methyldopa, and sulfamethoxazole [9].

ITP is characterized by antiplatelet antibodies that lead to destruction of platelets and impair production. Harrington and colleagues demonstrated the first evidence of ITP being caused by platelet antibodies in 1951. In their landmark experiment, normal volunteers, including the author, were infused with plasma from ITP patients, resulting in thrombocytopenia in the recipients [10]. Platelets labeled with antibodies are cleared by macrophages in the spleen, which leads to a decrease in platelet count. This was first demonstrated in the 1960s by Shulman who showed that splenic clearance was a major mechanism of thrombocytopenia in ITP, which led to splenectomy as a treatment for ITP [11]. By the 1980s and 1990s, assays were developed that showed that more than 80% of antibodies in patients with ITP were directed against GPIIb/IIIa, while the remaining were directed against GPIb/IX, GPIa/IIa, and GPIV. These antibodies provide targets for future drug development in ITP [12,13].

More recently it has been discovered that a decrease in circulating thrombopoietin (TPO) caused by decreased platelets leads to inhibition of megakaryocyte differentiation. This will further drop the platelet count leading to megakaryocyte hyperplasia in the bone marrow. The new mechanism of decreased platelet production in ITP secondary to TPO has led to the development of new directed therapies for ITP that will be discussed later [14–16].

Primary ITP in adults

Recently, the ITP adult and pediatric expert international working group panel provided statements on terminology, definitions, and outcome criteria for ITP. Primary ITP is defined as thrombocytopenia with a platelet count less than 100×10^9/L in the absence of other causes or disorders that were associated with thrombocytopenia [4]. ITP presents in multiple forms ranging from no symptoms or minimal bruising to life-threatening bleeding. In a systemic review, the fatal hemorrhage risk in patients with platelet counts less than 30,000/L was between 0.02 and 0.04 cases per patient year [17]. Serious bleeding occurs in many and may include gastrointestinal, mucosal, or intracranial hemorrhage. The international consensus report (ICR) on ITP states that the bleeding risk can be correlated to the severity of thrombocytopenia [1]. In those individuals with platelet counts lower than 30,000/L, a systematic review showed that predicted 5-year mortality rates ranged from 2.2% for patients younger than 40 years to 47.8% for those older than 60 years, advocating an active therapeutic approach [17,18].

A detailed history and physical examination should be performed to assess bleeding risk, prior episodes of bleeding or bruising, medication history, history of other disorders including malignancy and autoimmune disorders, family history of platelet disorders, infections, and exposures to substances that may lower platelets. During the physical examination, it is important to assess for petechiae, purpura, ecchymoses, and gross bleeding. Splenomegaly is usually not present.

Laboratory workup

Laboratory workup should include a complete blood count to assess for isolated thrombocytopenia. The American Society of Hematology (ASH) and ITP Consensus Report guidelines recommend that all patients have their peripheral smear reviewed to rule out other causes of thrombocytopenia. Evidence for bone marrow biopsy evaluation is controversial. Consensus guidelines agree that bone marrow biopsy should not be performed in those under the age of 60 with typical features of ITP; however, in those older than 60, the 2011 ASH consensus group do not recommend a bone marrow biopsy while the ICR consensus group does [1,9]. Each patient should be evaluated and bone marrow biopsy should be considered on a case-by-case basis. Viral testing is recommended in all patients, including HIV status and hepatitis C. *H. pylori* testing can be done if infection is suspected, though it is not recommended by consensus groups because clinical trial data has not been validated. Testing for lupus anticoagulant, antiphospholipid antibody, thyroid function, and urine analysis should be carried out if clinically indicated [1,9,19–25]. Table 11.1 summarizes diagnostic workup recommendations.

Table 11.1 Diagnostic workup for ITP in children and adults, recommended by both ASH and ICR consensus groups. Source: Provan et al. 2009 [1], Neunert et al. 2011 [9].

Initial evaluation	Other tests to consider
Patient history	*H. pylori* antigen
Family history	Thyroid-stimulating hormone (TSH)
Medication history	Antinuclear antibody (ANA)
Physical examination	Antiphospholipid antibody
Complete blood counts	Urine analysis
Bone marrow biopsy in selected cases	Liver function testing
HIV test	
Hepatitis C virus testing	
Peripheral smear review	

Management

The goal of treatment in patients with ITP is not to normalize the platelet count, but to achieve a platelet count that will prevent major bleeding. Since most patients with ITP are diagnosed incidentally, observation is usually considered appropriate therapy. Although there is no consensus concerning the platelet count at which to start treatment, most experts consider that patients with consistent platelet counts in excess of 50×10^9/L can be observed. These patients are at low risk for bleeding and can tolerate invasive procedures. In those individuals with platelet counts between 30 and 50×10^9/L, careful follow-up is indicated to ensure no bleeding complications. Using the Grading of Recommendations Assessment, Development, and Evaluation (GRADE) system of evidence, the ASH consensus guidelines show grade 2C (weak recommendation, low quality of evidence) for initiating treatment when the platelet count is below 30×10^9/L [1,21–24,26–30]. A treatment flow sheet is shown in Figure 11.1 to further guide clinicians in treatment choices.

Initial treatment

Glucocorticoids

Initial treatment of newly diagnosed ITP should include corticosteroids. Glucocorticoids have been widely accepted as the initial treatment for ITP. Glucocorticoids improve platelet count by decreasing platelet antibody, reducing platelet destruction by macrophages, and improving platelet production. Responses usually occur within 2–3 weeks but are usually transient, with one study showing that 60% of patients relapsed within 33 months of treatment [31]. Multiple studies and both the ASH and ICR consensus groups recommend corticosteroids as initial treatment. Prednisone at 0.5–2 mg/kg/day has been used until the platelet count increases to >30–50,000/L which may take weeks to month to be effective. Dexamethasone at 40 mg/day for 4 days has been shown to produce a sustained response in 50–86% of patients [32]. One study showed sustained responses during a 2–5-year follow-up period in 50% of patients treated [32,33]. Intravenous high-dose methylprednisolone has been used for a short-term response. Glucocorticoid therapy is limited by side effects including facial swelling, weight gain, hyperglycemia, cataracts, osteoporosis, infection risk, and psychologic disturbances [1,9,23,24,26, 34–36].

Intravenous immunoglobulin

Intravenous immunoglobulin (IVIg) has been shown to temporarily normalize platelets counts within 24 hours, with peak time to response

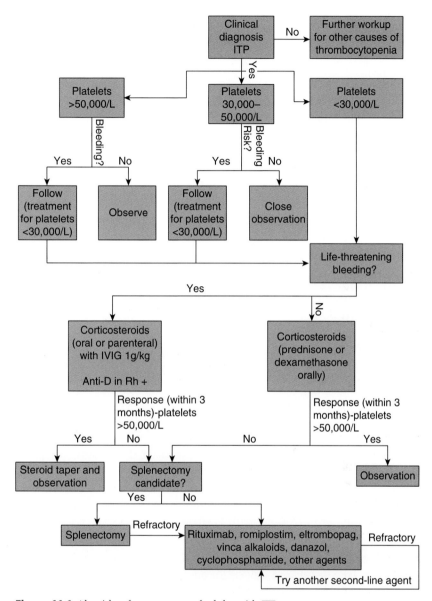

Figure 11.1 Algorithm for treatment of adults with ITP.

48–72 hours after administration. Both the ASH and ICR consensus groups recommend that IVIg be used with corticosteroids when a more rapid increase in platelet counts is required, such as in an emergency, prior to surgery, or during pregnancy [1,9,30]. The effect is transient and usually does not last more than a few weeks. The recommended dose of

IVIg is a total of 1 g/kg, either given in divided doses over 2 days or 0.4 g/kg per day for 4 days [26,37]. Side effects include headache, body aches, nausea, fever, alloimmune hemolysis, hepatitis, renal failure, and thrombosis.

Anti-D immunoglobulin

In Rh-positive, non-splenectomized patients with ITP, multiple consensus groups recommend the use of anti-D immunoglobulin in addition to corticosteroids in situations where an immediate rise in platelets is necessary [1,9,23,29]. Anti-D can work as well as IVIg in patients who need an acute increase in their platelet counts, but does not produce long-term responses. Anti-D carries a risk of severe hemolysis, and thus hemoglobin/hematocrit should be monitored after its use.

Patients who relapse or are refractory to corticosteroids
Surgical treatment
Splenectomy

In patients with glucocorticoid-refractory ITP, multiple second-line agents have been investigated. Splenectomy has been used in refractory ITP since the early 1900s. Splenectomy is indicated in patients with a platelet count less than 30×10^9/L despite adequate medical treatment and is an accepted treatment in those with refractory ITP [21,38,39]. In a systematic review by Kojouri et al. of 2,623 patients, 1,731 had a platelet response defined as a normal platelet count after splenectomy (66%). Median follow-up was 29 months [39]. Based on this review, using the GRADE system of evidence, the ASH consensus group gave splenectomy a grade 1B (strong recommendations with moderate quality of evidence) for use in ITP that was corticosteroid refractory [9]. Thus, splenectomy should be offered to patients with corticosteroid-refractory ITP who are medically fit.

Complications of splenectomy include bleeding, infection, thrombosis, cardiovascular disease, and a need for additional intervention. Kojouri et al. found that 12.9% of patients who underwent laparotomy and 9.6% who underwent laparoscopy had complications from splenectomy. Mortality was 1% with laparotomy and 0.2% with laparoscopy [38–41]. To prevent infection, post-splenectomy patients need to be given prophylactic polyvalent pneumococcal, meningococcal, and *H. influenzae* B vaccines at least 2 weeks prior to splenectomy. Some authors recommend that splenectomized patients have a home supply of antibiotics (e.g., levofloxacillin) for use in case of a febrile illness, and be educated to go to an emergency room with any true fever (101.4 F°) while carrying an alert that they are asplenic [1,9].

Medical treatment or treatment in those that are splenectomy refractory

Rituximab

Rituximab, a monoclonal anti-CD20 antibody, has been shown to improve platelet count in patients with ITP. Arnold et al., in a systematic review of 313 patients, showed complete response rate in 46.3% and a partial response rate in 24% of pooled patients with median follow-up of 9.5 months [42]. Several studies state that the response generally occurs between 1 and 8 weeks of treatment [21,41,43,44]. Based on an open-label phase 2 clinical trial, dosing is recommended at 375 mg/m^2 [44]. A phase III clinical trial combining dexamethasone and rituximab showed that 63% of patients had a platelet count over 50,000/L. At median follow-up of 20 months half of those patients continued to have a platelet count above 50,000/L [45]. From this literature the ASH consensus group gave grade 2C (weak recommendation, low quality of evidence) evidence that rituximab may be used as a second-line agent in ITP [9]. Rituximab should not be used in patients with hepatitis B infection because of reactivation of the virus. Other side effects include anaphylaxis and progressive multifocal leukoencephalopathy, although more data is needed on long-term adverse effects of this agent.

TPO-mimetic agents

Recently, two new agents have come to the forefront of treatment in refractory ITP. Both romiplostim and eltrombopag stimulate platelet production by activating the TPO receptor. Both drugs have been shown to be effective in raising the platelet count in patients with ITP while reducing bleeding risks in post-splenectomy patients. In the romiplostim phase III parallel, placebo-controlled double-blind randomized trial, romiplostim was given to 63 splenectomized and 62 non-splenectomized patients over a 6-month period [46]. Platelet response rate with platelet count greater than 50×10^9/L was seen in 79% and 88% of the splenectomized and non-splenectomized romiplostim patients, respectively, compared with 0% and 14% in the placebo arms [46]. In a follow-up study, non-splenectomized chronic ITP patients were randomized in a two to one fashion to romiplostim or standard care, with outcomes of splenectomy rates and treatment failure; 11% of patients on romiplostim compared to 30% of patients with standard care had treatment failure, while only 9% of patients on romiplostim vs 36% of patients on standard care went on to splenectomy [47]. In addition, 59% of patients treated with eltrombopag compared with 16% of placebo-treated patients had a platelet count greater than 50×10^9/L on day 43 of treatment [48]. When pooling all available data, a recent Cochrane review of eight clinical trials using TPO-mimetic agents did not show a difference in bleeding rates for patients when compared to controls, although patients receiving TPO-mimetic agents had a higher platelet count [49].

Based on these clinical trials, there is a weak recommendation with low quality of evidence to support use of TPO-mimetic agents in splenectomy-refractory ITP and in those cases where splenectomy is contraindicated [9]. Currently, it is recommended that romiplostim is administered as a weekly subcutaneous injection at 1–10 μg/kg to achieve a platelet count greater than $50 \times 10^9/L$ [46,47]. Eltrombopag is given orally at 25, 50, or 75 mg daily dosing [27,48,50,51]. Effect on platelets ceases once either drug is stopped and lifelong treatment is necessary to sustain a response.

Side effects from either agent are rare, although long-term side effects have not been established. Romiplostim has been shown to increase bone marrow reticulan formation in very few patients [47,51]. Eltrombopag has been associated with adverse liver function test results, and possibly to cause liver failure in rare cases [48,52].

Vinca alkaloids

Vinca alkaloids are thought to bind to platelet microtubules and inhibit destruction in the spleen while also promoting thrombopoiesis. Platelet counts transiently rise in most individuals but only result in a sustained remission in fewer than 10% of patients. Only small clinical trials have shown efficacy in those treated and sustained response is limited to less than 10% of patients. The recommended dose of vincristine is 1–2 mg and of vinblastine is 0.1 mg/kg (maximum dose 10 mg) by injection weekly for at least three doses. Peripheral neuropathy, neutropenia, hair loss, and constipation are common complications [53–55].

Danazol

Danazol is a synthetic androgen that antagonizes estrogens and is postulated to decrease Fc receptor numbers on phagocytic cells. In one study, out of 96 patients, 61% had a response to danazol with time to response at 3 months. Another study showed similar responses with 27 patients (46%) remaining in remission at a median of 119 ± 45 months [56]. In this study the highest rate of response was found in older females and splenectomized patients [57,58]. Danazol should be used in refractory disease, but there is a lack of a large clinical trial to establish its use in ITP. Side effects include weight gain, fluid retention, acne, and hepatotoxicity. It should not be used in pregnant women.

Cyclophosphamide

Cyclophosphamide improves platelet counts in ITP by immunosuppression. There is very limited data on the use of cyclophosphamide in ITP. Cyclophosphamide can be administered either orally (1–2 mg/kg) or intravenously in a pulse fashion (0.3–1 g/mg) for 1–3 doses for 2–4 weeks. Major complications include bone marrow suppression, hemorrhagic cystitis, infertility, development of acute myeloid leukemia, and alopecia [1,9,41].

Other agents

The ICR consensus group lists multiple other agents that have been used in refractory ITP, including azathioprine, interferon-alpha, dapsone, cyclosporine, ascorbic acid, colchicine, and combination chemotherapy including cyclophosphamide, vincristine, and prednisone. None of these therapies has clearly demonstrated effectiveness in large clinical trials [1].

ITP in children

Presentation in children is usually acute with bruising and purpura being present. All of the causes discussed in adult ITP diagnosis should be excluded in children. Full workup is similar to that in adults including a detailed history and physical examination, infection history, exposure history, medication history, and blood counts [1,7,9].

Management differs in children from that in adults, due to the fact that only 3% of children will have clinically significant symptoms. Important factors used to decide whether or not to treat children with ITP include bleeding symptoms, platelet count, and lifestyle issues, including activity level. Hospitalization should only occur in those with severe bleeding, and a watch-and-wait approach can be taken in those without overt bleeding. In children with moderate to severe bleeding symptoms, treatment should be initiated.

IVIg raises platelet counts in 80% of children and does so more quickly than corticosteroids. A single dose of 0.8–1 g/kg has been shown to be the best dose with the least side effects (headache, fever, nausea/vomiting) in children. Prednisone at a dose of 1–2 mg/kg/day can be used for 14 days or 4 mg/kg/day for 3–4 days has also been shown to improve platelet counts in children. Corticosteroid usage for longer than 2 weeks is not recommended because of the serious side effects in children. In life-threatening bleeding, a large dose of platelets with IVIg should be infused. High-dose intravenous corticosteroids can be used as well [7,8].

In children with chronic ITP, medications similar to those in adults have been used. Dexamethasone and high-dose methylprednisolone have both been shown to improve platelet counts in children with refractory or chronic ITP. Rituximab has also been used, resulting in an overall response rate between 31 and 68%. TPO-receptor agonists have not been analyzed in a clinical trial in children. Since their long-term safety profile is unclear, they should not be used in children at this time. With an extremely low likelihood of death from childhood ITP (<0.5%), splenectomy is rarely recommended, as the risk of sepsis is five times higher than in non-splenectomized children [1,8,9].

Treatment of ITP in emergency

Urgent increase in platelet count may be required in those patients requiring surgery, at high risk of bleeding, or with active central nervous system, gastrointestinal, or genitourinary bleeding that cannot be controlled. Consensus guidelines suggest combination therapy with intravenous corticosteroids and IVIg. In patients with extremely low platelets and bleeding, platelet transfusions can produce a transient rise in platelets to help with hemostasis. Antiplatelet therapies and other medications affecting platelet counts should be discontinued. Antifibrinolytic agents such as tranexamic acid and aminocaproic acid may be useful in preventing recurrent bleeding and may be of value in those patients requiring dental or surgical procedures [1,9,30].

ITP in pregnancy

The workup of ITP in a pregnant patient is the same as in a non-pregnant patient, with the addition of ruling out gestational thrombocytopenia, preeclampsia, HELLP syndrome, disseminated intravascular coagulation, folate deficiency, and massive obstetrical hemorrhage in pregnant patients with thrombocytopenia. Treatment in those with ITP is based on risk of maternal hemorrhage. Treatment should commence when the patient is symptomatic (bleeding), when platelet counts fall below 20–30,000/L or an increase in platelets is necessary for a procedure such as surgery or spinal or epidural anesthesia. Generally, platelet counts greater than 75,000/L are required for spinal or epidural anesthesia while platelet counts greater than 50,000/L are needed for cesarean section. Delivery of the fetus is based on obstetric indications and not the severity of ITP [9].

First-line treatments recommended by the ASH and ICR consensus groups are minimum dose corticosteroids to produce a response, or IVIg. Combination therapy has been shown to work in the refractory setting. Medications such as rituximab, TPO-receptor agonists, danazol, vinca alkaloids, and most immunosuppressive drugs should be avoided. Azathioprine has been shown to be safe in pregnancy and can be used as a second-line agent [1,9,28].

References

1. Provan D, Stasi R, Newland AC, et al. International consensus report on the investigation and management of primary immune thrombocytopenia. *Blood* 2010; 115:168–86.

2. McCrae K. Immune thrombocytopenia: no longer 'idiopathic'. *Cleve Clin J Med* 2011;78:358–73.

3. Ruggeri M, Fortuna S, Rodeghiero F. Heterogeneity of terminology and clinical definitions in adult idiopathic thrombocytopenic purpura: a critical appraisal from a systematic review of the literature. *Haematologica* 2008;93:98–103.

4. Rodeghiero F, Stasi R, Gernsheimer T, et al. Standardization of terminology, definitions and outcome criteria in immune thrombocytopenic purpura of adults and children: report from an international working group. *Blood* 2009;113:2386–93.

5. Neylon AJ, Saunders PW, Howard MR, et al. Clinically significant newly presenting autoimmune thrombocytopenic purpura in adults: a prospective study of a population-based cohort of 245 patients. *Br J Hematol* 2003;122:966–74.

6. Frederiksen H, Schmidt K. The incidence of idiopathic thrombocytopenic purpura in adults increases with age. *Blood* 1999;94:909–13.

7. Bolton-Maggs PH, Moon I. Assessment of UK practice for management of acute childhood idiopathic thrombocytopenic purpura against published guidelines. *Lancet* 1997;350:620–3.

8. Kuhne T, Buchanan GR, Zimmerman S, et al. A prospective comparative study of 2540 infants and children with newly diagnosed idiopathic thrombocytopenic purpura (ITP) from the Intercontinental Childhood ITP Study Group. *J Pediatr* 2003;143:605–8.

9. Neunert C, Lim W, Crowther M, et al. The American Society of Hematology 2011 evidence-based practice guideline for immune thrombocytopenia. *Blood* 2011; 117:4190–207.

10. Harrington WJ, Minnich V, Hollingsworth JW, Moore CV. Demonstration of a thrombocytopenic factor in the blood of patients with thrombocytopenic purpura. *J Lab Clin Med* 1951;38:1–10.

11. Shulman NR, Weinrach RS, Libre EP, Andrews HL. The role of the reticuloendothelial system in the pathogenesis of idiopathic thrombocytopenic purpura. *Trans Assoc Am Physicians* 1965;78:374–90.

12. He R, Reid DM, Jones CE, Shulman NR. Spectrum of Ig classes, specificities, and titers of serum antiglycoproteins in chronic idiopathic thrombocytopenic purpura. *Blood* 1994;83:1024–32.

13. Kiefel V, Santoso S, Kaufmann E, Mueller-Eckhardt C. Autoantibodies against platelet glycoprotein Ib/IX: a frequent finding in autoimmune thrombocytopenic purpura. *Br J Hematol* 1991;79:256–62.

14. Pan R, Wang J, Nardi MA, Li Z. The inhibition effect of anti-GPIIIa49-66 antibody on megakaryocyte differentiation. *Thromb Haemost* 2011;106:484–90.

15. Kuter DJ. Biology and chemistry of thrombopoietic agents. *Semin Hematol* 2010;47:243–8.

16. Nugent D, McMillan R, Nichol JL, Slichter SJ. Pathogenesis of chronic immune thrombocytopenia: increased platelet destruction and/or decreased platelet production. *Br J Hematol* 2009;146:585–96.

17. Cohen YC, Djulbegovic B, Shamai-Lubovitz O, Mozes B. The bleeding risk and natural history of idiopathic thrombocytopenic purpura in patients with persistent low platelet counts. *Arch Int Med* 2000;160:1630–8.

18. Djulbegovic B, Cohen Y. The natural history of refractory idiopathic thrombocyto-penic purpura. *Blood* 2001;98:2282–3.

19. Andemariam B, Bussel J. New therapies for immune thrombocytopenic purpura. *Curr Opin Hematol* 2007;14:427–31.

20. Arkfeld DG, Weitz IC. Immune thrombocytopenia in patients with connective tissue disorders and the antiphospholipid antibody syndrome. *Hematol Oncol Clin North Am* 2009;23:1239–49.

21. Cines DB, Bussel JB. How I treat idiopathic thrombocytopenic purpura (ITP). *Blood* 2005;106:2244–51.

22. Cines DB, Bussel JB, Liebman HA, Luning Prak ET. The ITP syndrome: pathogenic and clinical diversity. *Blood* 2009;113:6511–21.

23. George JN. Management of immune thrombocytopenia–something old, something new. *New Engl J Med* 2010;363:1959–61.

24. Stasi R, Evangelista ML, Stipa E, et al. Idiopathic thrombocytopenic purpura: current concepts in pathophysiology and management. *Thromb Haemost* 2008;99:4–13.

25. Toltl LJ, Arnold DM. Pathophysiology and management of chronic immune throm-bocytopenia: focusing on what matters. *Br J Hematol* 2011;152:52–60.

26. Bussel J. Treatment of immune thrombocytopenic purpura in adults. *Sem Hematol* 2006;43(3 Suppl 5):S3–10; discussion S8–9.

27. Bussel JB. Traditional and new approaches to the management of immune throm-bocytopenia: issues of when and who to treat. *Hematol Oncol Clin North Am* 2009;23:1329–41.

28. Cines DB, McMillan R. Management of adult idiopathic thrombocytopenic purpura. *Annu Rev Med* 2005;56:425–42.

29. George JN, Woolf SH, Raskob GE, et al. Idiopathic thrombocytopenic purpura: a practice guideline developed by explicit methods for the American Society of Hema-tology. *Blood* 1996;88:3–40.

30. Provan D. Characteristics of immune thrombocytopenic purpura: a guide for clinical practice. *Eur J Haematol Suppl* 2009;71:8–12.

31. Pamuk GE, Pamuk ON, Baslar Z, et al. Overview of 321 patients with idiopathic thrombocytopenic purpura. Retrospective analysis of the clinical features and response to therapy. *Ann Hematol* 2002;81:436–40.

32. Mazzucconi MG, Fazi P, Bernasconi S, et al. Therapy with high-dose dexamethasone (HD-DXM) in previously untreated patients affected by idiopathic thrombocyto-penic purpura: a GIMEMA experience. *Blood* 2007;109:1401–7.

33. Cheng Y, Wong RS, Soo YO, et al. Initial treatment of immune thrombocy-topenic purpura with high-dose dexamethasone. *New Engl J Med* 2003;349: 831–6.

34. Naithani R, Mahapatra M, Kumar R, et al. High dose dexamethasone therapy shows better responses in acute immune thrombocytopenia than in chronic immune thrombocytopenia. *Platelets* 2010;21:270–3.

35. Arruda VR, Annichino-Bizzacchi JM. High-dose dexamethasone therapy in chronic idiopathic thrombocytopenic purpura. *Ann Hematol* 1996;73:175–7.

36. Ozsoylu S. High-dose methylprednisolone for chronic idiopathic thrombocytopenic purpura. *Acta Hematol* 1988;79:55–6.

37. Imbach P. Immune thrombocytopenic purpura and intravenous immunoglobulin. *Cancer* 1991;68(6 suppl):1422–5.

38. McMillan R. Diagnostic approach to immune thrombocytopenia. *Prog Clin Biol Res* 1978;28:215–27.

39. Kojouri K, Vesely SK, Terrell DR, George JN. Splenectomy for adult patients with idiopathic thrombocytopenic purpura: a systematic review to assess long-term platelet count responses, prediction of response, and surgical complications. *Blood* 2004;104:2623–34.

40. Mikhael J, Northridge K, Lindquist K, et al. Short-term and long-term failure of laparoscopic splenectomy in adult immune thrombocytopenic purpura patients: a systematic review. *Am J Hematol* 2009;84:743–8.

41. Vesely SK, Perdue JJ, Rizvi MA, et al. Management of adult patients with persistent idiopathic thrombocytopenic purpura following splenectomy: a systematic review. *Ann Intern Med* 2004;140:112–20.

42. Arnold DM, Dentali F, Crowther MA, et al. Systematic review: efficacy and safety of rituximab for adults with idiopathic thrombocytopenic purpura. *Ann Intern Med* 2007;146:25–33.

43. Ling HT, Field JJ, Blinder MA. Sustained response with rituximab in patients with thrombotic thrombocytopenic purpura: a report of 13 cases and review of the literature. *Am J Hematol* 2009;84:418–21.

44. Godeau B, Porcher R, Fain O, et al. Rituximab efficacy and safety in adult splenectomy candidates with chronic immune thrombocytopenic purpura: results of a prospective multicenter phase 2 study. *Blood* 2008;112:999–1004.

45. Zaja F, Baccarani M, Mazza P, et al. Dexamethasone plus rituximab yields higher sustained response rates than dexamethasone monotherapy in adults with primary immune thrombocytopenia. *Blood* 2010;115:2755–62.

46. Kuter DJ, Bussel JB, Lyons RM, et al. Efficacy of romiplostim in patients with chronic immune thrombocytopenic purpura: a double-blind randomised controlled trial. *Lancet* 2008;371:395–403.

47. Kuter DJ, Rummel M, Boccia R, et al. Romiplostim or standard of care in patients with immune thrombocytopenia. *New Engl J Med* 2010;363:1889–99.

48. Bussel JB, Provan D, Shamsi T, et al. Effect of eltrombopag on platelet counts and bleeding during treatment of chronic idiopathic thrombocytopenic purpura: a randomised, double-blind, placebo-controlled trial. *Lancet* 2009;373:641–8.

49. Zeng Y, Duan X, Xu J, Ni X. TPO receptor agonist for chronic idiopathic thrombocytopenic purpura. *Cochrane Database Syst Rev* (Online)2011;(7):CD008235.

50. Bussel JB, Kuter DJ, George JN, et al. AMG 531, a thrombopoiesis-stimulating protein, for chronic ITP. *N Engl J Med* 2006;355:1672–81.

51. Bussel JB, Kuter DJ, Pullarkat V, et al. Safety and efficacy of long-term treatment with romiplostim in thrombocytopenic patients with chronic ITP. *Blood* 2009;113:2161–71.

52. Cheng G, Saleh MN, Marcher C, et al. Eltrombopag for management of chronic immune thrombocytopenia (RAISE): a 6-month, randomised, phase 3 study. *Lancet* 2011;377:393–402.

53. Sikorska A, Slomkowski M, Marlanka K, et al. The use of vinca alkaloids in adult patients with refractory chronic idiopathic thrombocytopenia. *Clin Lab Hematol* 2004;26:407–11.

54. Bonnotte B, Gresset AC, Chvetzoff G, et al. Efficacy of colchicine alone or in combination with vinca alkaloids in severe corticoid-resistant thrombocytopenic purpura: six cases. *Am J Hematol* 1999;107:645–6.

55. Facon T, Caulier MT, Wattel E, et al. A randomized trial comparing vinblastine in slow infusion and by bolus i.v. injection in idiopathic thrombocytopenic purpura: a report on 42 patients. *Br J Haematol* 1994;86:678–80.

56. Maloisel F, Andres E, Zimmer J, et al. Danazol therapy in patients with chronic idiopathic thrombocytopenic purpura: long-term results. *Am J Med* 2004;116: 590–4.
57. Stasi R, Provan D. Management of immune thrombocytopenic purpura in adults. *Mayo Clin Proc* 2004;79:504–22.
58. Ahn YS, Rocha R, Mylvaganam R, et al. Long-term danazol therapy in autoimmune thrombocytopenia: unmaintained remission and age-dependent response in women. *Ann Intern Med* 1989;111:723–9.

CHAPTER 12

Disseminated Intravascular Coagulation: Diagnosis and Management

Stephanie J. Davis[1] and Craig M. Kessler[2]
[1]Department of Internal Medicine, University of North Carolina Hospitals, Chapel Hill, NC, USA
[2]Division of Laboratory Medicine, Lombardi Comprehensive Cancer Center, Georgetown University Medical Center, Washington, DC, USA

Introduction

Disseminated intravascular coagulation (DIC) has been defined by the International Society on Thrombosis and Haemostasis (ISTH) Scientific Subcommittee on DIC as "an acquired syndrome characterized by the intravascular activation of coagulation with loss of localization arising from different causes. It can originate from and cause damage to the microvasculature, which if sufficiently severe, can produce organ dysfunction" [1]. DIC is marked by both thrombotic and hemorrhagic phenotypes, either or both of which may predominate at any time. The downstream consequences of DIC may consist of life-threatening hemorrhage or multisystem organ failure from microvascular thrombosis, which may contribute to high morbidity and mortality. Traditionally, DIC has been depicted as a dire complication of various conditions. As the understanding of coagulation and its modulators has advanced, this concept warrants updating. The object of this chapter is to characterize DIC as a unique disease entity; it is not simply the physiologic response to a pathologic condition, such as sepsis, trauma, or some systemic insult. DIC is a multifaceted disorder with a myriad of triggers, ranging from cytokine release secondary to sepsis or systemic inflammation, the circulation of cancer procoagulants in malignancy, or perturbation of the vascular endothelium with tissue injury. Through the mechanism of tissue factor elaboration, as well as platelet and endothelial activation, DIC is set in motion.

The challenge of diagnosing DIC in the clinical setting is twofold. First, the syndrome must be recognized even before it evolves into a fulminant

Hemostasis and Thrombosis: Practical Guidelines in Clinical Management, First Edition.
Hussain I. Saba and Harold R. Roberts.
© 2014 John Wiley & Sons, Ltd. Published 2014 by John Wiley & Sons, Ltd.

condition. Second, the clinician must then assess the particular phenotype the patient is expressing – thrombotic, hemorrhagic, or both – and direct appropriate therapy or supportive care toward reversing that phenotype. The approach to treatment of the disease state(s) underlying the DIC also may influence the way DIC presents and how it progresses, making it critical for the clinician to be aware of the clinical scenarios that have a high potential to precipitate DIC. Once the diagnosis has been suspected, confirmation by laboratory testing in a timely manner is paramount; however, DIC is a moving target. Unfractionated heparin has long been the mainstay and most widely used standard therapy, but the improved understanding of the triggers and downstream consequences of DIC has yielded many new pathways to exploit. Various potential therapies discussed in this chapter include commercial concentrates of antithrombin, activated protein C, recombinant tissue factor pathway inhibitor, and recombinant human factor VIIa. There has also been interest in administering adjunctive therapies, such as the antifibrinolytic agents ε-aminocaproic acid and tranexamic acid, and monoclonal anti-tissue factor IgG antibody. As the pharmacologic armamentarium for DIC expands, it is incumbent on the physician to appreciate when and if these new therapies can be useful and the inherent risks associated with each.

Etiology

The most commonly occurring clinical etiology of DIC is infection, followed by trauma, surgery, and malignancy. A 1978 series of 118 symptomatic patients with laboratory-confirmed DIC reported the following generalized associations: approximately 40% of cases occurred in the setting of systemic infection, 24% in the setting of trauma or surgery, 7% in malignancy, and 29% in miscellaneous settings [2]. A subsequent large review in 1980 characterized 346 patients with laboratory-confirmed DIC and found that 26% of patients had systemic infection, 24% had malignancy, 19% were post-surgical or trauma patients, 8% had severe liver disease, and 23% had miscellaneous causes [3].

The varying hierarchy of disease states leading to DIC may reflect the sensitivity and specificity of the diagnostic laboratory methods of the time, as well as referral patterns. With the advent of improved D-dimer assays and wider use of computed tomography (CT) scans, DIC is diagnosed more rapidly and therapeutic intervention initiated before fulminant disease manifestations develop. Thus, in a more recent review from 2000 of 204 symptomatic patients with laboratory-confirmed DIC, 46.5% had underlying malignancy – 33.8% with solid tumors and 12.7% with hematologic malignancies, 10.8% had aortic aneurysms (pre- or post-dissection not specified), 6.4% had systemic infections (type unspecified), 4.4% of patients had postoperative hemorrhagic complications, 2.9% had severe liver disease, 2.5% had obstetric complications, and 26.5 % had other miscellaneous underlying causes [4].

One can speculate that advances in antimicrobial therapy and early intervention in treating sepsis account for the declining incidence of DIC associated with infection in the last four decades. Nevertheless, recent studies still estimate that 35% of patients with severe sepsis[1] will develop DIC, with Gram-negative sepsis being the most classic precipitant [5]. However, DIC can be seen in a range of infections, including those due to Gram-positive bacteria, viruses, rickettsia, fungi, and protozoa (Table 12.1) [6–9].

Malignancy is another well-established cause of DIC, and this does not correlate with tumor bulk; in fact, DIC may develop in the presence of microscopic tumors [5]. It is estimated that up to 20% of patients with cancer, especially metastatic adenocarcinomas or lymphoproliferative malignancies, develop DIC [5]. The DIC of solid tumors is more frequently chronic and is associated with arterial and/or venous thrombotic events [10]. Venous events can present as deep vein thrombosis (DVT), pulmonary embolism, or superficial migratory thrombophlebitis, as originally defined by Trousseau. Arterial clots tend to occur as embolic events from nonbacterial thrombotic endocarditis (NBTE) and often present as digit ischemia or cerebral vascular accidents (CVA) [10]. In contrast, hematologic malignancies are more often associated with acute DIC presenting with hemorrhage, the most classic scenario being acute promyelocytic leukemia (APL) [11]. APL has a particularly high incidence of DIC-related hemorrhage, thought to be secondary to hyperfibrinolysis induced by excessive tissue factor elaboration and thrombin generation [11]. This coagulopathy is often abated by the early initiation of all-trans-retinoic acid (ATRA), which, by inducing promyelocyte differentiation, downregulates the synthesis of tissue factor or cysteine protease, the latter of which directly activates factor X [11].

---

[1] Severe sepsis is defined as 1) meeting two of four criteria for systemic inflammatory response syndrome (SIRS); 2) the presence of infection; and 3) evidence of end-organ dysfunction such as altered mental status, renal insufficiency, or coagulopathy. SIRS criteria are as follows: 1) temperature >38°C or <36°C; 2) heart rate > 90 beats per minute; 3) respiratory rate greater than 20 or arterial carbon dioxide tension ($PaCO_2$) less than 32 mmHg; or 4) white blood cell count greater than 12,000/μL or less than 4,000/μL or at least 10% bands [12].

Table 12.1 Conditions associated with DIC. Source: Adapted from Greer et al. 2004 [9]. Reproduced with permission of Lippincott, Williams & Wilkins.

Infection

Bacterial: Gram-positive bacteremia (*Staphylococcus aureus, Streptococcus pneumoniae, Streptococcus pyogenes, Clostridium perfringens*), Gram-negative bacterermia (*Neisseria meningitidis*, various Gram-negative rods)

Viral: herpes virus infection, acute viral hepatitis, dengue fever, Hanta virus

Spirochetes: leptospirosis, borreliosis

Rickettsial: Rocky Mountain spotted fever

Mycotic: histoplasmosis, aspergillosis

Protozoal: malaria (*P. falciparum*), trypanosomiasis, babesiosis

Obstetric emergencies

Amniotic fluid embolism

Abruptio placentae

Placenta previa

HELLP syndrome

Severe preeclampsia/eclampsia

Acute fatty liver of pregnancy

Septic abortion

Dead fetus syndrome

Chorioamnionitis

Malignancy

Solid tumors: lung most common (~24% postmortem [13]), adenocarcinoma of GI tract, prostate, breast

Hematologic malignancies: acute leukemia (particularly myeloid leukemia, APL most commonly)

Other malignancies: metastatic carcinoid, neuroblastoma, rhabdomyosarcoma

Tumor lysis syndrome (associated with tumor bulk and iatrogenesis)

Trauma

Penetrating trauma

Blunt trauma

Burns

Crush injuries

Major surgeries

Closed head trauma

Hypoxia, hypoperfusion

Cardiac arrest

Cardiogenic shock

Anaphylactic shock

Massive pulmonary embolism

Fat embolism

Adult respiratory distress syndrome (ARDS)

Fulminant intravascular hemolysis

Acute hemolytic transfusion reaction

Paroxysmal nocturnal hemoglobinuria (PNH)

Drug-induced hemolysis (most commonly in G6PD deficiency)

Sickle cell anemia

Freshwater submersion

Liver disease

Fulminant hepatic failure

Cirrhosis with end-stage liver disease

Reperfusion of orthotopic liver transplant

Environmental exposures

Hypothermia

Heat stroke

Snake bite (particularly rattlesnakes and vipers)

Vascular malformations

Aneurysms (stable or unstable/dissecting)

Takayasu arteritis

Coarctation of the aorta, other large vessels

Giant hemangiomas (Kasabach-Merritt syndrome)

Transplant rejection

Allograft rejection

Graft-versus-host disease (GVHD)

Table 12.1 (*Continued*)

Drug-induced	Other
Cytotoxic chemotherapy	Vasculitis
Monoclonal antibody chemotherapeutic agents (rituximab)	Acute pancreatitis
	Status epilepticus
High-dose Intravenous Immunoglobulin (IVIg)	Diabetic ketoacidosis
Recombinant Factor VIIa	
Parenteral iron therapy (acute iron toxicity)	
Rh$_0$(D) Immune Globulin Intravenous (WinRho)	
Recreational drugs (cocaine, amphetamines)	
Unfractionated heparin (via heparin-induced thrombocytopenia with thrombosis)	
Activated prothrombin complex concentrate (FEIBA)	

Hematologic conditions
Homozygous protein C/S deficiency
  (purpura fulminans)
Catastrophic antiphospholipid antibody
  syndrome (APLS)

Pathophysiology

The normal process of hemostasis is achieved through a tight balance between endogenous procoagulants and the naturally-circulating thrombotic modulators to allow for balanced thrombin generation, localized fibrin formation, and regulated fibrinolysis. At the surface of the tissue factor (TF)-expressing cells, such as monocytes or tumor cells, TF complexes with activated factor VII (VIIa) (Figure 12.1) [14]. This complex has two key downstream effects: the activation of factor X and the activation of factor IX [14]. Factor Xa remains at the surface of the TF-expressing cell while factor IXa travels to the platelet surface. At the TF-expressing cell, Factor Xa complexes with Factor Va, and this complex converts prothrombin to thrombin. This thrombin generation is modest and is adequate to activate factor XI, which in turn boosts factor IXa generation in the intrinsic clotting pathway. At the platelet surface, factor IXa interacts with factor VIIIa, and then, on a phospholipid platform, activates the zymogen factor X to Xa. Factor Xa then joins its cofactors calcium and factor Va on a phospholipid platform to create the prothrombinase complex to set up a "thrombin burst". This thrombin burst sets off a series of critical reactions. Fibrinogen is proteolyzed by thrombin to yield fibrin monomers.

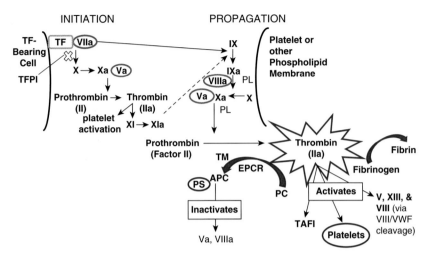

Figure 12.1 A cell-based model of coagulation. Source: Adapted from Roberts et al. 2006 [14], Monroe et al. 2002 [15]. APC, activated protein C; EPCR, endothelial protein C receptor; PC, protein C; PL, phospholipid cofactor; PS, protein S; TAFI, thrombin-activated fibrinolytic inhibitor; TF, tissue factor; TFPI, tissue factor pathway inhibitor; TM, thrombomodulin (membrane-based); V, VIII, etc., inactive factor V, VIII, etc.; Va, VIIa, etc., activated factor V, VII, etc.

Subsequently, these monomers cross-link into a tensile fibrin clot due to the action of factor XIII, which itself is activated by thrombin. In the presence of membrane-based thrombomodulin (TM) and endothelial protein C receptor (EPCR), thrombin activates protein C (PC). Activated protein C (APC) is then able to act in conjunction with protein S (PS) to inactivate factors Va and VIIIa, acting as built-in modulators of the coagulation system. Thrombin also activates thrombin-activatable fibrinolytic inhibitor (TAFI), an inherent upregulator of the system [14]. Lastly, the thrombin burst activates platelets, factors V, VIII, and XIII in a self-perpetuating, reinforcing manner. Activation of factor VIII occurs via factor VIII protein cleavage from von Willebrand factor (VWF), which chaperones factor VIII in its inactive state in the plasma circulation.

DIC results from a loss of the procoagulant/antithrombotic balance in the setting of sustained, systemic activation of the coagulation cascade by sepsis, cancer, trauma, or other injury [16]. The primary driving force in DIC is the overwhelming generation of tissue factor by endotoxin, cancer cells, or tissue injury [5]. As thrombin generation is enhanced, it is able to overcome its natural circulating inhibitors, and the overabundant fibrin formation becomes inappropriately deposited in the microvasculature [5,9]. This intravascular fibrin causes a "clothes-lining" effect on circulating erythrocytes in an area of high shear. This phenomenon results in intravascular hemolysis and red cell fragmentation, which is recognized in approximately 50% of DIC cases [9]. In response to ongoing fibrin generation, compensatory fibrinolysis is continuously stimulated, leading to the generation of fibrin degradation products (FDPs) and D-dimers (proteolyzed fragments emanating from cross-linked fibrin) [9]. With the upregulated activation of the coagulation cascade, clotting factors and platelets become consumed and are eventually depleted, as are the endogenous inhibitors of coagulation [9]. This can be detected in the coagulation laboratory (see Diagnosis below).

Thus, with sustained overstimulation, this normally finely tuned process becomes unregulated. Overproduction of fibrin leads to unchecked thrombosis, and excessive fibrinolysis leads to unchecked bleeding; this yields hemorrhage and microvascular thrombosis, respectively [16]. Hypoperfusion results and creates tissue ischemia, leading to end-organ damage, particularly in areas rich in microvascular beds, such as the kidneys and the lungs [9].

This loss of balance is corroborated by immunohistochemical staining of tissue biopsies of purpura fulminans, a type of extreme tissue ischemia seen in DIC [17,18]. It has been shown that these cells demonstrate a decreased expression of activated protein C receptors, thrombomodulin, and endothelial protein C receptors on their surfaces [18]. Downregulation of activated protein C receptors yields reduced protein C activity and, thus, less inhibition of coagulation, explaining some of the thrombotic phenotype seen in purpura fulminans [18].

Thrombin production in sepsis is ultimately tied to toxin release by the infectious organism and cytokine production by the host [5]. In Gram-negative sepsis, bacterial membrane lipopolysaccharide (LPS) acts as an endotoxin and increases tissue factor expression by host monocytes and granulocytes, while in Gram-positive sepsis, endotoxins such as staphylococcal alpha toxin increase tissue factor expression by host cells [5,18,19]. Furthermore, endotoxins are also known to activate the vascular endothelium, providing a second mechanism of coagulation activation in Gram-negative sepsis [9]. Proinflammatory cytokines released in sepsis, such as interleukin-6 (IL-6) and tumor necrosis factor (TNF), have been shown to augment this process by increasing tissue factor expression by host immune cells [17].

Thrombin production in malignancy is multifactorial. Cancer cells express an exaggerated amount of tissue factor as well as cancer procoagulant, a cysteine protease unique to some malignant cells (predominantly derived from gastrointestinal cancers), which is able to directly activate factor X in a tissue factor-independent mechanism [20–24].

Many obstetric emergencies activate coagulation by release of fetal tissue or amniotic fluid into the maternal circulation, such as in abruptio

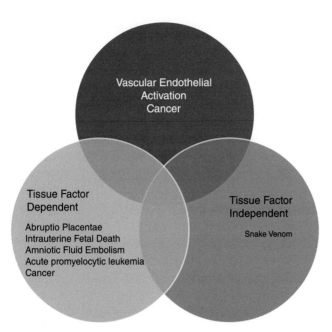

Figure 12.2 The multifactorial nature of the various etiologies of disseminated intravascular coagulation [14].

placentae and amniotic fluid embolism, which act as a strong stimulant of tissue factor expression and, therefore, upregulated coagulation [5].

Trauma causes DIC by a similar mechanism: tissue injury results in release of tissue thromboplastin and other substances which stimulate coagulation through tissue factor [5]. Trauma that includes injury to the vasculature has an additional stimulating effect by activating the vascular endothelium [9]. Blood loss with hypoperfusion will also contribute to the process.

The mechanisms by which snake venoms activate coagulation vary as well. Some venom contains a substance able to directly activate factor X while other venoms act locally at the bite site to cause injury to, and therefore activate, the vascular endothelium [25]. Aneurysms and giant hemangiomas also cause injury to the vascular endothelium and platelet activation sufficient to cause DIC despite the seemingly more benign settings (Figure 12.2) [9].

Diagnosis

Acute DIC is typically diagnosed in the presence of a predisposing condition and in association with concurrent thrombocytopenia with a platelet count less than 100,000/μL; a prolonged prothrombin time (PT) and activated partial thromboplastin time (aPTT) due to clotting factor deficiency from consumption; fibrinogen levels less than 100 mg/dL; elevated D-dimers, reflecting the degradation of cross-linked fibrin and generation of other fibrin (-ogen) degradation products by accelerated fibrinolysis; and increased thrombin time [26]. Thrombocytopenia is largely due to rapid intravascular consumption of platelets that results in a net deficiency despite accelerated platelet generation. Fibrin strands deposited within the microvasculature result in hemolysis and fragmentation of red blood cells, creating microangiopathic hemolytic anemia. This can be confirmed by the presence of schistocytes and red cell fragments on a peripheral smear in approximately 50% of patients with DIC [9].

As clotting factors are consumed, the liver eventually becomes unable to compensate for the increased synthetic demand, resulting in a net deficiency of these proteins, particularly fibrinogen (factor I) and factor V [9]. DIC is also notable for more rapid consumption of the endogenous modulators of coagulation than the liver can generate. Protein C and antithrombin (AT) activity levels detectable in plasma are therefore typically reduced in DIC; the deficiency of protein S activity is typically due to both consumption and binding to the acute phase reactant inflammatory complement component C4-binding protein [1,26].

Chronic DIC, such as that seen in malignancy, can be present even in the absence of absolute thrombocytopenia or PT/aPTT increases [27]. When the process is less fulminant, the bone marrow can increase thrombopoiesis and maintain a normal or near-normal platelet count. The liver, too, has compensatory mechanisms to upregulate clotting protein production to keep up with consumption. The fibrinogen level in inflammatory states such as malignancy is typically very elevated at baseline as an acute phase reactant; thus, a net decrease in fibrinogen may result in a level that is still normal or high by laboratory standards [27]. In early DIC, low levels of thrombin may activate FVIII and thus keep the aPTT in the normal range whereas, with more fibrinolytic activation, FVIII activity decreases. Acute and chronic DIC cannot be differentiated by the presence of schistocytes and elevated FDPs, including elevated D-dimers [27].

The Scientific Subcommittee on DIC of the ISTH has developed a scoring system for what is characterized as "overt" (or acute) DIC and "non-overt" (or evolving) DIC [26]. Overt DIC is defined only in the setting of a known predisposing condition and has been shown to correlate with higher 28-day mortality [26,28]. Scores of 0–3 are given for the degree of aberration of each of the following components: a depressed platelet count, elevated fibrin markers (soluble fibrin monomers or fibrin degradation products; FDPs), a prolonged prothrombin time (PT), and a reduced

Table 12.2 Scoring system for overt disseminated intravascular coagulation. Source: Toh 2007 [29]. Reproduced with permission of John Wiley & Sons, Ltd.

Risk assessment	Does the patient have an underlying disorder known to be associated with overt DIC?
	Yes: Proceed
	No: Do not use this algorithm
Laboratory studies to order	Platelet count, fibrin-related marker, prothrombin time (PT), fibrinogen
Laboratory marker	**Points assigned (0, 1, 2, or 3)**
Platelet count	>100,000 = 0; <100,000 = 1; <50,000 = 2
Elevated fibrin-related marker (D-dimer, FDPs)	No increase = 0; moderate increase = 2; strong increase = 3
Prolonged prothrombin time (PT)	<3 sec = 0; >3 sec but <6 sec = 1; >6 sec = 2
Fibrinogen level	>1.0 g/L = 0; <1.0 g/L = 1
Calculate score	>5: Compatible with overt DIC; repeat score daily
	≤5: Suggestive (not affirmative) for non-overt DIC; repeat score in 1–2 days

Table 12.3 Scoring system for non-overt disseminated intravascular coagulation. Source: Toh 2007 [29]. Reproduced with permission of John Wiley & Sons, Ltd.

Risk assessment	Does the patient have an underlying disorder known to be associated with overt DIC?
	Yes = 2 points assigned
	No = 0 points assigned
Laboratory studies to order	For major criteria: platelet count, fibrin-related marker, prothrombin time (PT)
	For specific criteria: antithrombin (AT), protein C
Laboratory marker	**Points assigned (−1, 0, or 1)**
Platelet count	>100,000 = 0; <100,000 = 1
	Rising = −1; stable = 0; falling = 1
Prolonged prothrombin time (PT)	<3 sec = 0; >3 sec = 1
	Falling = −1; stable = 0; rising = 1
Elevated fibrin-related marker (D-dimer, FDPs)	Normal = 0; raised = 1
	Falling = −1; stable = 0; rising = 1
Antithrombin (AT, or ATIII)	Normal = −1; low = 1
Protein C	Normal = −1; low = 1
Thrombin–antithrombin (TAT) complexes	Normal = −1; abnormal = 1
Calculate score	≥5: Compatible with non-overt DIC

fibrinogen level (Table 12.2) [26,29]. A score of 5 or more is consistent with overt DIC while a score less than 5 suggests evolving or "non-overt" DIC [26,29]. It is recommended that this scoring be repeated daily in patients with confirmed overt DIC and daily or every other day in patients with non-overt DIC [26,29]. Scoring of non-overt DIC (Table 12.3) does not require a known underlying condition and scores platelet counts, prothrombin times, and fibrin degradation markers [26,29]. These scoring criteria, however, also include score adjustments based on trends, for instance, whether these values are stable, rising, or falling [26,29]. The non-overt scoring system, in contrast to the overt DIC scoring criteria, also takes into account the decreased activity levels of antithrombin and protein C as well as the increased levels of thrombin–antithrombin (TAT) complexes [26,29]. Although evaluating non-overt DIC is less precise, it provides a way to potentially detect a developing coagulopathy early enough to intervene. The ISTH scoring system for overt DIC has an estimated diagnostic sensitivity of 91% and specificity of 97%, compared to blinded expert assessment for DIC [28]. Unfortunately, the scoring systems are somewhat cumbersome tools for most clinicians to utilize.

Clinical consequences

DIC is associated with a significant mortality rate, estimated at approximately 50% [2]. Patients may experience bleeding and potentially life-threatening hemorrhage [2]. The percentage of patients with this outcome seems to vary with the underlying condition: only about 15% of patients with DIC and sepsis incur bleeding, but almost all patients with DIC as a result of obstetric complications experience bleeding [9]. Major organ dysfunction is also common but seems to vary with the underlying cause as well. Approximately 20% of patients with DIC due to obstetric catastrophes experience major organ dysfunction compared to 76% of patients with DIC secondary to sepsis [9]. The most common outcomes seen are renal failure, liver failure, respiratory compromise, and central nervous system (CNS) dysfunction [2,9]. Acute renal failure can occur directly through renal thrombotic microangiopathy or indirectly via acute tubular necrosis (ATN) secondary to hypotension and shock [2]. Acute liver failure occurs from hepatocellular injury also as a result of hypotension and shock [2]. Respiratory failure can occur from acute lung injury secondary to pulmonary infarct or adult respiratory distress syndrome (ARDS), frequently requiring mechanical ventilation [2]. Many of the same conditions that promote DIC cause concurrent ARDS, namely trauma, septic shock, and burns [2]. CNS complications are also seen in DIC and may manifest as altered mental status that is mild, such as disorientation or delirium, or profound, such as obtundation or coma [2,9]. Furthermore, patients may experience stroke or transient ischemic attack (TIA) from cerebral vascular microthrombi from NBTE and hemorrhage [2].

Treatment modalities and evolving therapeutics

As DIC is usually attributable to a serious underlying condition, treatment of this underlying condition remains the most effective treatment for DIC [9]. However, concurrent supportive care is often needed, and patients may require aggressive replacement of blood, plasma clotting components, and platelets while awaiting resolution of the underlying disorder using conventional treatment strategies (i.e., antibiotics, chemotherapy, delivery of the fetus, IV fluid resuscitation, etc.). Thrombotic complications of DIC occasionally need to be addressed and, for this, graduated low-dose continuous infusion of unfractionated heparin (UFH) has remained the cornerstone of therapy. In this schema, initial UFH doses may begin with a 3000 U bolus and a 300 U/hour infusion, monitoring platelets and fibrinogen levels every 2–4 hours. UFH doses can be increased according to the laboratory data until one notes a consistent rise in platelets and/or fibrinogen. This mitigates the potential to induce overt bleeding due to "over" anticoagulation in the context of clotting factor deficiencies and thrombocytopenia.

Therapeutic doses of low-molecular-weight heparin (LMWH) have been recommended for patients with DIC complicated by arterial or venous thromboembolism, purpura fulminans, or vascular skin infarction (Grade C, Level IV) [30]. UFH or LMWH is recommended for venous thromboembolism prophylaxis in patients at risk for DIC who are not experiencing bleeding (Grade A, Level 1B) [30].

The use of blood products must be dictated by the clinical scenario and not simply to normalize abnormal laboratory test results. For patients with DIC and active bleeding or those who are at high risk for bleeding, platelet transfusions are recommended to sustain the platelet count over 50,000 (Grade C, Level IV) [30]. Performing invasive diagnostic or therapeutic procedures in patients with overt DIC and abnormal coagulation testing is fraught with high risk and should not be considered lightly. Fresh frozen plasma may be used (Grade C, Level IV) but more efficient to correct severe hypofibrinogenemia (fibrinogen level <100) is the administration of fibrinogen concentrate (as off-label use) or cryoprecipitate (Grade C, Level IV) [30].

Recombinant human factor VIIa (rFVIIa) has been used off-label by the military for life-threatening bleeding due to penetrating injuries and has, at times, been considered a last resort in DIC-related hemorrhage.

A prospective controlled clinical trial for severe traumatic bleeding in a civilian scenario demonstrated no improved survival benefit [31]. Anecdotally, rFVIIa has been reported to successfully reverse severe bleeding complications; however, the safety and efficacy of rFVIIa in DIC remain unclear. A systematic review recently reported a clinical benefit for the use of rFVIIa in bleeding patients with DIC secondary to postpartum hemorrhage, trauma, sepsis, malignancy, or liver failure [32]. However, there have been reports of thromboembolic complications and death associated with the administration of rFVIIa when used in patients with laboratory and clinical evidence of pre-existing DIC [33]. Thus, in the absence of clinical benefit ascertained from randomized controlled trials, rFVIIa should be used judiciously in patients with DIC and, perhaps, at doses much lower than recommended for bleeding hemophilia patients with alloantibody inhibitors (i.e., 10–20 μg/kg IV bolus rather than 90 μg/kg every 2–3 hours). Prior placebo controlled studies in non-coagulopathic individuals have reported dose-related arterial thromboembolic complications after rFVIIa therapy [34].

The use of antithrombin (AT) concentrates has also been subjected to limited clinical trials but to date has demonstrated little clinical benefit in DIC or in clinical settings frequently associated with DIC, such as severe sepsis. The KyberSept trial was a double-blind, placebo-controlled, multicenter phase III clinical trial in patients with severe sepsis to determine whether high-dose intravenous AT concentrate (plasma-derived) improved mortality [35]. There was no difference in all-cause mortality at 28 days between the treatment and placebo groups and, when used in conjunction with heparin, there was a significant increase in bleeding complications in patients receiving high doses of AT [35]. Recombinant AT concentrate is currently available but has not been evaluated in large populations with DIC.

Activated protein C (rhAPC) concentrate or drotrecogin alpha (activated) (DrotAA), previously marketed as Xigris by Eli Lilly in 2001, initially demonstrated promise to modulate overt DIC. The PROWESS study, a phase III randomized double-blind multicenter trial, reported that patients receiving rhAPC had a 28-day all-cause mortality rate of 24.7%, compared to 30.8% in the placebo group [36]. However, there was a nonsignificant increased incidence of bleeding observed in the treatment arm versus placebo [36]. Due to controversy surrounding its efficacy, the PROWESS-Shock trial was launched in 2011 focusing on the patient cohort who benefited the most in PROWESS retrospective subgroup analysis, namely those in shock with multisystem organ failure [37,38]. In this study, DrotAA did not reduce the rate of death from septic shock at 28 and 90 days and, subsequently, Xigris was withdrawn from the market in October 2011 [37,38].

Recombinant tissue factor pathway inhibitor (TFPI) has been examined in coagulopathy and initially showed benefit in animal models and human phase I and II trials [39,40]. When studied on a larger scale in the OPTIMIST trial, a multicenter, randomized, placebo-controlled trial, recombinant TFPI, or tifacogin, failed to demonstrate an improvement in 28-day all-cause mortality of patients with severe sepsis and coagulopathy [39,40]. Notably, there was an increased risk of bleeding in the tifacogin group when compared to placebo [39,40].

Use of antifibrinolytic agents such as ε-aminocaproic acid (Amicar®) and tranexamic acid (TXA), while used for other causes of bleeding, are not generally recommended in DIC [39]. Tranexamic acid has shown a limited role in conditions where DIC is associated with hyperfibrinolysis, such as in AML and advanced prostate cancer [29]. The CRASH2 trial demonstrated that tranexamic acid can be used to control the excessive bleeding which induces or results from DIC in severe trauma patients (Grade A, Level 1b) [41]. There was a significant reduction in overall mortality (relative risk 0.91, 95% CI 0.85–0.97) and specific mortality due to bleeding (RR 0.85, 95% CI 0.76–0.96) [42]. Further examination of the data indicated that the benefits of tranexamic acid were dependent on the promptness of drug initiation [42]. Thus, therapeutic advantage was observed only if tranexamic acid (intravenous loading dose 1 g over 10 min followed by infusion of 1 g over 8 h) was administered within 3 hours of onset of bleeding [42]. The proportion of individuals who benefited from tranexamic acid treatment was reduced with as little as a 1-hour delay [43]. The relative risk of death from bleeding with tranexamic acid was estimated in the CRASH-2 trial as 0.85 (95% CI 0.76–0.96) compared to 0.96 (95% CI 0.86–1.08) if treatment was delayed by 1 hour [43].

Evolving therapeutics

While yet to be studied in DIC, CNTO 859, an emerging humanized anti-tissue factor monoclonal antibody has therapeutic implications worth investigating [44]. CNTO 859 was shown in xenograft models to inhibit breast cancer metastasis and tumor growth in vitro [44]. Being an agent directed against tissue factor, it is reasonable to extrapolate the use of this agent to DIC, a process largely driven by tissue factor.

Lepirudin and argatroban, parenteral direct thrombin inhibitors used to prevent or treat thrombosis in heparin-induced thrombocytopenia (HIT), are not well studied in DIC at this time but have been shown in limited case studies to improve the coagulopathy and laboratory parameters of DIC in patients with HIT [45]. Dabigatran, the first oral specific anti-IIa (thrombin) anticoagulant, is approved in the US for prevention of non-valvular atrial fibrillation-induced embolic stroke and for venous thromboembolism (VTE) prevention after total hip and knee replacement surgery [46]. Its theoretical potential benefit for prevention or reversal of DIC in critical clinical scenarios remains to be established or evaluated in clinical trials.

Rivaroxaban, an oral direct factor Xa inhibitor approved for the treatment of VTE, stroke prevention in non-valvular atrial fibrillation, and secondary prevention of coronary events in patients with acute coronary syndrome, may also have potential benefit in the treatment of DIC but has yet to be studied for this indication [47]. Parenteral administration of the indirect factor Xa inhibitor fondaparinux is currently approved for VTE prophylaxis in orthopedic and abdominal surgeries and for the treatment of VTE in place of heparin; this drug is now being considered for management of acute coronary syndrome as well [48]. Fondaparinux was shown in a case report to successfully treat Trousseau's syndrome as a manifestation of DIC in malignancy when heparin was ineffective [49].

While many of these agents show promise in preventing and treating VTE, further evaluation of their role in DIC is required before these drugs can be recommended in the treatment of DIC.

References

1. Taylor FB, Jr, Toh CH, Hoots WK, et al. Towards definition, clinical and laboratory criteria, and a scoring system for disseminated intravascular coagulation on behalf of the Scientific Subcommittee on Disseminated Intravascular Coagulation (DIC) of the International Society on Thrombosis and Haemostasis (ISTH). *Thromb Haemost* 2001;86:1327–30.
2. Seigal T, Seligsohn U, Aghai E, Modan M. Clinical and laboratory aspects of disseminated intravascular coagulation (DIC): a study of 118 cases. *Thromb Haemost* 1978;39:122.
3. Spero JA, Lewis JH, Hasiba U. Disseminated intravascular coagulation: findings in 346 patients. *Thromb Haemost* 1980;43:28.
4. Okajima K, Sakamoto Y, Uchiba M. Heterogeneity in the incidence and clinical manifestations of disseminated intravascular coagulation: a study of 204 cases. *Am J Hematol* 2000;65:215–22.
5. Levi M. Disseminated intravascular coagulation. *Crit Care Med* 2007;35:2191–6.
6. Murray HW, Tuazon CU, Sheagren JN. Staphylococcal septicemia and disseminated intravascular coagulation: *Staphylococcus aureus* endocarditis mimicking meningococcemia. *Arch Intern Med* 1977;137:844.
7. Stossel TP, Levy R. Intravascular coagulation associated with pneumococcal bacteremia and symmetrical peripheral gangrene. *Arch Intern Med* 1970;125:876.
8. de Virgilio C, Klein S, Chang L, et al. Clostridial bacteremia: implications for the surgeon. *Am Surg* 1991;57:388.

9. Greer JP, Foerster J, Lukens JM, et al. *Wintrobe's Clinical Hematology*, 11th edition. Philadelphia: Lippincott Williams & Wilkins, 2004;1430–40.

10. Sack GH, Jr, Levin J, Bell WR. Trousseau's syndrome and other manifestations of chronic disseminated coagulopathy in patients with neoplasms: Clinical, pathophysiologic, and therapeutic features. *Medicine (Baltimore)* 1977;56:1–37.

11. Barbui T, Finazzi G, Falanga A. The impact of all-trans-retinoic acid on the coagulopathy of acute promyelocytic leukemia. *Blood* 1998;91:3093.

12. Septic Shock. Pinsky, MR. *Medscape Reference*. Updated Aug 13, 2012. Accessed Sept 1, 2012. http://emedicine.medscape.com/article/168402-overview.

13. Kramer J, Otten HM, Levi M, ten Cate H. The association of disseminated intravascular coagulation with specific diseases. *Réanimation* 2002;11:575–83.

14. Roberts HR, Hoffman M, Monroe DM. A cell-based model of thrombin generation. *Semin Thromb Hemost* 2006;2(suppl 1):32–8.

15. Monroe DM, Hoffman M, Roberts HR. Platelets and thrombin generation. *Arterioscler Thromb Vasc Biol* 2002;22:1381–9.

16. Toh CH. Diagnosis and treatment of disseminated intravascular coagulation: bleeding complications in cancer patients. *6th International Conference on Thrombosis and Hemostasis Issues in Cancer*, April 21, 2012.

17. Jansen PM, Pixley RA, Brouwer M, et al. Inhibition of factor XII in septic baboons attenuates the activation of complement and fibrinolytic systems and reduces the release of interleukin-6 and neutrophil elastase. *Blood* 1996;87:2337.

18. Faust SN, Levin M, Harrison OB, et al. Dysfunction of endothelial protein C activation in severe meningococcal sepsis. *N Eng J Med* 2001;345: 408–16.

19. Levi M, van der Poll T, ten Cate H, van Deventer SJ. The cytokine-mediated imbalance between coagulant and anticoagulant mechanisms in sepsis and endotoxaemia. *Eur J Clin Invest* 1997;27:3.

20. Edwards RL, Rickles FR. Macrophage procoagulants. *Prog Hemost Thromb* 1984; 7:183.

21. Rickles FR, Levin M, Edwards RL. Hemostatic alterations in cancer patients. *Cancer Metastasis Rev* 1992;11:237.

22. Rao LV. Tissue factor as a tumor procoagulant. *Cancer Metastasis Rev* 1992;11: 249.

23. Gordon SG, Mielicki WP. Cancer procoagulants: a factor X activator, tumor marker and growth factor from malignant tissue. *Blood Coagul Fibrinolysis* 1997;8:73.

24. Gordon SG, Franks JJ, Lewis B. Cancer procoagulant: a factor X activating procoagulant from malignant tissue. *Thromb Res* 1975;6:127.

25. Tun P. Heparin therapy in Russell's viper bite victims with disseminated intravascular coagulation: a controlled trial. *Southeast Asian J Trop Med Public Health* 1992;23: 282.

26. Leclerc F, Hazelzet J, Jude B, et al. Protein C and S deficiency in severe infectious purpura of children: a collaborative study of 40 cases. *Intensive Care Med* 1992;18:202–5.

27. Leung L, Mannucci PM. Clinical features, diagnosis, and treatment of disseminated intravascular coagulation in adults. *Uptodate*. Updated April 2, 2012. Accessed Sept 1, 2012. http://www.uptodate.com/contents/clinical-features-diagnosis-and-treatment-of-disseminated-intravascular-coagulation-in-adults?source=search_result&search=DIC&selectedTitle=1%7E150.

28. Bakhtiari K, Meijers JCM, de Jonge E, Levi M. Prospective validation of the International Society of Thrombosis and Haemostasis scoring system for disseminated intravascular coagulation. *Crit Care Med* 2004;32:2416.

29. Toh CH, Hoots WK. The scoring system of the Scientific and Standardisation Committee on Disseminated Intravascular Coagulation of the International Society on Thrombosis and Haemostasis: a 5-year overview. *J Thromb Hemost* 2007;5: 604–6.

30. Levi M, Toh CH, Thachil J, Watson HG. Guidelines for the diagnosis and management of disseminated intravascular coagulation. *Br J Hematol* 2009;145:24–33.

31. Hauser CJ, Boffard K, Dutton R, et al. Results of the CONTROL Trial: efficacy and safety of recombinant activated factor VII in the management of refractory traumatic hemorrhage. *J Trauma* 2010;69:489–500.

32. Franchini M, Manzato F, Salvagno GL, Lippi G. Potential role of recombinant activated factor VII for the treatment of severe bleeding associated with disseminated intravascular coagulation: a systematic review. *Blood Coagul Fibrinolysis* 2007;18:589.

33. O'Connell KA, Wood JJ, Wise RP, Lozier JN, Braun MM. Thromboembolic adverse events after use of recombinant human coagulation factor VIIa. *JAMA* 2006; 295:293–8.

34. Levi M, Levy J, Anderson H, Truloff D. Safety of recombinant activated factor VII in randomized clinical trials. *N Engl J Med* 2010;363:1791–800.

35. Warren BL, Eid A, Singer P, et al. Caring for the critically ill patient. High dose antithrombin III in severe sepsis: a randomized controlled trial. *JAMA* 2001;286: 1869–78.

36. Bernard GR, Vincent JL, Laterre PF, et al. Efficacy and safety of recombinant human activated protein C for severe sepsis. Recombinant Human Activated Protein C Worldwide Evaluation in Severe Sepsis (PROWESS) Study Group. *N Eng J Med* 2001;344:699–709.

37. Ranieri VM, Thompson BT, Barie PS, et al. Drotrecogin Alfa (Activated) in adults with septic shock. *N Eng J Med* 2012;366:2055–64.

38. Poole D, Bertolini G, Garattini. Withdrawal of "Xigris" from the market: old and new lessons. *J Epidemiol Community Health* 2012;66:571–2.

39. Hook KM, Abrams CS. The loss of homeostasis in hemostasis: new approaches in treating and understanding acute disseminated intravascular coagulation in critically ill patients. *Clin Trans Sci* 2012;5:85–92.

40. Abraham E, Reinhart K, Opal S, et al. Efficacy and safety of tifacogin (recombinant tissue factor pathway inhibitor) in severe sepsis. *JAMA* 2003;290:238–247.

41. Mannucci PM, Levi M. Prevention and treatment of major blood loss. *N Eng J Med* 2007;356:2301–11.

42. Ker K, Kiriya J, Perel P, et al. Avoidable mortality from giving tranexamic acid to bleeding trauma patients: an estimation based on WHO mortality data, a systemic literature review and data from the CRASH-2 trial. *BMC Emerg Med* 2012;12:3.

43. Roberts I, Prieto-Merino D, Shakur H, et al. Effect of consent rituals on mortality in emergency care research. *Lancet* 2011;377:1071–2.

44. Ngo CV, Picha K, McCabe F, et al. CNTO 859, a humanized anti-tissue factor monoclonal antibody, is a potent inhibitor of breast cancer metastasis and tumor growth in xenograft models. *Int J Cancer* 2007;120:1261–7.

45. Mukundan S, Zeigler ZR. Direct antithrombin agents ameliorate disseminated intravascular coagulation in suspected heparin-induced thrombocytopenia thrombosis syndrome. *Clin Appl Thromb Hemost* 2002;8:287–9.

46. Blommel ML, Blommel AL. Dabigatran etexilate: a novel oral direct thrombin inhibitor. *Am J Health Syst Pharm* 2011;68:1506–19.

47. Turpie AG, Kreutz R, Llau J, et al. Management consensus guidance for the use of rivaroxaban: an oral, direct factor Xa inhibitor. *Thromb Haemost* 2012;108: 876–86.
48. Sharma T, Mehta P, Gajra A. Update on fondaparinux: role in management of thromboembolic and acute coronary events. *Cardiovasc Hematol Agents Med Chem* 2010;8:96–103.
49. Kitchens CS. Thrombocytopenia and thrombosis in disseminated intravascular coagulation (DIC). *Hematology Am Soc Hematol Educ Program* 2009;240–6.

CHAPTER 13

Mechanisms of Fibrinolysis and Basic Principles of Management

John W. Weisel and Rustem I. Litvinov

Department of Cell and Developmental Biology, University of Pennsylvania Perelman School of Medicine, Philadelphia, PA, USA

Biochemical process of fibrinolysis and its regulation

After a clot or thrombus is formed, it is normally dissolved by the fibrinolytic system [1,2]. The central enzyme in fibrin lysis is plasmin (Pn), a serine protease derived from its inactive precursor, plasminogen (Plg), by the action of activators. Pn also cleaves a variety of other substrates including extracellular matrix proteins, and activates other proteases and growth factors. As a result, in addition to fibrinolysis, Plg and Pn are involved in a number of other physiologic and pathophysiologic processes such as cell migration, wound healing, inflammation, embryogenesis, ovulation, angiogenesis, tumor growth and metastasis, and atherosclerosis.

Fibrinolysis occurs first by the conversion of Plg to Pn by a Plg activator, primarily on fibrin, and then by the degradation of fibrin by Pn. Any Pn that comes off fibrin is rapidly inactivated by inhibitors. Attachment of Plg and tissue-type plasminogen activator (t-PA) to a clot is mediated by the C-terminal lysine residues on fibrin and the specific lysine-binding sites on the Plg and t-PA molecules.

There is a complex system of biochemical reactions comprising fibrinolysis and its regulatory mechanisms (Figure 13.1). Most Pn activity is generated on the fibrin fibers after formation of the ternary complex of fibrin, t-PA, and Plg. Because Pn cleaves at lysine residues, the new C-terminal lysines become exposed and provide additional binding sites for Plg and t-PA, as a positive feedback mechanism. As a consequence, the fibrin network is degraded to soluble fibrin degradation products (FDP).

There are a number of mechanisms to moderate the activity of the primary profibrinolytic components, such as Plg activator inhibitor-1

Hemostasis and Thrombosis: Practical Guidelines in Clinical Management, First Edition.
Hussain I. Saba and Harold R. Roberts.
© 2014 John Wiley & Sons, Ltd. Published 2014 by John Wiley & Sons, Ltd.

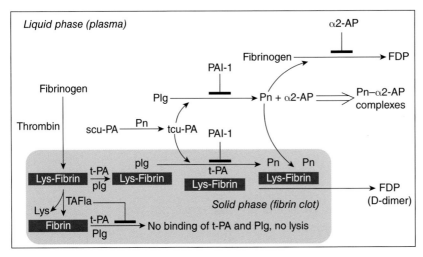

Figure 13.1 Schematic representation of the major reactions of fibrinolysis and their regulation on a fibrin clot surface and in the surrounding plasma milieu. The highlighted area represents a fibrin clot surface (solid phase) surrounded by the blood plasma (liquid phase). Black arrows show the biochemical conversions involving proteolytic cleavage. *T*-like symbols indicate inhibitory effects. Lys-Fibrin, C-terminal lysine residues on fibrin to which Plg and t-PA bind selectively; Plg, plasminogen, bound to the C-terminal lysine residues on fibrin and free in plasma; Pn, plasmin, formed on fibrin (by the action of t-PA) and in plasma (by the action of tcu-PA) from Plg. Pn cleaves fibrin and fibrinogen, activates scu-PA and TAFI (not shown); t-PA, tissue-type Plg activator, fibrin selective Plg activator, bound to fibrin via the C-terminal lysine residues on fibrin; scu-PA, single-chain urokinase-type Plg activator (inactive); tcu-PA, two-chain uPA (active), non-fibrin-selective Plg activator; PAI-1, plasminogen activator inhibitor-1, blocks both t-PA and tcu-PA; TAFIa, thrombin-activatable fibrinolysis inhibitor (enzymatically active form) that splits off the C-terminal lysine residues from fibrin, thus preventing binding of Plg and t-PA to fibrin; α_2-AP, α_2-antiplasmin, direct Pn inhibitor, forms circulating Pn–α_2-AP complexes; FDP, fibrin(ogen) degradation products, resulting from cleavage of fibrin or fibrinogen by Pn; D-dimer, a proteolytic fragment (degradation product) that is formed by Pn only from cross-linked fibrin.

(PAI-1), a potent inhibitor of t-PA and u-PA, and α_2-antiplasmin (α_2-AP), which directly inhibits Pn (Figure 13.1). A thrombin-activatable fibrinolysis inhibitor (TAFI or TAFIa after activation) cleaves C-terminal lysine residues from partially degraded fibrin and thus inhibits fibrinolysis by preventing the lysine-dependent binding of Plg on fibrin. Lipoprotein(a) [Lp(a)] has a structural homology with Plg and, therefore, may compete with Plg for binding to lysine residues and impair fibrinolysis [3].

Plasminogen and plasmin

Plasminogen (Plg) is a 92-kDa glycoprotein in blood plasma at a concentration of about 0.2 mg/mL (2 μM) [4]. Native human Plg, called Glu-Plg because it has glutamate at the N-terminus, comprises the N-terminal ("preactivation") peptide (residues Glu1–Lys77), five homologous kringle domains (K1-K5), and the catalytic protease domain (residues Val562-Asn791). The kringle domains mediate Plg binding to various substrates, cofactors, and receptors, including fibrin(ogen). Kringles 1 and 4 exhibit the strongest affinities for lysine residues, physiologically relevant for binding to fibrin, to extracellular matrix components, and to cells. The conversion of inactive Plg to proteolytically active plasmin (Pn) involves cleavage of the Arg561-Val562 bond near kringle 5. Another reaction concomitant with Plg activation is the Pn-catalyzed cleavage at Lys62, Arg68, or Lys77 residues, which yields the truncated forms, referred to as Lys-Plg. Native Glu-Pg is a compact molecule with intramolecular interactions between the N-terminal and the C-terminal region, arranged in a spiral-type conformation [5], and Glu-Plg to Lys-Plg conversion results in transition from compact to an extended open conformation, which becomes more readily activated [6]. Because of improved fibrin binding and activation of Lys-Plg compared to Glu-Plg, the formation of Lys-Plg within a clot is a positive feedback mechanism that can further stimulate the activation of Plg by t-PA.

Plasminogen activators

The activators of plasminogen (Plg) are the serine proteases t-PA or u-PA and bacterial proteins that acquire proteolytic activity after the interaction with human Plg or Pn, streptokinase (SK), and staphylokinase (SAK). t-PA and SAK are fibrin-selective, remaining bound to fibrin and protected from rapid inhibition, while SK and two-chain u-PA are non-fibrin-selective enzymes, activating both Plg in the circulating blood and fibrin-bound Plg.

Tissue-type Plg activator

Tissue-type Plg activator (t-PA) is a 70-kDa glycoprotein with a circulating level in plasma of about 5 ng/mL (70 pM) [4]. It consists of finger, epidermal growth factor-like, two kringle, and C-terminal trypsin-like catalytic domains. The single-chain t-PA (sct-PA) can be converted to the two-chain form (tct-PA) by Pn-catalyzed cleavage, but the single-chain form itself exhibits considerable catalytic activity. Both sct-PA and tct-PA act by forming a ternary complex with fibrin and Plg, undergoing conformational changes, and catalyze the conversion of Plg to active Pn by cleaving the Arg561-Val562 bond. Binding of t-PA to fibrin has been mainly localized to the finger and the kringle 2 domains, while in fibrin there are high-affinity Lys-dependent t-PA binding sites in the compact portion of fibrin(ogen) αC region and low-affinity Lys-independent t-PA binding sites located in the $\gamma 312$-324 region, all of which are cryptic in fibrinogen and become exposed in fibrin. Because t-PA and Plg bind to the same sets of sites, the zymogen and its activator are brought into close proximity, which results in efficient local generation of Pn.

Urokinase-type Plg activator

Urokinase-type Plg activator (u-PA) is a 53-kDa glycoprotein, with concentrations in plasma of 2–4 ng/mL [7], and it is also found in urine. The single-chain inactive form (pro-u-PA or scu-PA) is converted to a two-chain active enzyme (tcu-PA) by Pn and other proteases. tcu-PA activates both circulating and fibrin-bound Plg by cleaving the Arg561-Val562 bond with a similar rate [8]. u-PA consists of an amino-terminal growth factor domain, a kringle domain, and a C-terminal serine protease domain.

Streptokinase

Streptokinase (SK) is a 47 kDa protein produced by various strains of β-hemolytic *Streptococci*. Unlike u-PA and t-PA, which possess proteolytic activity themselves, SK is not an enzyme but acquires the ability to activate human Plg indirectly by forming a 1:1 complex with Plg or Pn, in which the zymogen catalytic site is activated non-proteolytically by an intramolecular cleavage of the Arg560-Val561 bond. The resultant activator complex is a highly specific enzyme, which binds free Plg and converts it into Pn by proteolytic cleavage. In addition, Pn cleaves the SK molecule, generating the N-terminal 59-residue fragment, which remains covalently attached to the rest of the molecule, precluding binding of the SK–Plg complex with fibrin [9].

Staphylokinase

Staphylokinase (SAK) is a 15.5-kDa protein produced by *Staphylococcus aureus* that does not possess enzymatic activity but forms a 1:1 complex with trace amounts of Pn on fibrin that activates other Plg molecules [10]. In plasma, in the absence of fibrin the trace amounts of free Pn and the Plg activator activity in the SAK–Pn complex are rapidly inhibited by α_2-AP, but in the presence of fibrin, generation of the active SAK–Pn complex is facilitated because the initial trace amounts of fibrin-bound Pn are protected from α_2-AP and inhibition of the complex at the clot surface is greatly delayed and Plg activation is enhanced.

Modulators of fibrinolysis

The effectiveness of fibrinolysis results from the combination of regulated enzymatic activity and the physical characteristics of the fibrin scaffold, such as the density of fibers and branch points, pore size, and fiber diameter. In general, the rate of lysis appears to be faster for clots made up of thicker fibers than for clots made up of thinner fibers, but this also depends on other biophysical properties of the clot [11]. In addition, platelet aggregation and clot retraction have dramatic effects on fibrinolysis [12]. Stretching also affects the rate of lysis of clots [13].

The fibrinolytic system is regulated by a number of proteins, either directly inhibiting proteolytic activity or modulating the substrate-binding interactions that affect specificity and activation/inactivation rates of the fibrinolytic enzymes.

Thrombin-activatable fibrinolysis inhibitor

Thrombin-activatable fibrinolysis inhibitor (TAFI) is a 60-kDa procarboxypeptidase that in the active form (TAFIa) becomes an effective regulator of fibrinolysis through removal of surface-exposed C-terminal lysine residues from degrading fibrin, thus eliminating Plg- and t-PA-binding sites. In addition, TAFIa eliminates Pn binding sites, shortening its half-life and slows down the conversion of Glu-Plg to Lys-Plg by Pn. The enzymatic activity of TAFIa is remarkably unstable, with a half-life of minutes. Thrombin is a relatively weak activator of TAFI, but in the presence of thrombomodulin the activation by thrombin is enhanced more than 1000-fold [14].

Plasminogen activator inhibitors 1 and 2

Plasminogen activator inhibitor 1 (PAI-1), a 50-kDa glycoprotein, which is the major inhibitor of u-PA and t-PA, belongs to the serpin (*serine protease inhibitor*) superfamily of proteins. Its normal plasma concentration is only about 0.4 nM [15], but in platelet-rich thrombi the local concentration of PAI-1 can be high due to its continuous synthesis in platelets, and it can be accumulated at the sites of vascular injury due to interactions with vitronectin, to protect the developing thrombus from premature lysis. Plasminogen activator inhibitor 2 (PAI-2) is a serpin that is thought to be a modulator of intracellular proteolytic events not related to fibrinolysis.

α₂-Antiplasmin

α_2-Antiplasmin (α_2-AP), or α_2-plasmin inhibitor, a 63-kDa serpin, is the primary physiologic inhibitor of Pn, circulating at a concentration of about 1 μM (70 μg/mL) [16]. It forms a very stable inactive Pn–α_2-AP complex, it can be covalently cross-linked to fibrin, making it more resistant to lysis, and it can competitively inhibit Plg interactions with fibrin due to the presence of exposed lysine residues.

Lipoprotein (a)

Lipoprotein (a) [Lp(a)] is a plasma lipoprotein similar in structure to low-density lipoprotein, in that it is composed of a core of apolar lipid enclosed in a predominantly phospholipid monolayer with associated glycoproteins. The apo(a) glycoprotein has a strong structural homology with Plg and it exists in several isoforms, containing from 12 to 51 Plg kringle 4-like units as well as a Plg kringle 5-like unit and an inactive protease region homologous to that in Plg [17]. Due to structural homology of the kringles, Lp(a) may interfere with Plg binding to lysine residues in fibrin and in cell receptors and, thereby, impair fibrinolysis and pericellular proteolysis.

α₂-Macroglobulin

α_2-Macroglobulin (α_2-MG) with a molecular weight of ~725 kDa is found in circulation at a concentration of about 3 μM (2.5 mg/mL) [18] and can bind to different proteases and their complexes with inhibitors. Under certain conditions Pn and Plg activators may react with α_2-MG followed by relatively slow inhibition of their activity. Cell- and fibrin-bound Pn is protected from α_2-MG.

Other modulators of fibrinolysis

Some other inhibitors, such as PAI-3 (protein C inhibitor), neuroserpin, histidine-rich glycoprotein, and protease nexin have been shown to have minor, local, and/or uncertain effects on the activity of components of human fibrinolytic system.

Cell surface "fibrinolytic" receptors

The Plg activation system appears to be widely involved in many physiologic and pathologic processes other than fibrinolysis via Pn generation on the cell surface. Therefore, there are many cellular binding sites or receptor molecules for Plg and its activators.

Plg receptors

Binding of Plg to cells is mediated by a heterogeneous population of Plg receptors. Interaction of Plg with the cell-surface binding sites accelerates conversion of Plg to Pn, enhances the catalytic activity of Pn itself, and protects bound Pn from inactivation by inhibitors. Plg receptors are present on platelets, monocytes, macrophages, neutrophils, endothelial cells, and some nonvascular cells [19].

u-PA receptor

The 55-kDa u-PA receptor (u-PAR) is essential for Plg activation on the cell surface, mediated by strong binding of its specific ligand, u-PA. The binding results in a strong enhancement of cell surface Plg activation, the effect being dependent on the simultaneous binding of pro-uPA to u-PAR and of Plg to its cell surface receptors. In addition to binding to u-PAR, u-PA can cleave intact three-domain u-PAR(I–III) molecules, releasing the ligand-binding domain I and leaving the cleaved form of u-PAR, uPAR(II–III), on the cell membrane. This cleavage inactivates the binding potential of u-PAR toward u-PA and vitronectin. PAI-1 can couple to u-PAR-bound uPA, inhibiting degradation of the extracellular matrix proteins initiated by cell-associated u-PA. The inhibitory effect of PAI-1 can be abrogated either by u-PA-induced cleavage and inactivation or by formation of a quaternary complex of (u-PAR)-(u-PA)-(PAI-1) with α_2-MG, which is then internalized and digested, while u-PAR is recycled to the cell surface [20].

t-PA receptors

Binding of t-PA along with Plg to cells can lead to accelerated Pn generation. Monocytes and monocytoid cells bind t-PA and are able to stimulate t-PA enzyme activity up to around 20-fold. The role of t-PA is mainly in fibrinolysis and that of u-PA in pericellular proteolysis, cell migration, adhesion, invasion, and other cell-related processes and functions.

Pathologic fibrinolysis

Although the process of fibrinolysis described above is an important protective mechanism aimed at recanalizing blood vessels, in vivo it may be excessive (hyperfibrinolysis) or insufficient (hypofibrinolysis), contributing to bleeding and thrombotic disorders and, thus, complicating many pathologic conditions of various etiology (Figure 13.2).

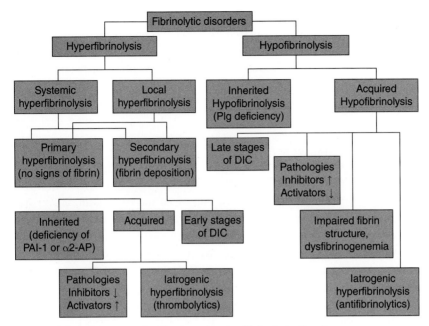

Figure 13.2 Pathogenetic classification of major fibrinolytic disorders.

Hyperfibrinolysis

Increased activation of the fibrinolytic system that causes and or sustains a bleeding tendency has been conditionally segregated into primary and secondary hyperfibrinolysis (frequently referred to as "primary and secondary fibrinolysis"). The term "primary fibrinolysis" implies excessive fibrinolytic activity generated without or with a minor apparent association with a hypercoagulable or thrombotic state, whereas "secondary fibrinolysis" designates a fibrinolytic response to intravascular thrombin generation and fibrin deposition. Because primary fibrinolysis is assumed to develop in the absence of fibrin and results in cleavage of fibrinogen, it can be termed "primary fibrinogenolysis."

Primary (hyper)fibrinolysis

Primary fibrinolysis can be caused by hereditary or acquired disorders. Inherited hyperfibrinolysis is rare and results mainly from a deficiency of α2-AP [21,22] or PAI-1 [23]. Acquired primary fibrinolysis is more common, but its mechanisms are not clear and may be determined by an underlying disease and depend on its pathogenesis. Chronic liver disease is known to be associated with fibrinolysis and its incidence correlates with disease severity [24]. In end-stage liver cirrhosis, which is often associated with mucocutaneous and gastrointestinal bleeding, the fibrinolytic system is strongly activated by an increased endothelial release and decreased hepatic clearance of t-PA, decreased activity of TAFIa, and decreased synthesis of α2-AP and PAI-1 [25–27]. There are alternative notions pointing at endotoxinemia or ascites fluid as the main source of hyperfibrinolysis in liver cirrhosis [28] that have been a matter of debate [29]. During orthotopic liver transplantation, the imbalanced fibrinolytic activity in underlying chronic liver disease is shifted toward hyperfibrinolysis mainly by high concentrations of t-PA released from graft liver endothelial cells perturbed by hypoxia and acidosis [30,31]. Other surgical procedures, such as cardiopulmonary bypass in cardiac surgery, may be followed by increased t-PA levels and hyperfibrinolysis [32]. Severe trauma is also accompanied by remarkable hyperfibrinolysis coincident with coagulopathy and bleeding, which has been attributed to primary fibrinolysis [33]. However, in massive tissue damage, fulminant disseminated intravascular coagulation (DIC) followed by hyperfibrinolysis is more likely [34]. Acute promyelocytic leukemia associated with life-threatening hemorrhage has been traditionally accounted for by excessive fibrinolysis associated with DIC. Yet, leukemic cells were found to express high levels of annexin II, a protein with high affinity for Plg and t-PA and a cofactor for Plg activation. These mechanisms may lead to enhanced generation of surface-bound α2-AP-protected Pn activity and play a role in exacerbating hyperfibrinolysis and bleeding independently of DIC [35]. In patients with benign prostatic hyperplasia, undergoing transurethral resection of the prostate, postoperative blood loss was shown to depend on local increase of the urinary fibrinolytic activity caused by u-PA highly expressed in prostatic tissues [36]. Increased levels of u-PA in blood in prostate cancer in association with postoperative bleeding have also been reported [37]. Systemic and local primary hyperfybrinolysis seems to contribute significantly to menorrhagia of various etiologies that are managed successfully by antifibrinolytic medications [38].

Secondary (hyper)fibrinolysis

The vast majority of acquired hyperfibrinolytic situations occur as a consequence of intravascular activation of the blood coagulation system and fibrin formation. Clinically delayed bleeding after primary hemostasis or a thrombotic event is typical for secondary hyperfibrinolysis. However, most often hypercoagulability and hyperfibrinolysis develop concurrently, which makes discrimination between primary and secondary fibrinolysis difficult. Intravascular activation of the coagulation system ranges from a small subclinical hypercoagulability to severe thrombotic events. Accordingly, the compensatory fibrinolytic response should be proportional to the extent to which fibrin has spread in the vasculature. Local thrombosis usually does not affect significantly the overall fibrinolytic potential in blood, while pronounced systemic hyperfibrinolysis accompanies early stages of DIC, which is characterized by widespread microvascular fibrin deposition, impairing blood supply to various tissues and causing multiple organ failure. DIC is a life-threatening syndrome, complicating a variety of disorders, most commonly severe infection or inflammation, trauma, burns, cancer, as well as many other diseases and pathologic states [39–42].

The initiation of massive thrombin generation in DIC is mediated by the tissue factor pathway. The source of tissue factor and the amount exposed to the blood depends on the underlying disease and extent of tissue injury and/or tissue factor expression on cells, such as monocytes and vascular endothelium, in response to cytokines and other pathologic stimuli. In DIC, in addition to strong tissue factor-induced procoagulant activity, all major anticoagulants, such as antithrombin III, the protein C system, and tissue factor pathway inhibitor, are markedly reduced due to consumption, impaired or downregulated synthesis, and proteolytic degradation. All these processes exaggerate diffuse obstruction of the microvascular bed, resulting in progressive organ dysfunction. The ongoing and diffuse activation of the coagulation system results also in depletion of procoagulants and platelets, which may cause severe bleeding, named consumption coagulopathy. Hyperfibrinolysis exacerbates the hemorrhage observed in DIC by breaking down fibrin and fibrinogen, and generating fibrin(ogen) degradation products (FDP) with remarkable anticoagulant and antiplatelet properties. FDP comprise fibrin(ogen) fragments with incomplete sets of binding sites that inhibit competitively fibrin polymerization and fibrin(ogen)-mediated platelet adhesion and aggregation. The fibrinolytic potential in DIC is determined mainly by the relative concentrations of t-PA and PAI-1, both of which increase significantly due to secretion and release from activated and or damaged vascular endothelial cells and platelets, as reflected by the elevated concentrations of the t-PA–PAI-1 complex [43]. Following a transient hyperfibrinolytic reaction, the fibrinolytic system in DIC is largely suppressed at the time of maximal activation of coagulation, leading to hypofibinolysis that aggravates intravascular fibrin deposition (see below).

Laboratory tests for (hyper)fibrinolysis

Laboratory assessment of the fibrinolytic system is performed in combination with methods to analyze coagulation and anticoagulant proteins as well as platelets. These laboratory tests help to examine bleeding tendency and confirm or rule out hyperfibrinolysis due to inherited deficiency of α2-AP and or PAI-1. The challenge of distinguishing between primary fibrinolysis and DIC can prove crucial for guiding appropriate treatment. In hypercoagulable and thrombotic states, the testing would assess fibrinolytic potential and, along with clinical judgment, would help in making an informed decision on patient management, including thrombolytic therapy. A modern comprehensive fibrinolysis panel includes the following tests: euglobulin lysis time, which is a modified plasma clot lysis time; thromboelastography and thromboelastometry; D-dimer, fibrinogen concentration and FDP, α2-AP activity, PAI-1, Plg, t-PA, u-PA (all activity and antigen), Pn–α2-AP complex, and TAFI (antigen). Some of the tests have become more or less routine (euglobulin lysis time, thromboelastography/thromboelastometry, D-dimer, fibrinogen, and FDP), while others are used mainly for research purposes and their interpretations and prognostic values have been a matter of discussion [44].

Euglobulin lysis time and thromboelastography are used first to reveal hyperfibrinolysis, since they detect increased Plg activation and subsequent accelerated fibrin clot lysis, but they miss the interactions between Plg, Plg activators, inhibitors, and fibrin that in aggregate determine increased Pn activity. Despite wide application, the use of thromboelastography and thromboelastometry provoke discussions regarding their effective utilization [45]. The FDP assay measures amounts of cleavage products of either fibrinogen or fibrin and therefore cannot discriminate between primary and secondary fibrinolysis. D-dimer is produced exclusively from cross-linked fibrin, which makes a high level of D-dimer with low fibrinogen level and platelet count in combination with prolonged PT and PTT indicative of DIC. However, for the diagnosis of DIC, time-dependent changes are necessary. A negative D-dimer test is most commonly used to rule out specific diagnoses.

Primary fibrin(ogen)olysis is likely when hemorrhage is associated with hypofibrinogenemia without an increase or with a disproportionally minor elevation of D-dimer in combination with normal or subnormal platelet count. Other common laboratory signs of primary and secondary hyperfibrinolysis include elevation of t-PA associated with a decrease of Plg and an increase of Pn–α2-AP complexes.

Treatment of (hyper)fibrinolysis

When severe bleeding is attributed to hyperfibrinolysis, the use of an antifibrinolyic agent may be appropriate to alleviate hemorrhage. The drugs used most frequently to reduce increased fibrinolytic activity are lysine analogs, ε-aminocaproic acid and tranexamic acid. They both act by binding to Plg and blocking the interaction of Plg and Pn with fibrin, thereby preventing Plg activation and dissolution of the fibrin clot.

Until recently, a powerful antiplasmin agent, aprotinin, was used extensively over many years during surgical procedures, most often in orthotopic liver transplantation. After a 2008 trial in patients undergoing coronary artery bypass grafting showed a significantly higher mortality rate in the group that received aprotinin [46], this medication was withdrawn from the market by the US Food and Drug Administration. A recent retrospective analysis has confirmed aprotinin's efficacy in preventing blood loss during liver transplantation [47]. In February 2012, the European Medicines Agency found that the benefits of aprotinin in preventing blood loss outweigh its risks in patients undergoing isolated heart bypass surgery and recommended lifting the suspension of aprotinin for this group of patients in the European Union.

It is noteworthy that the benefits of reduction of bleeding associated with the use of antifibrinolytics go together with the potential risk of hypofibrinolysis and thrombotic complications. Therefore, administration of antifibrinolytics must be carefully correlated with other therapies, especially with replacement with whole blood and its components. Needless to say, elimination of the primary cause of a hemostatic disorder must be a strategic priority.

Hypofibrinolysis

Reduction of fibrinolytic activity has been associated with various thrombotic disorders or thrombophilia, accompanying diabetes and insulin resistance, coronary artery disease, ischemic stroke, venous thromboembolism (deep vein thrombosis/pulmonary embolism), preeclampsia, etc. Established mechanisms of fibrinolysis impairment include inherited dysfunction and deficiency of Plg, increased levels of PAI-1, α2-AP or impaired release of t-PA or u-PA [48,49], as well as low TAFIa levels [50]. In addition, delayed fibrinolysis is correlated with abnormal structure and increased stiffness of fibrin clots in patients with premature coronary atherothrombosis [51]. Some dysfibrinogenemias can cause delayed fibrinolysis, resulting in thrombosis [52]. Profound suppression of fibrinolysis is associated with later stages of DIC, and, at the time of maximal activation of coagulation, the fibrinolytic system is largely inactive because of a sustained increase in plasma levels of PAI-1 [53]. During DIC in sepsis, fibrinolysis is attenuated by formation of Pn–α2-AP complexes and blockage of Plg activators, both t-PA and u-PA, by PAI-1 released from endothelial cells and perhaps platelets in response to TNF-α and endotoxin [54]. Suppression of fibrinolysis in sepsis is also augmented by thrombin-induced activation of TAFI [55]. Strongly elevated PAI-1 levels in patients with severe sepsis is a negative prognostic sign [56]. Infusion of exogenous fibrinolytic medications may be the only way to overcome hypo- or afibrinolysis and restore the potential of effective dissolution of obstructive thrombi, of course in combination with all means to abolish the origin of the disorder.

Thrombolytic therapy

Therapeutic thrombolysis or thrombolytic therapy, the dissolution of thrombi by the delivery of exogenous Plg activators into the circulation, such as those listed below, is a common treatment for acute myocardial infarction and stroke [57,58].

Alteplase, reteplase, duteplase, tenecteplase, lanoteplase, monteplase, and pamiteplase

Recombinant t-PA, rt-PA, alteplase (Activase®), is almost identical to wild-type t-PA [59]. During standard thrombolytic therapy, plasma concentrations of about 4000 ng/mL are achieved, an almost 1000-fold increase over physiologic values. Reteplase (Retavase®, Rapilysin®) is a single-chain non-glycosylated deletion mutant of rt-PA consisting only of the kringle 2 and the catalytic domain that has a similar plasminogenolytic activity as wild-type rt-PA, but its binding to fibrin is fivefold lower. Duteplase is a double-chain rt-PA analog and it has been studied in myocardial infarction. Tenecteplase (TNK-rt-PA) is a mutated variant of rt-PA such that deletion of a glycosylation site results in a longer half-life and increases the resistance to PAI-1, while maintaining the fibrin-binding properties. Lanoteplase (n-PA) is a deletion and single Asn117→Gln point mutation variant of rt-PA lacking the finger region and the epidermal growth factor domain, with an increased plasma half-life compared to alteplase. Monteplase is a mutant of tPA that has a prolonged biologic half-life. Pamiteplase is a t-PA mutant that produces a longer half-life and improved fibrin binding.

Streptokinase and anistreplase

Streptokinase (SK), the first enzyme to be used as a thrombolytic agent, is low in cost, but may cause immunologic complications and produces generalized proteolysis with an associated bleeding tendency. Anistreplase or acylated Plg-SK activator complex is a derivative of SK that has a longer plasma half-life.

Urokinase and saruplase

The active form of u-PA (tcu-PA), now produced recombinantly, is used as a thrombolytic agent, as is the recombinant pro-urokinase or scu-PA (saruplase).

Desmoteplase

Desmoteplase is a Plg activator originally from the saliva of the vampire bat *Desmodus rotundus* that lacks the second kringle site and the Pn-sensitive cleavage site of t-PA, and is extremely fibrin-dependent and fibrin-specific.

Plasmin
Plasmin and a truncated form microplasmin, are being considered as direct thrombolytic agents.

Staphylokinase
Recombinant staphylokinase (SAK) has been shown to be more fibrin-specific than rt-PA in patients with evolving myocardial infarction but can induce an immune reaction.

Substances that stimulate release of endogenous t-PA
A promising aspect of thromboprophylaxis and therapeutic thrombolysis is the use of substances that stimulate release of endogenous t-PA, such as a derivative of vasopressin (desmopressin), some acylated dipeptides, and a pyrimidine derivative.

References

1. Greenberg CS, Lai T-S, Ariens RAS, Weisel JW, Grant PJ. *Biology and disorders of fibrinogen and factor XIII.* In: Handin RI, Lux SE, Stossel TP (eds), *Blood Principles and Practice of Hematology*, 2nd edition. Philadelphia: Lippincott Williams & Wilkins, 2003;1225–48.
2. Weisel JW. Fibrinogen and fibrin. *Adv Protein Chem* 2005;70:247–99.
3. Angles-Cano E, de la Pena Diaz A, Loyau S. Inhibition of fibrinolysis by lipoprotein(a). *Ann N Y Acad Sci* 2001;936:261–75.
4. Booth NA, Bennett B. Fibrinolysis and thrombosis. *Baillieres Clin Haematol* 1994;7:559–72.
5. Weisel JW, Nagaswami C, Korsholm B, et al. Interactions of plasminogen and polymerizing fibrin and its derivatives monitored with a photoaffinity cross-linker and electron microscopy. *J Mol Biol* 1994;235:1117–35.
6. Fredenburgh JC, Nesheim ME. Lys-plasminogen is a significant intermediate in the activation of glu-plasminogen during fibrinolysis in vitro. *J Biol Chem* 1992;267: 26150–6.
7. Darras V, Thienpont M, Stump DC, Collen D. Measurement of urokinase-type plasminogen activator (u-PA) with an enzyme-linked immunosorbent assay (ELISA) based on three murine monoclonal antibodies. *Thromb Haemost* 1986;56:411–14.
8. Fears R. Binding of plasminogen activators to fibrin: characterization and pharmacological consequences. *Biochem J* 1989;261:313–24.
9. Reed GL, Houng AK. The contribution of activated factor XIII to fibrinolytic resistance in experimental pulmonary embolism. *Circulation* 1999;99:299–304.
10. Lijnen HR, Van Hoef B, De Cock F, et al. On the mechanism of fibrin-specific plasminogen activation by staphylokinase. *J Biol Chem* 1991;266:11826–32.
11. Weisel JW. Structure of fibrin: impact on clot stability. *J Thromb Haemost* 2007;5(suppl 1):116–24.
12. Collet J-P, Montalescot G, Lesty C, Weisel JW. A structural and dynamic investigation of the facilitating effect of glycoportein IIb/IIIa inhibitors in dissolving platelet-rich clots. *Circ Res* 2002;90:428–34.

13. Varju I, Sotonyi P, Machovich R, et al. Hindered dissolution of fibrin formed under mechanical stress. *J Thromb Haemost* 2011;9:979–86.
14. Heylen E, Willemse J, Hendriks D. An update on the role of carboxypeptidase U (TAFIa) in fibrinolysis. *Front Biosci* 2011;17:2427–50.
15. Fay WP, Murphy JG, Owen WG. High concentrations of active plasminogen activator inhibitor-1 in porcine coronary artery thrombi. *Arterioscler Thromb Vasc Biol* 1996;16:1277–84.
16. Collen D, Wiman B. Turnover of antiplasmin, the fast-acting plasmin inhibitor of plasma. *Blood* 1979;53:313–24.
17. Weisel JW, Nagaswami C, Woodhead JL, et al. The structure of lipoprotein(a) and ligand-induced conformational changes. *Biochemistry* 2001;40:10424–35.
18. Sottrup-Jensen L. Alpha-macroglobulins: structure, shape, and mechanism of proteinase complex formation. *J Biol Chem* 1989;264:11539–42.
19. Plow EF, Herren T, Redlitz A, Miles LA, Hoover-Plow JL. The cell biology of the plasminogen system. *Faseb J* 1995;9:939–45.
20. Del Rosso M, Margheri F, Serrati S, et al. *Curr Pharm Des* 2011;17:1924–43.
21. Aoki N. Discovery of alpha2-plasmin inhibitor and its congenital deficiency. *J Thromb Haemost* 2005;3:623–31.
22. Carpenter SL, Mathew P. Alpha2-antiplasmin and its deficiency: fibrinolysis out of balance. *Haemophilia* 2008;14:1250–4.
23. Iwaki T, Tanaka A, Miyawaki Y, et al. Life-threatening hemorrhage and prolonged wound healing are remarkable phenotypes manifested by complete plasminogen activator inhibitor-1 deficiency in humans. *J Thromb Haemost* 2011;9:1200–6.
24. Bennani-Baiti N, Daw HA. Primary hyperfibrinolysis in liver disease: a critical review. *Clin Adv Hematol Oncol* 2011;9:250–2.
25. Leebeek FW, Kluft C, Knot EA, et al. A shift in balance between profibrinolytic and antifibrinolytic factors causes enhanced fibrinolysis in cirrhosis. *Gastroenterology* 1991;101:1382–90.
26. Hu KQ, Yu AS, Tiyyagura L, et al. Hyperfibrinolytic activity in hospitalized cirrhotic patients in a referral liver unit. *Am J Gastroenterol* 2001;96:1581–6.
27. Ferro D, Celestini A, Violi F. Hyperfibrinolysis in liver disease. *Clin Liver Dis* 2009;13:21–31.
28. Agarwal S, Joyner KA, Jr., Swaim MW. Ascites fluid as a possible origin for hyperfibrinolysis in advanced liver disease. *Am J Gastroenterol* 2000;95:3218–24.
29. Piscaglia F, Donati G, Giannini R, Bolondi L. Liver cirrhosis, ascites, and hyperfibrinolysis. *Am J Gastroenterol* 2001;96:3222.
30. Porte RJ, Bontempo FA, Knot EA, et al. Systemic effects of tissue plasminogen activator-associated fibrinolysis and its relation to thrombin generation in orthotopic liver transplantation. *Transplantation* 1989;47:978–84.
31. Segal HC, Hunt BJ, Cottam S, et al. Fibrinolytic activity during orthotopic liver transplantation with and without aprotinin. *Transplantation* 1994;58:1356–60.
32. Vanek T, Jares M, Snircova J, Maly M. Fibrinolysis in coronary artery surgery: detection by thromboelastography. *Interact Cardiovasc Thorac Surg* 2007;6:700–4.
33. Kashuk JL, Moore EE, Sawyer M, et al. Primary fibrinolysis is integral in the pathogenesis of the acute coagulopathy of trauma. *Ann Surg* 2010;252:434–42; discussion 43–4.
34. Hayakawa M, Sawamura A, Gando S, et al. Disseminated intravascular coagulation at an early phase of trauma is associated with consumption coagulopathy and excessive fibrinolysis both by plasmin and neutrophil elastase. *Surgery* 2011;149:221–30.

35. Stein E, McMahon B, Kwaan H, et al. The coagulopathy of acute promyelocytic leukaemia revisited. *Best Pract Res Clin Haematol* 2009;22:153–63.
36. Nielsen JD, Gram J, Holm-Nielsen A, et al. Post-operative blood loss after transurethral prostatectomy is dependent on in situ fibrinolysis. *Br J Urol* 1997;80:889–93.
37. Kohli M, Kaushal V, Mehta P. Role of coagulation and fibrinolytic system in prostate cancer. *Semin Thromb Hemost* 2003;29:301–8.
38. Gleeson NC. Cyclic changes in endometrial tissue plasminogen activator and plasminogen activator inhibitor type 1 in women with normal menstruation and essential menorrhagia. *Am J Obstet Gynecol* 1994;171:178–83.
39. Slofstra SH, Spek CA, ten Cate H. Disseminated intravascular coagulation. *Hematol J* 2003;4:295–302.
40. Levi M. Disseminated intravascular coagulation: What's new? *Crit Care Clin* 2005;21:449–67.
41. Levi M. Disseminated intravascular coagulation. *Crit Care Med* 2007;35:2191–5.
42. Lippi G, Ippolito L, Cervellin G. Disseminated intravascular coagulation in burn injury. *Semin Thromb Hemost* 2010;36:429–36.
43. Fukao H, Ueshima S, Okada K, et al. Tissue-type plasminogen activator, type 1 plasminogen activator inhibitor and their complex in plasma with disseminated intravascular coagulation. *Thromb Res* 1992;68:57–65.
44. Gorog DA. Prognostic value of plasma fibrinolysis activation markers in cardiovascular disease. *J Am Coll Cardiol* 2010;55:2701–9.
45. Bluth MH, Kashuk JL. Whole blood thromboelastometry: another Knight at the Roundtable? *Crit Care* 2011;15:1021.
46. Fergusson DA, Hebert PC, Mazer CD, et al. A comparison of aprotinin and lysine analogues in high-risk cardiac surgery. *N Engl J Med* 2008;358:2319–31.
47. Trzebicki J, Kosieradzki M, Flakiewicz E, et al. Detrimental effect of aprotinin ban on amount of blood loss during liver transplantation: single-center experience. *Transplant Proc* 2011;43:1725–7.
48. Lau HK, Teitel JM, Cheung T, et al. Hypofibrinolysis in patients with hypercoagulability: the roles of urokinase and of plasminogen activator inhibitor. *Am J Hematol* 1993;44:260–5.
49. Schuster V, Hugle B, Tefs K. Plasminogen deficiency. *J Thromb Haemost* 2007;5:2315–22.
50. Meltzer ME, Doggen CJ, de Groot PG, et al. Low thrombin activatable fibrinolysis inhibitor activity levels are associated with an increased risk of a first myocardial infarction in men. *Haematologica* 2009;94:811–18.
51. Collet JP, Allali Y, Lesty C, et al. Altered fibrin architecture is associated with hypofibrinolysis and premature coronary atherothrombosis. *Arterioscler Thromb Vasc Biol* 2006;26:2567–73.
52. Soria J, Soria C, Caen P. A new type of congenital dysfibrinogenaemia with defective fibrin lysis: Dusard syndrome: possible relation to thrombosis. *Br J Haematol* 1983;53:575–86.
53. Deitch EA. Animal models of sepsis and shock: a review and lessons learned. *Shock* 1998;9:1–11.
54. Hack CE. Fibrinolysis in disseminated intravascular coagulation. *Semin Thromb Hemost* 2001;27:633–8.
55. Zeerleder S, Schroeder V, Hack CE, et al. TAFI and PAI-1 levels in human sepsis. *Thromb Res* 2006;118:205–12.
56. Raaphorst J, Johan Groeneveld AB, Bossink AW, Hack CE. Early inhibition of activated fibrinolysis predicts microbial infection, shock and mortality in febrile medical patients. *Thromb Haemost* 2001;86:543–9.

57. Kiernan TJ, Gersh BJ. Thrombolysis in acute myocardial infarction: current status. *Med Clin North Am* 2007;91:617–37; x.

58. Meretoja A, Tatlisumak T. Thrombolytic therapy in acute ischemic stroke: basic concepts. *Curr Vasc Pharmacol* 2006;4:31–44.

59. Bell WR. Present-day thrombolytic therapy: therapeutic agents: pharmacokinetics and pharmacodynamics. *Rev Cardiovasc Med* 2002;3(suppl 2):S34–44.

CHAPTER 14

Post-thrombotic Syndrome

Jean-Philippe Galanaud[1] and Susan R. Kahn[2]

[1]Department of Internal Medicine, Montpellier University Hospital, Montpellier, France
[2]Division of Internal Medicine and Lady Davis Institute, Jewish General Hospital, Montreal QC, Canada

Definition and diagnosis of post-thrombotic syndrome

Post-thrombotic syndrome (PTS) refers to chronic clinical manifestations of venous insufficiency following a deep vein thrombosis (DVT). The spectrum of post-thrombotic manifestations is wide, ranging from minor signs and symptoms (e.g., slight pain and swelling, hyperpigmentation, venous ectasia) to severe manifestations such as venous claudication and leg ulcers [1]. The clinical picture of PTS is nonspecific and conditions other than DVT such as primary venous insufficiency, chronic congestive heart failure, or trauma may produce similar symptoms or signs in the lower extremities [2]. Post-thrombotic syndrome is termed a "syndrome" because its symptoms and clinical signs typically vary from one patient to another. It is not a static process and it can wax and wane over time.

Post-thrombotic syndrome is primarily diagnosed on clinical grounds. As initial pain and swelling associated with acute DVT may not resolve before 3 months or so, PTS should not be definitively diagnosed before this time [3].

Six different clinical scales have been used to define PTS in clinical trials, which limits comparison of results between studies [3]. In order to improve standardization of the diagnosis of PTS, international guidelines now recommend assessing PTS and grading its severity with the Villalta scale. The components of the Villalta scale and its scoring algorithm are shown in Table 14.1. This scale has proven inter-observer reliability and is responsive to clinical change [4,5]. However, this scale does not provide information about the anatomic distribution of the original DVT, whether there is

---

Hemostasis and Thrombosis: Practical Guidelines in Clinical Management, First Edition.
Hussain I. Saba and Harold R. Roberts.
© 2014 John Wiley & Sons, Ltd. Published 2014 by John Wiley & Sons, Ltd.

Table 14.1 Villalta scale for the assessment of post-thrombotic syndrome.

Symptoms, self-reported by patient	Clinical signs, assessed by clinician on examination of the leg
Heaviness	Pretibial edema
Pain	Skin induration
Cramps	Hyperpigmentation
Pruritus	Venous ectasia
Paresthesia	Redness
	Pain during calf compression
	Ulcer

Symptoms are self-rated by the patient and clinical signs are rated by the clinician as 0 (absent), 1 (mild), 2 (moderate), or 3 (severe), except ulcer, which is rated by the clinician as present or absent. All numeric points are summed to yield a total score: a score of 0–4 indicates the absence of PTS; 5–9, mild PTS; 10–14, moderate PTS; and ≥15 or the presence of an ulcer, severe PTS.

residual thrombosis with obstruction or reflux on ultrasonographic exploration, and the presence of healed ulcer is not considered independently of the six clinical signs that are assessed as part of the scale. These important ancillary features are reported in the CEAP (clinical, etiologic, anatomic, pathophysiologic) classification that can be used for research purposes jointly with the Villalta scale for PTS evaluation [3,6].

Incidence

Post-thrombotic syndrome is the most frequent complication of DVT [2]. Estimates of the incidence of PTS vary across studies due to the utilization of different diagnostic approaches and definitions of PTS [7]. It is generally acknowledged that after a proximal DVT, even when adequate anticoagulation therapy is prescribed, 20–50% of patients will develop PTS and 5–10% will go on to severe PTS [1,8,9].

Most cases of PTS develop within 2 years of acute DVT [8,10–12]. However, two studies demonstrated a gradual increase in PTS incidence during the first 4 or 5 years after DVT [9,13] whereas another one found no further increase in the overall incidence of PTS after 1 year, but a gradual increase in PTS severity over time [14].

With regard to venous ulcer, its incidence usually ranges from 1 to 2% after 2–5 years of follow-up [8,9,12,15]. Ulceration has been observed in approximately 2–10% of patients up to 10 years after DVT, with a gradual increase in incidence over time [16,17].

Pathophysiology

The pathophysiology of PTS still remains unclear. Its development after DVT is believed to be the consequence of venous hypertension which leads to impaired venous return, reduced calf muscle perfusion, and abnormal function of the microvasculature with increased tissue permeability, which together pave the way for the characteristic clinical manifestations of PTS. Two main mechanisms are thought to be associated with PTS: persistent (residual) venous obstruction and valvular reflux [2]. After acute DVT, residual venous thrombosis persists in many patients [17]. Indeed, standard anticoagulant treatment of DVT prevents thrombus extension and embolization to pulmonary arteries but does not lyse the thrombus. Valvular reflux, reflecting damages to venous valves, is also frequent after DVT. Reflux could be the consequence of thrombus-induced activation of inflammation, fibrous scarring associated with acute and resolving thrombosis, or venous dilation distal to the obstructed venous segment [2] (Figure 14.1).

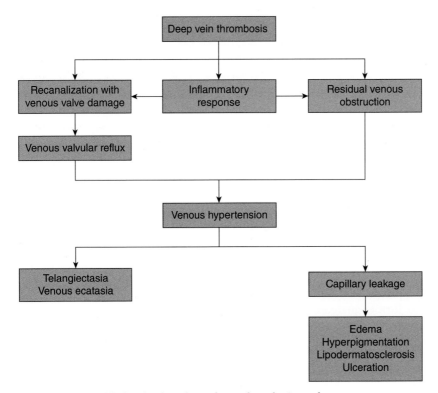

Figure 14.1 Simplified pathophysiology of post-thrombotic syndrome.

Risk factors for post-thrombotic syndrome

A number of clinical, biologic, and ultrasonographic risk factors for PTS have been identified. Among these, proximal location of initial DVT (e.g., iliofemoral) and a history of previous ipsilateral DVT appear to be the strongest and most unquestionable ones [1,2,8,15,18–21].

Numerous other risk factors have been inconsistently reported, and their association with PTS is probably milder, e.g., older age [9,16,18], higher body mass index [8,9,21], varicose veins [11,19], persistence of leg symptoms and signs at 1 month after DVT [8], elevated D-dimer early after DVT or after anticoagulant withdrawal, and elevated markers of inflammation (intracellular adhesion molecule 1, interleukin-6, and C-reactive protein) [2].

Conversely, the risk of PTS does not appear to be influenced by inherited thrombophilia (factor V Leiden or the prothrombin mutation) or by the circumstances of the initial DVT (i.e., unprovoked vs result of reversible risk factors vs cancer related) [2]. Although ipsilateral DVT recurrence was found to increase the risk of developing PTS, duration of anticoagulation in itself had no effect on risk of PTS [12,15,16]. However, the quality of anticoagulant treatment could play an important role, as one study found that patients with DVT who had subtherapeutic international normalized ratios (INR) more than half of the time during the initial 3 months of treatment with vitamin K antagonists (VKA) had a threefold higher risk of developing PTS [9]. This finding has been confirmed in the REVERSE cohort [22] and underlines the importance of close INR monitoring after DVT to ensure an adequate intensity of oral anticoagulation.

Finally, the risk of PTS after isolated distal DVT, which represents up to half of all lower limb DVT, is relatively unstudied [23]. Recent data suggests that the risk could be only 30% lower than that of proximal DVT [19], but development of severe PTS may be less common [24].

Socioeconomic impact

Impact on quality of life

Post-thrombotic syndrome severely impacts the quality of life of affected individuals. In the VETO multicenter cohort study that recruited 357 patients with acute DVT, PTS was the principal determinant of health-related quality of life at 2 years' follow-up [25]. Patients with DVT who had not developed PTS could expect that, at 2 years, their quality of life would be similar to that of the general population. On the contrary, patients who developed PTS had generic quality of life scores that were similar to that reported for patients with arthritis, chronic lung disease, hearing impairment, or diabetes. In addition, general and disease-specific quality of life worsened significantly with increasing severity of PTS. Patients with severe PTS had generic quality of life scores that were comparable to published norms for persons with severe chronic diseases, such as angina, cancer, or congestive heart failure [25].

Economic burden

After DVT, PTS is not only the main determinant of quality of life, but also an important predictor of healthcare costs. Retrospective administrative claims database analyses as well as Markov modeling underlined the substantial impact of the development of PTS on medical costs [17]. However, there are also important indirect costs associated with lost productivity, loss of functional independence, and forced retirement that were not taken into account in those studies. In the cost analysis of the prospective VETO study conducted in Canada, medical and total costs associated with DVT during the 2 years after diagnosis were C$5,180 (95% CI $4344, $6017), with a full 51.6% of costs being attributable to non-medical resource use [26]. Furthermore, medical and total costs of patients who developed PTS during follow-up were 35–45% higher than those of patients without PTS, and PTS was an important independent predictor of overall costs. These results suggest that use of measures to prevent PTS have the potential to substantially decrease overall costs of DVT.

In summary, PTS reduces quality of life of affected patients and significantly increases costs associated with DVT.

Therapeutic management of post-thrombotic syndrome

Prevention of post-thrombotic syndrome

In the absence of effective treatment, the cornerstones of management of PTS mainly rely on prevention of its occurrence through the prevention of DVT and the prevention of PTS after an episode of DVT.

Prevention of deep vein thrombosis

Hospitalization for acute medical illness is associated with an eightfold increased risk of venous thromboembolism (VTE) in the absence of thromboprophylaxis [27]. The risk of VTE is even greater in surgical patients. The risk of developing PTS after DVT may be significant even in case of asymptomatic DVT, which represents the majority of DVT in an inpatient setting: a meta-analysis of surgical patients reported that the risk of developing a PTS was 60% higher in those with asymptomatic DVT compared to patients without DVT (RR 1.6 [1.2–2.0]) [28,29]. In addition, data suggests low rates of adherence to recommended thromboprophylaxis strategies, especially in medical inpatients, which could be improved with a wider use of multi-component approaches, audit and feedback, and use of automatic reminders [27]. Appropriate use of thromboprophylaxis in high-risk patients has, therefore, the potential to decrease PTS incidence.

Therapeutic thromboprophylactic options available are the use of pharmacologic thromboprophylaxis with prophylactic doses of anticoagulants and mechanical thromboprophylaxis with graduated compression stockings and intermittent pneumatic compression [27].

Prevention of post-thrombotic syndrome after deep vein thrombosis

Even when appropriate thromboprophylaxis is used, the risk of DVT is not eliminated (reduced by ~50–60%) and one-half of VTE occur unpredictably [2,29]. After DVT, a number of treatments may be effective in preventing the development of PTS. Of note, the impact of such treatments on the risk of PTS after DVT has not been assessed.

Elastic compression stockings

Graduated elastic compression stockings (ECS) which reduce venous hypertension, decrease edema, and improve tissue microcirculation appear to prevent PTS [2]. In a meta-analysis of five randomized trials of compression stockings versus control published to date, Musani reported that venous compression, usually with below-knee ECS (91% of the 338 treated patients) reduced the average risk of overall PTS by 46% and severe PTS by 62% [30]. Although the authors concluded that venous compression seems indicated after DVT, they also underlined important differences in the design of analyzed studies, such as wide variation in type of stockings used, time interval from diagnosis to application of stockings, and duration of ECS treatment. Thus, the most recent ACCP guidelines suggest, rather than recommend, prescribing ECS for 2 years after DVT to prevent PTS (Grade 2B) [31]. An ongoing double-blind trial of active vs placebo ECS should provide important information on the value of using ECS after DVT [32].

When prescribing ECS to prevent PTS after DVT, Prandoni and colleagues recently reported that below-knee ECS were as effective as and better tolerated than thigh-length ECS [33]. Indeed, compliance is the Achilles heel of compression therapy and, in order to improve compliance, several strategies have been tested and showed promising results:
- Patient education: use of a health belief model may encourage patients to comply with recommendations to wear ECS [34];
- Individual tailored duration of ECS.

In a prospective management study 6 months after a proximal DVT, patients with a negative PTS assessment using the Villalta scale and no venous reflux on duplex testing, or patients with two consecutive negative PTS assessments from 6 months onward if reflux was present at 6 months were allowed to discontinue compression therapy [11]. At 2 years, the cumulative incidence of PTS with this management strategy was similar to that of the compression stockings arm of trials testing 2 or more years' use of ECS (29.6% vs 26%, respectively). Furthermore, this strategy allowed discontinuing compression therapy in 17% of patients at 6 months and in 48% at 1 year. The authors concluded that individualized tailored duration of ECS therapy based on Villalta clinical scores might be a safe management option, but that randomized trials of this strategy are needed.

Another therapeutic option which is currently under evaluation is to use lighter compression strength (20–30 mmHg) ECS, instead of the 30–40 mmHg ECS that are currently suggested.

Pharmacologic strategies to prevent PTS

By preventing DVT recurrence, a strong predictor of PTS, optimal and/or prolonged anticoagulant treatment has the potential to influence PTS occurrence. In one recent meta-analysis, treatment of DVT with low-molecular-weight heparin (LMWH) monotherapy compared with long-term treatment with VKA was reported to reduce the rate of self-reported leg ulcers by 87%, of signs and symptoms of PTS by 23%, and improved recanalization [35]. If confirmed, underlying mechanisms could be an anti-inflammatory effect of LMWH or more predictable quality of thera-peutic anticoagulation than VKA, thus preventing subclinical DVT recur-rence. This latter argument suggests that the new oral anticoagulants (e.g., direct thrombin inhibitors, Xa inhibitors) might be of interest to prevent PTS [17]; however, this has not been studied to date.

Endovascular strategies

Some studies, mainly patient series, have reported that systemic throm-bolytic therapy and catheter-directed thrombolysis (including mechanical thrombectomy with thrombus fragmentation and or aspiration) in patients with acute proximal DVT might prevent PTS by accelerating removal of thrombus and increasing venous patency [36]. The recent randomized controlled CaVenT Study, that compared additional catheter-directed thrombolysis to conventional treatment with anticoagulants and compres-sion stockings in patients with iliofemoral DVT, found that catheter-directed thrombolysis significantly reduced the rate of PTS at 2 years by 14.4% (incidence of PTS: 41.1% in catheter-directed thrombolysis group versus 55.6% in control group) [37]. However, because of the very low rate of severe PTS in the studied population (1/209), it was not possible to determine the impact of catheter-directed thrombolysis to prevent severe PTS; 3/101 patients experienced a major bleeding episode related to thrombolysis. In the absence of strong evidence to support the effectiveness, safety, and cost-effectiveness of these techniques, and pending the results of the ongoing multicenter ATTRACT Study (clinical trials ID NCT00790335), the latest ACCP guidelines suggest to not routinely use catheter-directed thrombolysis, systemic thrombolysis, or operative venous thrombectomy as a means of preventing PTS after acute proximal DVT [31].

Treatment of established post-thrombotic syndrome
Conservative treatment
Exercise training

Exercise training is an effective treatment for symptomatic arterial claudication. A recent pilot study of 39 patients with PTS conducted in two centers in Canada found that 6 months of intensive exercise training reduced the severity of PTS symptoms and signs and improved quality of life [38]. Potential underlying physiologic mechanisms could be improved endurance, reduced muscular effort from improved strength, reduced swelling and discomfort via improved function of the calf muscle pump, and improved musculoskeletal function via increased flexibility of ankle and knee joints. These promising results need to be confirmed by a larger study.

Compression therapy

In routine clinical practice, use of compression stockings from morning to bedtime and frequent leg elevation constitute the cornerstones of managing established PTS, although this management regimen has not to date been validated by a clinical trial [2,31]. A recent systematic review found only low-quality evidence in favor of a true and sustained benefit of compression stockings to treat PTS: of note, none of the trials included in the review reported significant changes in symptom relief, calf or ankle circumference, or ulcer healing [7]. Intermittent compression devices have been shown to be effective in improving PTS symptoms, PTS severity, and quality of life. Such devices could be tried in patients with moderate to severe PTS that is not adequately relieved with compression stockings [7,31].

Pharmacologic therapies

Three "venoactive" drugs have been evaluated in four studies to treat PTS: rutosides, defibrotide, and hidrosmina [7]. In a recent meta-analysis, use of venoactive medications was associated with a small and non-significant increased likelihood of symptomatic relief but also an increased likelihood of adverse effects (RR 1.1 [0.9–1.5] and RR 2.0 [0.8, 5.5], respectively). In addition, these studies did not assess quality of life improvement or potential long-term benefit (or harm). Given the low-quality evidence to date for the effectiveness of these drugs in patients with PTS, their use is not suggested for PTS treatment [31].

Surgical treatment

In cases of moderate or severe PTS not adequately relieved with conservative treatment, various surgical treatments (including vein dilation and stent placement, venous bypass grafting, endophlebectomy with reconstruction, valve reconstruction/transplant, and interruption of perforating veins) have been developed and reported [39]. Except for transplantation of cryopreserved venous valve allografts, a variety of surgical procedures may be of promise for the treatment of PTS, with overall clinical improvement and ulcer healing rates of 50% or more during follow-up in comparison to presurgical healing rates [39]. Thus, surgical treatments may have the potential to be effective where conservative and medical treatments have failed, but multicenter randomized trials with adequate control groups, sufficient follow-up time, and systematic reporting of operative adverse events are needed.

In summary, the management of PTS primarily relies on its prevention, by preventing DVT with the use of thromboprophylaxis in patients at high risk of VTE and preventing PTS with the use of ECS (ankle pressure 30–40mmHg) for 2 years after acute proximal DVT. In the case of established PTS, conservative management with daily wearing of ECS stockings can be prescribed and exercise training recommended. In the absence of symptomatic relief with this approach, intermittent pneumatic devices or, in the case of severe PTS, expert surgical consultation can be considered.

References

1. Prandoni P, Kahn SR. Post-thrombotic syndrome: prevalence, prognostication and need for progress. *Br J Haematol* 2009;145:286–95.
2. Kahn SR. How I treat postthrombotic syndrome. *Blood* 2009;114:4624–31.
3. Kahn SR, Partsch H, Vedantham S, et al. Definition of post-thrombotic syndrome of the leg for use in clinical investigations: a recommendation for standardization. *J Thromb Haemost* 2009;7:879–83.
4. Kahn SR. Measurement properties of the Villalta scale to define and classify the severity of the post-thrombotic syndrome. *J Thromb Haemost* 2009;7:884–8.
5. Rodger MA, Kahn SR, Le Gal G, et al. Inter-observer reliability of measures to assess the post-thrombotic syndrome. *Thromb Haemost* 2008;100:164–6.
6. Kolbach DN, Neumann HA, Prins MH. Definition of the post-thrombotic syndrome, differences between existing classifications. *Eur J Vasc Endovasc Surg* 2005;30: 404–14.

7. Cohen JM, Akl EA, Kahn SR. Pharmacologic and compression therapies for post-thrombotic syndrome: a systematic review of randomized controlled trials. *Chest* 2012;141:308–20.

8. Kahn SR, Shrier I, Julian JA, et al. Determinants and time course of the postthrombotic syndrome after acute deep venous thrombosis. *Ann Intern Med* 2008;149: 698–707.

9. van Dongen CJ, Prandoni P, Frulla M, et al. Relation between quality of anticoagulant treatment and the development of the postthrombotic syndrome. *J Thromb Haemost* 2005;3:939–42.

10. Prandoni P, Lensing AW, Cogo A, et al. The long-term clinical course of acute deep venous thrombosis. *Ann Intern Med* 1996;125:1–7.

11. Ten Cate-Hoek AJ, Ten Cate H, Tordoir J, et al. Individually tailored duration of elastic compression therapy in relation to incidence of the postthrombotic syndrome. *J Vasc Surg* 2010;52:132–8.

12. Kahn SR, Kearon C, Julian JA, et al. Predictors of the post-thrombotic syndrome during long-term treatment of proximal deep vein thrombosis. *J Thromb Haemost* 2005;3:718–23.

13. Prandoni P, Villalta S, Bagatella P, et al. The clinical course of deep-vein thrombosis. Prospective long-term follow-up of 528 symptomatic patients. *Haematologica* 1997; 82:423–8.

14. Roumen-Klappe EM, den Heijer M, Janssen MC, et al. The post-thrombotic syndrome: incidence and prognostic value of non-invasive venous examinations in a six-year follow-up study. *Thromb Haemost* 2005;94:825–30.

15. Stain M, Schonauer V, Minar E, et al. The post-thrombotic syndrome: risk factors and impact on the course of thrombotic disease. *J Thromb Haemost* 2005;3:2671–6.

16. Schulman S, Lindmarker P, Holmström M, et al. Post-thrombotic syndrome, recurrence, and death 10 years after the first episode of venous thromboembolism treated with warfarin for 6 weeks or 6 months. *J Thromb Haemost* 2006;4:734–42.

17. Prandoni P. Healthcare burden associated with the post-thrombotic syndrome and potential impact of the new oral anticoagulants. *Eur J Haematol* 2012;88:185–94.

18. Prandoni P, Lensing AW, Prins MH, et al. Below-knee elastic compression stockings to prevent the post-thrombotic syndrome: a randomized, controlled trial. *Ann Intern Med* 2004;141:249–56.

19. Tick LW, Kramer MH, Rosendaal FR, et al. Risk factors for post-thrombotic syndrome in patients with a first deep venous thrombosis. *J Thromb Haemost* 2008;6: 2075–81.

20. Ashrani AA, Heit JA. Incidence and cost burden of post-thrombotic syndrome. *J Thromb Haemost* 2009;28:465–76.

21. Asbeutah AM, Riha AZ, Cameron JD, et al. Five-year outcome study of deep vein thrombosis in the lower limbs. *J Vasc Surg* 2004;40:1184–9.

22. Chitsike RS, Rodger MA, Kovacs MJ, et al. Risk of post-thrombotic syndrome after subtherapeutic warfarin anticoagulation for a first unprovoked deep vein thrombosis: Results from the REVERSE cohort study. *J Thromb Haemost* 2012;10:2039–44.

23. Palareti G, Schellong, S. Isolated Distal DVT: what we know and what we are doing. *J Thromb Haemost* 2012;10:11–19.

24. Masuda E.M, Kistner R.L, Musikasinthorn C, et al. The controversy of managing calf vein thrombosis. *J Vasc Surg* 2012;55:550–61.

25. Kahn SR, Shbaklo H, Lamping DL, et al. Determinants of health-related quality of life during the 2 years following deep vein thrombosis. *J Thromb Haemost* 2008;6: 1105–12.

26. Guanella R, Ducruet T, Johri M, et al. Economic burden and cost determinants of deep venous thrombosis during two years following diagnosis: a prospective evaluation. *J Thromb Haemost* 2011;9:2397–405.

27. Kahn SR, Lim W, Dunn AS, et al. Prevention of VTE in Nonsurgical Patients: Antithrombotic Therapy and Prevention of thrombosis, 9th ed: American College of Chest Physicians Evidence-Based Clinical Practice Guidelines. *Chest* 2012;141(S2): 195–226.

28. Wille-Jørgensen P, Jorgensen LN, Crawford M. Asymptomatic postoperative deep vein thrombosis and the development of postthrombotic syndrome. a systematic review and meta-analysis. *Thromb Haemost* 2005;93:236–41.

29. Lloyd NS, Douketis JD, Moinuddin I, et al. Anticoagulant prophylaxis to prevent asymptomatic deep vein thrombosis in hospitalized medical patients: a systematic review and meta-analysis. *J Thromb Haemost* 2008;6:405–14.

30. Musani MH, Matta F, Yaekoub AY, et al. Venous compression for prevention of postthrombotic syndrome: a meta-analysis. *Am J Med* 2010;123:735–40.

31. Kearon C, Akl EA, Comerota, AJ, et al. Antithrombotic Therapy for VTE Disease: Antithrombotic Therapy and Prevention of Thrombosis, 9th ed: American College of Chest Physicians Evidence-Based Clinical Practice Guidelines. *Chest* 2012; 141(S2):419–94.

32. Kahn SR, Shbaklo H, Shapiro S, et al. Effectiveness of compression stockings to prevent the post-thrombotic syndrome (the SOX Trial and Bio-SOX biomarker substudy): a randomized controlled trial. *BMC Cardiovasc Disord* 2007;24:21.

33. Prandoni P, Noventa F, Quintavalla R et al. on behalf of the Canano Investigators. Thigh-length versus below-knee compression elastic stockings for prevention of the postthrombotic syndrome in patients with proximal-venous thrombosis: a randomized trial. *Blood* 2012;119:1561–5.

34. Crumley C. Post-thrombotic syndrome: patient education based on the health belief model. *J Wound Ostomy Continence Nurs* 2011;38:648–54.

35. Hull RD, Liang J, Townshend G. Long-term low-molecular-weight heparin and the post-thrombotic syndrome: a systematic review. *Am J Med* 2011;124:756–65.

36. Vendantham S. Catheter-directed thrombolysis for deep vein thrombosis. *Curr Opin Hematol* 2010;17:464–8.

37. Enden T, Haig Y, Kløw NE, et al. CaVenT Study Group. Long-term outcome after additional catheter-directed thrombolysis versus standard treatment for acute iliofemoral deep vein thrombosis (the CaVenT study): a randomised controlled trial. *Lancet* 2012;379:31–8.

38. Kahn SR, Shrier I, Shapiro S, et al. Six-month exercise training program to treat post-thrombotic syndrome: a randomized controlled two-centre trial. *CMAJ* 2011;183:37–44.

39. Bond RT, Cohen JM, Comerota A, Kahn SR, et al. Surgical treatment of moderate-to-severe post-thrombotic syndrome. *Ann Thoracic Surg* 2013;27:242–58.

CHAPTER 15

Von Willebrand Disease: Clinical Aspects and Practical Management

Francesco Rodeghiero, Alberto Tosetto, and Giancarlo Castaman
Department of Cell Therapy and Hematology, Hemophilia and Thrombosis Center, San Bortolo Hospital, Vicenza, Italy

The von Willebrand factor and its laboratory measurement

Von Willebrand disease (VWD) is the most common hemorrhagic disorder, with an estimated prevalence approaching 1 in 100 individuals, without ethnic differences [1], caused by a quantitative or qualitative defect of von Willebrand factor (VWF). Von Willebrand factor is a large non-enzymatic, multimeric glycoprotein required for the adhesion of platelets to subendothelium, for platelet-to-platelet cohesion and aggregation and acting as the carrier of plasma factor VIII (FVIII), effectively increasing its concentration at the site of the formation of the hemostatic plug [2,3]. The VWF coding gene includes about 178 kilobases with 52 exons and is located at chromosome 12p13.2. The building block of VWF multimers is a dimer made by two single-chain pro-VWF molecules, joined through disulfide bonds within their C-terminal region. Von Willebrand factor multimers (up to 20,000 kDa) are formed within the Golgi apparatus by N-terminal joining of the basic dimer. Specific domains present in each VWF subunit allow interaction with platelet glycoproteins Ib and IIb/IIIa (Gp-Ib and Gp-IIb/IIIa), FVIII and subendothelial collagen. Platelet-subendothelium adhesion and platelet-to-platelet cohesion and aggregation in vessels with elevated shear stress is promoted by the interaction of a region of the A1 domain of VWF with platelet Gp-Ib. It is thought that high shear stress is able to activate the A1 domain of the collagen-bound VWF by stretching VWF multimers into a filamentous form. The interaction between Gp-Ib and VWF can be mimicked by the addition of the antibiotic ristocetin,

Hemostasis and Thrombosis: Practical Guidelines in Clinical Management, First Edition.
Hussain I. Saba and Harold R. Roberts.
© 2014 John Wiley & Sons, Ltd. Published 2014 by John Wiley & Sons, Ltd.

which promotes the binding of VWF to Gp-Ib present on fresh or formalin-fixed platelet suspensions. Aggregation of platelets within the growing hemostatic plug is promoted by the interaction with a second receptor on platelets, Gp-IIb-IIIa which after activation, binds to VWF and fibrinogen, recruiting more platelets into a stable plug. Von Willebrand factor is the carrier of FVIII in plasma, protecting it from proteolytic degradation, prolonging its half-life in the circulation and efficiently localizing it at the site of vascular injury (for review, see [4]).

VWF is synthesized by endothelial cells and megakaryocytes. Although VWF is secreted from cytoplasm of endothelial cells via a constitutive pathway, the more hemostatically efficient large multimers are released from specialized endothelial storage organelles called Weibel–Palade bodies through a stimuli-responsive pathway (either by physiologic agonists like adrenalin and thrombin or pharmacologic agents like desmopressin) [4]. The diverse multimer species observed in plasma are the result of VWF proteolysis by ADAMTS-13 [4].

The laboratory tests used for diagnosis of VWD usually explore only one of the above-mentioned VWF functions and, therefore, a single test is not sufficient to evaluate the full hemostatic role of VWF.

While *prothrombin time (PT)* is normal, *partial thromboplastin time (PTT)* may be prolonged as a result of low FVIII levels, which can be very low in severe quantitative VWF deficiencies.

The *bleeding time (BT)* roughly explores the VWF–Gp-Ib interaction and is usually prolonged, but may be normal in patients with mild forms of VWD especially when platelet VWF content is normal. Platelet function analyser (PFA) *closure time (CT)* allows rapid, non-invasive determination of VWF-dependent platelet function at high shear stress. This system was demonstrated to be sensitive and reproducible when screening for severe VWF deficiencies.

Measurement of *VWF antigen (VWF:Ag)* is useful to demonstrate quantitative deficiencies of VWF, and is nowadays available as latex immunoassay for most automated coagulometers, allowing a rapid and accurate quantitative measurement of VWF. The assay for *ristocetin cofactor activity (VWF:RCo)* explores the interaction of VWF with the platelet glycoprotein Ib/IX/V complex, and it is still the standard method for quantitative measurement of VWF platelet-dependent activity. It is based on the property of the antibiotic ristocetin to agglutinate formalin-fixed normal platelets in the presence of VWF. A new ELISA test exploiting the interaction of VWF with plate-immobilized recombinant Gp-Ibα in the presence of ristocetin seems to be very promising as a replacement for VWF:RCo, but it has not yet been fully validated [5].

Assays for *VWF:CB* are also available, and the ratio of VWF:CB to VWF:Ag levels appears to be useful for distinguishing between quantitative and qualitative defects. Finally, *electrophoretic VWF multimer analysis* allows full characterization of the multimer pattern, but this technique is usually available in specialized laboratories only and is not strictly necessary for the diagnosis and clinical management of patients.

Classification of von Willebrand disease

Von Willebrand disease is commonly classified into two distinct quantitative (type 1 and 3) and one qualitative (type 2) subtypes (Box 15.1) [6].

In patients with type 1 (quantitative defect) VWD, accounting for about 70% of all diagnosed cases, concomitantly reduced levels of VWF:RCo and VWF:Ag are observed, with a normal multimeric structure. Both VWF:Ag and VWF:RCo have wide variation in normal subjects, with blood group O individuals having VWF:Ag and VWF:RCo levels as low as 40 U/dL. However, VWD should be strongly suspected when VWF:Ag and VWF:RCo are below this cut-off, and the likelihood of VWD is particularly high only for values <30 U/dL.

In patients with type 2 VWD (qualitative defect), missense mutations may impair specific functional domains (2M, 2N) or may affect multimerization (2A) [6]. In both instances, the qualitative nature of the defect can be inferred from a greatly reduced VWF:RCo/VWF:Ag or VWF:CB/VWF:Ag ratio (type 2M and type 2A) or FVIII/VWF:Ag ratio (type 2N) [7]. Type 2B is characterized by gain-of-function mutations in the A1 domain causing increased affinity of VWF for platelet Gp-Ib. Large multimers

---

Box 15.1 Classification of von Willebrand disease. Source: Adapted from Sadler et al. 2006 [6]. Reproduced with permission of John Wiley & Sons, Ltd.

Quantitative deficiency of VWF
Type 1: Partial quantitative deficiency of VWF
Type 3: Virtually complete deficiency of VWF

Qualitative deficiency of VWF
Type 2: Qualitative deficiency of VWF
A) Type 2A: Qualitative variants with decreased platelet-dependent function associated with the absence of high- and intermediate-molecular-weight VWF multimers
B) Type 2B: Qualitative variants with increased affinity for platelet Gp-Ib, with the absence of high- molecular-weight VWF multimers
C) Type 2M: Qualitative variants with decreased platelet-dependent function not caused by the absence of high-molecular-weight VWF multimers
D) Type 2N: Qualitative variants with markedly decreased affinity for factor VIII

spontaneously bind to platelets with subsequent removal from circulation and increased proteolysis so that these patients have a decreased proportion of large multimers and variable thrombocytopenia [8].

Type 3 VWD is a recessive disease with very low prevalence (1–2 cases per million), characterized by the presence of no or only trace amounts of VWF in plasma and platelets and by FVIII <5 U/dL.

Clinical manifestations

Clinical expression of VWD is usually mild in type 1, with increasing severity in type 2 and type 3. In general, the severity of bleeding correlates with the degree of the reduction of FVIII. Mucocutaneous bleeding (epistaxis especially during childhood, menorrhagia, easy bruising) is a typical, prominent manifestation of the disease and may affect the quality of life. However, the rate of spontaneous bleeding may be low even in patients with severe VWF deficiency [9]. Bleeding after dental extraction is the most frequent postoperative bleeding manifestation. Since FVIII is usually only mildly reduced, manifestations of a severe coagulation defect (hemarthrosis, deep muscle hematoma) are rarely observed in type 1 VWD and are mainly post-traumatic. On the contrary, in type 3 VWD, the severity of bleeding may sometimes be similar to that of moderate hemophilia. Gastrointestinal bleeding may be particularly frequent and difficult to manage in elderly patients, especially those lacking high-molecular-weight multimers in plasma [10]. Bleeding after delivery is rarely observed in type 1 VWD since FVIII/VWF levels tend to correct at the end of pregnancy in mild type 1 cases, whereas females with types 2A, 2B, and 3 VWD usually need replacement therapy postpartum to prevent immediate or delayed bleeding. Postoperative bleeding may not occur even in more severely affected type 1 patients, whereas in type 3 prophylactic treatment is always required.

Diagnosis of von Willebrand disease

The diagnosis of VWD may be very challenging in patients who have mild forms (usually type 1) of the disease, because of the great clinical and laboratory phenotype overlap with otherwise normal subjects. A slightly reduced VWF level can be found even in normal subjects, and bleeding symptoms are also frequently reported by "normal" subjects [11–13]. For this reason, the patient should be interviewed about their bleeding history using a structured, written questionnaire to improve the quality of data collection and to reduce both intra- and inter-observer variability. Collected data must be unambiguously interpreted to verify if the bleeding history is compatible with a bleeding disease, and for this purpose a bleeding score (BS), accounting for both the number and the severity of the bleeding symptoms, may be useful. The BS is generated by summing the severity of all bleeding symptoms reported by a subject, and graded according to an "a priori" scale [11,14]. Previous experience from the International Multicenter Study suggests that a bleeding score ($\geq$3 or $\geq$5 in males and females, respectively) could be considered as a useful cut-off to identify adults with a bleeding diathesis in whom it is worthwhile to measure VWF-related activities [11]. The diagnosis of VWD is then based on the presence of reduced VWF:RCo (or VWF:CB) (<40 U/dL), with a further characterization of VWD type based on assessment of VWF:Ag, FVIII, and multimer pattern, as previously described. However, it should be always borne in mind that the identification of other relatives with low VWF is a crucial clue to the definite diagnosis [15]. Box 15.2 summarizes a diagnostic flowchart for VWD.

Box 15.2 Practical approach to the diagnosis of von Willebrand disease

1. Consider VWD diagnosis within the context of an appropriate personal and/or familial bleeding history.
2. Perform PFA-100 or BT, platelet count, APTT, PT to exclude other common hemostatic defects.
3. VWF:RCo assay should be done if personal* and/or familial bleeding history is significant. If not possible, VWF:Ag assay or VWF:CB assay should be performed. VWF:Ag <3 U/dL suggests type 3 VWD.
4. If any of these tests is below 40 U/dL, the diagnosis of VWD should be considered.
5. Other family members with possible bleeding history should be evaluated. Finding another member with bleeding and reduced VWF strongly supports the diagnosis.
6. VWF:Ag, VWF:RCo, and FVIII:C should be measured on the same sample to assess the presence of reduced ratio VWF:RCo/VWF:Ag (a ratio <0.6 suggests type 2 VWD) or FVIII:C/VWF:Ag (a ratio <0.6 suggests type 2N VWD, to be confirmed by binding study of FVIII:C to patient's VWF).
7. Aggregation of patient platelet-rich plasma in presence of increasing concentration of ristocetin (0.25, 0.5, 1.0 mg/mL, final concentration) should be assessed. Aggregation at low concentration ($\leq$0.5 mg/mL) suggests type 2B VWD.
8. Multimer pattern using a low resolution gel should be evaluated. Lack of high-molecular-weight multimers suggests type 2A and or 2B. Presence of full complement of multimers suggests type 1 (or 2N, 2M). Absence of multimers in type 3.
9. If bleeding history is clinically significant, carry out a test infusion with desmopressin. FVIII/VWF measurements should be evaluated at least at baseline, 60 and 240 minutes from the start of intravenous infusion or subcutaneous injection. If basally prolonged, bleeding time (or PFA-100 if available) should be measured at 60 and 240 minutes.

*The use of a structured bleeding evaluation questionnaire is advisable [11,14]. In an adult a bleeding score $\geq$3 or $\geq$5 in males and females, respectively, represents a cut-off for a significant bleeding history [10].

Management of patients with von Willebrand disease

The correction of low FVIII and VWF is the aim of treatment in VWD. Desmopressin and transfusional therapy with blood products represent the two treatments of choice in VWD [16]. Other forms of treatment can be considered as adjunctive or alternative to these two modalities.

Desmopressin

Desmopressin (1-deamino-8-D-arginine vasopressin, DDAVP), a synthetic analog of vasopressin, is the treatment of first choice in responsive patients with VWD. It is relatively cheap and carries no risk of transmitting blood-borne viruses. DDAVP is usually administered intravenously at a dose of 0.3 μg/kg diluted in 50–100 mL saline infused over 30 minutes or subcutaneously at the same dosage using a concentrated formulation. An intranasal preparation is also available; this route, however, is associated with erratic absorption and requires a greater dose.

Patients with type 1 VWD are the best candidates for DDAVP treatment [17]. In these patients FVIII, VWF and the BT (or PFA) are usually corrected within 30 minutes and remain normal for 6–8 hours. Response to DDAVP is assessed at least after 1 hour (peak) following the infusion and is defined as complete when FVIII and VWF:RCo attain levels ≥50 U/dL. Factor VIII and VWF:RCo plasma levels should also be measured at least 4 hours after infusion to identify patients with increased clearance who are possible candidates for alternative treatments [18].

In other VWD types, responsiveness to DDAVP is variable [19]. In type 2A, FVIII levels are increased by DDAVP but VWF:RCo usually remains low. Desmopressin is best avoided in type 2B, because of the transient appearance of thrombocytopenia. Platelet count should be checked during test infusion to unravel possible non-classical type 2B cases with thrombocytopenia occurring after infusion. Type 2M shows a higher level of VWF:Ag compared to VWF:RCo. In type 2N, relatively high levels of FVIII are observed following DDAVP, but released FVIII circulates for a shorter time period in patients' plasma because the stabilizing effect of VWF is impaired. Patients with type 3 VWD are usually unresponsive to DDAVP [19].

Since the responses in a given patient and within his/her family are consistent on different occasions, a test dose of DDAVP is required to establish the individual response pattern, and will facilitate the planning of future treatment. Infusions can be repeated every 12–24 hours depending on the type and severity of the bleeding episode. However, most patients treated repeatedly with DDAVP become less responsive to therapy, particularly after 3–4 closely spaced administrations.

Side effects of DDAVP may include mild tachycardia, headache, and flushing, which can be attenuated by slowing the rate of infusion [19]. Hyponatremia and volume overload due to the antidiuretic effects of DDAVP are relatively rare complications, primarily occurring in children <2 years who received closely repeated infusions. Even though no thrombotic episodes have been reported in patients with VWD treated with DDAVP, this drug should be used with caution in elderly patients with atherosclerotic disease.

Other non-transfusional therapies

Two other types of non-transfusional therapy are used in the management of VWD: antifibrinolytic amino acids and estrogens. *Antifibrinolytic amino acids* are synthetic drugs which interfere with the lysis of newly formed clots by saturating the binding sites on plasminogen, thereby preventing its attachment to fibrin and making plasminogen unavailable within the forming clot [20]. ε-Aminocaproic acid (50 mg/kg four times a day) and tranexamic acid (15–25 mg/kg three times a day) are the most frequently used antifibrinolytic amino acids. Both medications can be administered orally, intravenously, or topically and are useful alone or as adjuncts in the management of oral cavity bleeding, epistaxis, gastrointestinal bleeding, and menorrhagia [20]. *Estrogens* may be very useful in reducing the severity of menorrhagia in women with VWD, even type 3, despite the fact that FVIII/VWF levels are not modified [21].

Transfusional therapies

Transfusional therapy with virus-inactivated intermediate-purity concentrates containing FVIII/VWF, originally developed for the treatment of hemophilia A, is currently the treatment of choice in patients who are unresponsive to DDAVP [16]. Ideally, products labeled for VWF content and with a VWF/FVIII ratio higher than 1 are preferred [16]. A very high purity VWF concentrate, with very low content of FVIII, is also effective, but it is not yet available in North America. However, the very low content of FVIII in this concentrate requires the infusion of a supplemental dose of pure FVIII concentrate for the treatment of acute bleeding episodes and for emergency surgeries to ensure hemostasis. Thereafter, infused VWF stabilizes endogenously synthesized FVIII with normalization of FVIII levels after 6–8 hours, so that no further infusion of FVIII-containing concentrates is necessary. No concentrate contains a completely normal VWF multimer pattern, because VWF proteolysis occurs during purification due to the action of platelet and leukocyte proteases contaminating the plasma used for fractionation. However, high post-infusion levels of these moieties are consistently obtained. Several retrospective and prospective studies have documented an excellent or good hemostasis in >95% of cases [22]. A sustained rise in FVIII lasting for up to 24 hours, higher than predicted from the doses infused, is observed because of the stabilizing effect of exogenous VWF on endogenous FVIII, which is synthesized at a normal rate in these patients. Thus, very high FVIII levels may be observed when multiple infusions are given for severe bleeding episodes or to cover major surgery, and the occurrence of deep vein thrombosis has been reported in patients with VWD, especially following surgery [23].

The dosages of concentrates recommended for the control of bleeding episodes are summarized in Table 15.1.

Table 15.1 Doses of factor VIII in factor VIII–VWF concentrates recommended in patients with von Willebrand disease unresponsive to desmopressin.

Type of bleeding	FVIII:C dose* (U/kg)	Number of infusions	Objective
Major surgery	40–60	Once a day or every other day	Maintain FVIII 80–100 U/dL for the first 2 days and then >50 U/dL for 5–7 days
Minor surgery; caesarean section	30	Once a day or every other day	Maintain FVIII >30 U/dL for at least 5–7 days
Dental extractions	20–40	Single	Obtain FVIII >30–50 U/dL; subsequent infusions on clinical need
Delivery and/or epidural anesthesia	30–40	Single	Obtain FVIII >50 U/dL; subsequent infusions on clinical need
Spontaneous or post-traumatic bleeding	20–40	Single	Obtain FVIII >30–50 U/dL; subsequent infusions on clinical need
Severe frequent bleeding (gastrointestinal, menorrhagia, hemarthrosis)	20–40	Twice or thrice weekly	Short-term control: dose adjusted on the basis of clinical response. Lifelong prophylaxis: still experimental, to be adopted within clinical trials

*Prefer FVIII/VWF concentrates labeled for both FVIII:C and VWF:RCo content and with VWF/FVIII ≥1.

Platelet concentrates (at doses of $4 - 5 \times 10^{11}$ platelets) may be required in the rare situations where replacement treatment does not control bleeding. For the rare patients with type 3 VWD who develop anti-VWF alloantibodies after multiple transfusions, the infusion of VWF concentrates may not only be ineffective, but may also cause post-infusion life-threatening anaphylaxis due to the formation of immune complexes. Recombinant FVIII or activated FVII may be required in these patients [24,25].

Secondary long-term prophylaxis

Patients with severe forms of VWD may suffer from recurrent hemarthroses, severe epistaxis causing acute or chronic anemia, or gastrointestinal bleeding and may therefore benefit from secondary long-term prophylaxis. A report from Sweden (35 patients with severe VWD) and one summarizing results from Italy (12 patients) have both reported excellent results [26,27]. However, more prospective trials are needed to better evaluate the cost-effectiveness of this approach versus on-demand therapy.

Pregnancy in women with von Willebrand disease

Pregnant women with VWD may be at increased risk of postpartum hemorrhage if untreated [28]. However, in most patients with type 1 VWD, the levels of VWF and FVIII are normalized by the end of pregnancy and treatment is rarely required. Patients with the frequent VWD Vicenza and C1130F mutations show only a slight increase of these moieties during pregnancy, and treatment with desmopressin is required at delivery [29]. Patients with type 2N associated with the common R854Q mutation show a complete normalization of FVIII and no treatment is usually required [29]. In VWD type 2B the increase of the abnormal VWF can cause or worsen thrombocytopenia. In general, patients with VWD should be monitored for VWF:RCo and FVIII levels once during the third trimester of pregnancy and within 10 days of the expected delivery date. The risk of bleeding is minimal when FVIII:C and VWF:RCo levels are $\geq$50 U/dL. In type 1 VWD pregnant women with FVIII levels lower than 40 U/dL, desmopressin on the day of villocentesis, amniocentesis and of parturition, and for a couple of days thereafter, is advisable. In order to prevent late bleeding, VWF:RCo and FVIII levels should be checked and women monitored clinically for at least 2 weeks postpartum [23,29]. Oral tranexamic acid can be administered during this period. In women with type 3 VWD, VWF and FVIII do not increase during pregnancy and thus VWF/FVIII concentrates are required to cover delivery or cesarean section [29]. The latter should be reserved only for the usual obstetric indications. There is no apparent increased bleeding risk for neonates with VWD.

Conclusions

Von Willebrand disease is the most frequent inherited bleeding disorder. Definite diagnosis and characterization usually requires an array of tests and should be reserved to patients with a significant bleeding history. Nowadays, several safe and effective therapeutic options are easily available to prevent or control bleeding episodes which, however, rarely persistently affect the quality of life.

Acknowledgments

This work was supported by a grant from the Fondazione Progetto Ematologia (Hematology Project Foundation, Vicenza, Italy).

References

1. Castaman G, Rodeghiero F. The epidemiology of von Willebrand disease. In Federici AB, Lee CA, Berntorp EE, Lillicrap D, Montgomery RR (eds), *Von Willebrand Disease: Basic and Clinical Aspects*. Oxford: Wiley-Blackwell, 2011;86–90.
2. Wu YP, Vink T, Schiphorst M, et al. Platelet thrombus formation on collagen at high shear rates is mediated by von Willebrand factor-glycoprotein Ib interaction and inhibited by von Willebrand factor-glycoprotein IIb/IIIa interaction. *Arterioscler Thromb Vasc Biol* 2000;20:1661–7.
3. Reininger AJ, Heijnen HF, Schumann H, et al. Mechanism of platelet adhesion to von Willebrand factor and microparticle formation under high shear stress. *Blood* 2006;107:3537–45.
4. Montgomery RR, Haberichter S. *von Willebrand factor structure and function*. In Federici AB, Lee CA, Berntorp EE, Lillicrap D, Montgomery RR (eds), *Von Willebrand Disease: Basic and Clinical Aspects*. Oxford: Wiley-Blackwell, 2011;30–48.
5. Federici AB, Canciani MT, Forza I, et al. A sensitive ristocetin cofactor activity assay with recombinant glycoprotein Ib alpha for the diagnosis of patients with low von Willebrand factor levels. *Haematologica* 2004;89:77–85.
6. Sadler JE, Budde U, Eikenboom JC, et al. Working Party on von Willebrand Disease Classification. Update on the pathophysiology and classification of von Willebrand disease: a report of the Subcommittee on von Willebrand Factor. *J Thromb Haemost* 2006;4:2103–14.
7. Meyer D, Fressinaud E, Mazurier C. Clinical, laboratory, and molecular markers of type 2 von Willebrand disease. In Federici AB, Lee CA, Berntorp EE, Lillicrap D, Montgomery RR (eds), *Von Willebrand Disease: Basic and Clinical Aspects*. Oxford: Wiley-Blackwell, 2011;137–47.

8. Federici AB, Mannucci PM, Castaman G, et al. Clinical and molecular predictors of thrombocytopenia and risk of bleeding in patients with von Willebrand disease type 2B: a cohort study of 67 patients. *Blood* 2009;113:526–34.

9. Castaman G, Tosetto A, Federici AB, et al. Bleeding tendency and efficacy of anti-haemorrhagic treatments in patients with type 1 von Willebrand disease and increased von Willebrand factor clearance. *Thromb Haemost* 2011;105: 647–54.

10. Castaman G, Federici AB, Tosetto A, et al. Different bleeding risk in type 2A and 2M Von Willebrand disease: a 2-year prospective study in 107 patients. *J Thromb Haemost* 2012;10:632–8.

11. Rodeghiero F, Castaman G, Tosetto A, et al. The discriminant power of bleeding history for the diagnosis of type 1 von Willebrand disease: an international, multi-center study. *J Thromb Haemost* 2005;3:2619–26.

12. Wahlberg T, Blomback M, Hall P, et al. Application of indicators, predictors and diagnostic indices in coagulation disorders. I. Evaluation of a self-administered questionnaire with binary questions. *Methods Inf Med* 1980;19:194–200.

13. Sramek A, Eikenboom JC, Briet E, et al. Usefulness of patient interview in bleeding disorders. *Arch Intern Med* 1995;155:1409–15.

14. Tosetto A, Rodeghiero F, Castaman G. Bleeding scores in inherited bleeding disorders: clinical or research tools? *Haemophilia* 2008;14:415–22.

15. Tosetto A, Castaman G, Rodeghiero F. Evidence-based diagnosis of type 1 von Willebrand disease: a Bayes theorem approach. *Blood* 2008;111:3998–400.

16. Rodeghiero F, Castaman G, Tosetto A. How I treat von Willebrand disease. *Blood* 2009;114:1158–65.

17. Castaman G, Lethagen S, Federici AB, et al. Response to desmopressin is influenced by the genotype and phenotype in type 1 von Willebrand disease (VWD): results from the European Study MCMDM-1VWD. *Blood* 2008;111:3531–9.

18. Castaman G, Tosetto A, Rodeghiero F. Reduced von Willebrand factor survival in von Willebrand disease: pathophysiologic and clinical relevance. *J Thomb Haemost* 2009;7(suppl 1):71–4.

19. Lethagen S, Federici AB, Castaman G. *On the use of desmopressin in von Willebrand disease*. In Federici AB, Lee CA, Berntorp EE, Lillicrap D, Montgomery RR (eds), *Von Willebrand Disease: Basic and Clinical Aspects*. Oxford: Wiley-Blackwell, 2011; 186–99.

20. Mannucci PM. Hemostatic drugs. *N Engl J Med* 1998;339:245–53.

21. Foster PA. The reproductive health of women with von Willebrand disease unresponsive to DDAVP: results of an international survey. On behalf of the Subcommittee on von Willebrand Factor of the Scientific and Standardization Committee of the ISTH. *Thromb Haemost* 1995;74:784–90.

22. Makris M, Colvin B, Gupta V, et al. Venous thrombosis following the use of intermediate purity FVIII concentrate to treat patients with von Willebrand's disease. *Thromb Haemost* 2002;88:387–8.

23. Castaman G. Treatment of von Willebrand disease with FVIII/VWF concentrates. *Blood Transfus* 2011;9:s9–s13.

24. Ciavarella N, Schiavoni M, Valenzano E, Mangini F, Inchingolo F. Use of recombinant factor VIIa (NovoSeven) in the treatment of two patients with type III von Willebrand's disease and an inhibitor against von Willebrand factor. *Haemostasis* 1996;26:10–14.

25. Franchini M, Gandini G, Giuffrida A, De Gironcoli M, Federici AB. Treatment for patients with type 3 von Willebrand disease and alloantibodies: a case report. *Haemophilia* 2008;14:645–6.

26. Berntorp E, Petrini P. Long-term prophylaxis in von Willebrand disease. *Blood Coagul Fibrinolysis* 2005;16:S23–6.
27. Federici AB, Castaman G, Franchini M, et al. Clinical use of Haemate P in inherited von Willebrand disease: a cohort study on 100 Italian patients. *Haematologica* 2007;92:944–51.
28. Lee CA, Kadir R, Kouides PA. *Women with von Willebrand disease*. In Federici AB, Lee CA, Berntorp EE, Lillicrap D, Montgomery RR (eds), *Von Willebrand Disease: Basic and Clinical Aspects*. Oxford: Wiley-Blackwell, 2011;174–85.
29. Castaman G, Tosetto A, Rodeghiero F. Pregnancy and delivery in women with von Willebrand's disease and different von Willebrand factor mutations. *Haematologica* 2010;95:963–9.

CHAPTER 16

Platelets in Hemostasis: Inherited and Acquired Qualitative Disorders

Noman Ashraf[1] and Hussain I. Saba[2]

[1] Department of Hematology/Oncology, University of South Florida/James A. Haley VA Hospital, Tampa, FL, USA
[2] USF College of Medicine, Department of Malignant Hematology at Moffitt Cancer Center, University of South Florida, Tampa, FL, USA

Platelets are essential blood cells that interact with injured blood vessels and the coagulation system to establish hemostasis. Disorders affecting platelets are among the most frequently encountered hematologic problems and can lead to bleeding of varying severity. An understanding of the normal biology of platelets is imperative to diagnose and properly manage these conditions. In this chapter we will review the role of platelets in hemostasis, discuss diagnostic tests commonly employed to evaluate platelets, and describe some inherited and acquired platelet disorders along with their treatment.

Thrombopoiesis

Platelets are produced in the bone marrow by fragmentation of the megakaryocytic cytoplasm. During differentiation, megakaryocytes undergo endomitosis whereby DNA replicates in the absence of nuclear or cytoplasmic division, resulting in large cells with abundant cytoplasm and a multilobed polyploid nucleus [1]. As the megakaryocyte matures, secretory granules assemble in the cytoplasm and the plasma membrane invaginates to form a demarcation membrane system. In conjunction with microtubules, the membrane forms filamentous projections called proplatelets which then release platelets into the bloodstream. Each megakaryocyte gives rise to 1000–5000 platelets and this process takes about 10 days.

Hemostasis and Thrombosis: Practical Guidelines in Clinical Management, First Edition.
Hussain I. Saba and Harold R. Roberts.

Under normal circumstances, approximately 1×10^{11} platelets are produced every day. After circulating for 7–10 days, platelets lose their surface receptors (e.g., collagen receptor, GPVI, CD42b) and senescent platelets are removed by phagocytic cells of the reticuloendothelial system. Previously thought to be a passive process, senescence and apoptosis likely involve intrinsic signals as well [2]. Thrombopoiesis parallels consumption and is tightly regulated by cytokines such as thrombopoietin (TPO) and interleukins 6 and 11 (IL-6 and IL-11).

Thrombopoietin is the principal regulator of platelet production. Binding to its receptor c-Mpl, thrombopoietin promotes differentiation of megakaryocyte progenitors, endomitosis, and platelet production. Inherited defects in the c-Mpl receptor lead to a severe thrombocytopenic condition called congenital amegakaryocytic thrombocytopenia (CAMT). Similar to megakaryocytes, platelets also express c-Mpl and regulate free TPO levels by binding and removing it from the circulation. TPO is produced constitutively by the liver but circulating TPO levels depend on the platelet and megakaryocyte mass. When platelet counts are low, less TPO is removed and more is available to stimulate thrombopoiesis. The converse is true when platelet counts are high. Normal bone marrow has significant reserve and, if needed, platelet production can increase eightfold. Synthetic agonists of c-Mpl are now available and approved for treatment of immune thrombocytopenia (ITP).

Platelet structure

The deceptively simple-appearing platelets are minute anucleate blood cells measuring 1.5–2.5 μm. Their plasma membrane forms a unique open canalicular system by invaginating deep into the platelet. It provides a large surface area for adsorption and activation of the coagulation protein complexes (prothrombinase and Xase). Upon platelet activation, the negatively charged phospholipid, phosphatidylserine, translocates from the inner leaflet to the external surface to interact with the coagulation proteins. Embedded in the plasma membrane are the numerous glycoproteins including Gp-Ib/IX/V and integrin αIIb/β3 (formerly Gp-IIb/IIIa) involved in platelet adhesion and aggregation, respectively. Just beneath the plasma membrane lies an elaborate cytoskeleton responsible for maintaining the discoid shape of resting platelets and inducing shape change upon activation.

Platelets contain alpha-granules (α-), dense-granules (δ-), lysosomes, peroxisomes, and organelles such as mitochondria and the dense tubular system (DTS), a derivative of the smooth endoplasmic reticulum. The DTS sequesters intracellular calcium and is the major site of thromboxane production [3]. Once activated, platelet α- and δ-granules release their contents resulting in a secondary wave of amplified aggregation. Alpha-granules contain more than 280 proteins including von Willebrand factor (VWF), platelet-derived growth factor (PDGF), and the platelet-specific proteins – platelet factor 4 (PF4) and β-thromboglobulin [4]. Coagulation factors V, VII, and XIII and fibrinogen are also found in α-granules but, rather than being synthesized by platelets, they are endocytosed from the blood. Dense-granules contain adenosine diphosphate (ADP), adenosine triphosphate (ATP), serotonin, and calcium, responsible for the dense appearance on electron microscopy.

Platelet physiology

Primary hemostasis, the formation of a platelet plug at the site of endothelial injury, occurs in the following phases: adhesion and activation, aggregation, and release reaction (Figure 16.1).

Adhesion and activation

Platelets possess unique glycoproteins (Gp) that adhere to exposed subendothelium following vessel injury. The particular glycoprotein involved is dictated by blood flow patterns. Under high shear (e.g., in arterioles) VWF first coats exposed collagen. Platelet surface Gp-Ib/IX/V complex then binds collagen through VWF. Deficiency of either VWF (von Willebrand' disease; VWD) or Gp-Ib/IX/V (Bernard–Soulier syndrome) leads to a bleeding disorder. In addition to tethering the platelet, this interaction exposes and activates Gp-IIb/IIIa which then more firmly binds the platelet to collagen (also through VWF). Integrin α2β1 (formerly Gp-Ia/IIa) and Gp-VI further strengthen this interaction by directly binding collagen. In low flow states, Gp-Ia/IIa is primarily responsible for initiating adhesion and activation.

Once activated, the cytoskeleton induces a shape change and platelets become more flattened. They extend filopodia in an attempt to bridge the endothelial defect. The cytoskeleton later also mediates clot retraction.

Aggregation

Inactivated Gp-IIb/IIIa cannot bind circulating fibrinogen, but a conformational change during activation allows it to bind fibrinogen. As more platelets are activated they cross-link fibrinogen through Gp-IIb/IIIa and aggregate. The platelet plug is further strengthened after agonists are released from granules, more platelets are recruited, and the coagulation cascade is complete with formation of fibrin. Gp-IIb/IIIa is defective in

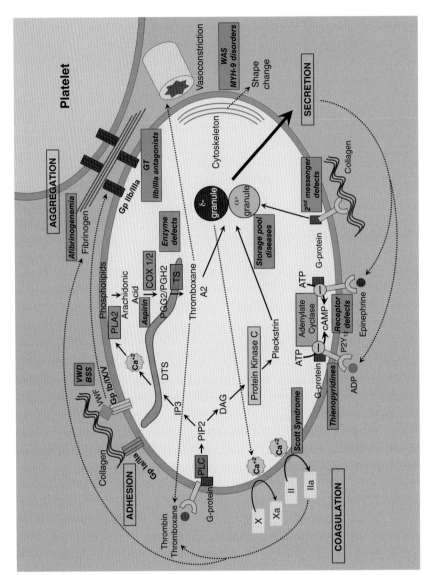

Figure 16.1 Normal platelet function and select functional disorders. ADP, adenosine diphosphate; ATP, adenosine triphosphate; BSS, Bernard–Soulier syndrome; cAMP, cyclic adenosine monophosphate; DAG, diacylglycerol; DT, dense tubular system; GT, Glanzmann's thrombasthenia; IP3, inositol 1,4,5-triphosphate; PGG2, prostaglandin G2; PGH2, prostaglandin H2; PIP2, phosphatidylinositol 4,5-bisphosphate; PLA2, phospholipase A2; PLC, phospholipase C; TS, thromboxane synthase; VWD, von Willebrand disease; VWF, von Willebrand factor; WAS, Wiskott–Aldrich syndrome. Source: Noman Ashraf MD. Reproduced with permission of Noman Ashraf MD. (See also Plate 16.1.)

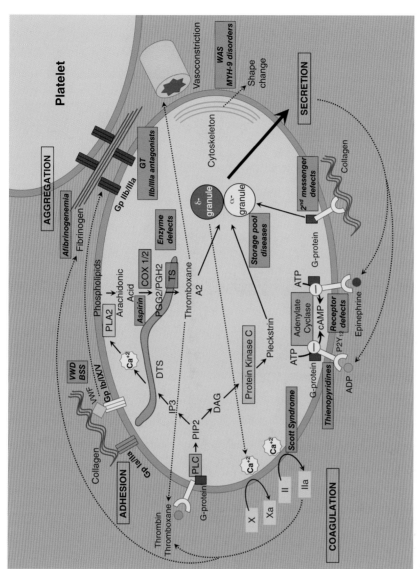

Plate 16.1 Normal platelet function and select functional disorders. ADP, adenosine diphosphate; ATP, adenosine triphosphate; BSS, Bernard–Soulier syndrome; cAMP, cyclic adenosine monophosphate; DAG, diacylglycerol; DT, dense tubular system; GT, Glanzmann's thrombasthenia; IP3, inositol 1,4,5-triphosphate; PGG2, prostaglandin G2; PGH2, prostaglandin H2; PIP2, phosphatidylinositol 4,5-bisphosphate; PLA2, phospholipase A2; PLC, phospholipase C; TS, thromboxane synthase; VWD, von Willebrand disease; VWF, von Willebrand factor; WAS, Wiskott–Aldrich syndrome. Source: Noman Ashraf MD. Reproduced with permission of Noman Ashraf MD. See also Figure 16.1.

Hemostasis and Thrombosis: Practical Guidelines in Clinical Management, First Edition.
Hussain I. Saba and Harold R. Roberts.
© 2014 John Wiley & Sons, Ltd. Published 2014 by John Wiley & Sons, Ltd.

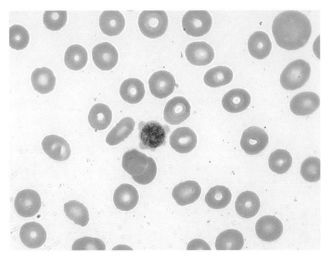

Plate 16.3 Macrothrombocyte: a platelet equal in size to a red blood cell. Image courtesy of Ling Zhang MD, Moffitt Cancer Center, Tampa, FL. See also Figure 16.3.

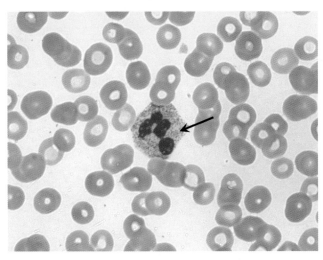

Plate 16.7 Döhle-like body (arrow). Image courtesy of Ling Zhang MD, Moffitt Cancer Center, Tampa, FL. See also Figure 16.7.

Glanzmann's thrombasthenia and a similar diathesis is iatrogenically induced by Gp-IIb/IIIa antagonists.

Release reaction

Upon activation, contents of platelet granules and other agonists are released into the open canalicular system. These agonists bind to specific receptors on platelets and further amplify the hemostatic response through second messengers. Most receptors are coupled with G-proteins and common intracellular signaling pathways which culminate in an increased synthesis of thromboxane A2 (TXA2), release of cytosolic calcium, and decreased production of cyclic adenosine monophosphate (cAMP).

Thrombin and TXA2 stimulate phospholipase C, which hydrolyzes phosphatidylinositol bisphosphate (PIP2) into inositol triphosphate (IP3) and diacylglycerol (DAG) [5]. IP3 releases cytosolic calcium from the DTS, which then mediates further degranulation and production of TXA2 through the phospholipase A2/cyclooxygenase pathway. In addition to platelet activation, TXA2 also causes vasoconstriction. Aspirin inhibits TXA2 production by irreversibly acetylating cyclooxygenase. DAG activates phosphokinases which further activate the platelet.

ADP released from dense-granules binds to its receptor $P2Y_{12}$ and inhibits adenylate cyclase, the enzyme responsible for cAMP production. Low cAMP levels activate platelets whereas high cAMP levels, induced by inhibitors like prostacyclin, inhibit platelets.

Fusion of α-granules with the plasma membrane also increases the number of available Gp-IIb/IIIa receptors and facilitates aggregation.

Role in coagulation

Platelets and the coagulation system are complementary. Calcium and coagulation factors released from platelets promote coagulation. More importantly, platelets provide the phospholipid, phosphatidylserine, for two rate-limiting steps of the coagulation cascade. In the presence of calcium, both Xase and prothrombinase adsorb to the surface of activated platelets to generate thrombin and fibrin. Thrombin in turn is a potent platelet agonist and fibrin strengthens the platelet plug.

Evaluation of platelet disorders

Although not mutually exclusive, platelet disorders can be quantitative (affecting platelet counts) or qualitative (affecting platelet function). The following assist in evaluation of platelet disorders.

History and examination

A detailed history and physical examination may be as effective as the bleeding time to diagnose platelet disorders [6]. Patients with mild platelet defects are often asymptomatic; however, those with severe disorders present at an early age with petechiae and mucocutaneous bleeding from the nose, gums, and genitourinary and gastrointestinal tracts. Some patients may not manifest until later when faced by a hemostatic challenge such as surgery, or menarche in females with congenital platelet disorders. Unlike hemophilia, bleeding is immediate and hemarthroses or deep hematomas are uncommon.

One must be cognizant that perception of bleeding is very subjective and 25% of patients with a self-reported bleeding history may not have a bleeding diathesis [7]. Criteria for significant bleeding proposed by the International Society on Thrombosis and Hemostasis may be useful (two or more sites, bleeding requiring hospitalization/transfusion, or bleeding from one site three times or more) [8]. To aid diagnosis, it is important to elicit a history of hemostatic challenges in the past, the need for transfusions, and a family history of bleeding/platelet disorders. Additionally, one must inquire about the use of over-the-counter medications and herbal remedies which often compromise platelet function.

Complete blood count and smear

A complete blood count (CBC) can readily establish the presence of thrombocytopenia and may even suggest an etiology (e.g., the presence of blasts). Most modern automated analyzers use electrical impedance or optical methods and are fairly accurate. However, a peripheral blood film must still be examined to confirm the platelet count. Immature large platelets may be underestimated by analyzers. EDTA-induced clumping can be corrected by analyzing blood in a citrated or heparinized tube [9]. Additionally, morphology of platelets and other blood cells on a smear is diagnostic in some inherited platelet disorders.

Coagulation studies

Prothrombin time (PT), activated partial thromboplastin time (aPTT), and thrombin time (TT) must always be performed to rule out clotting factor abnormalities. Clinically VWD, a more common condition, can be indistinguishable from qualitative platelet disorders. Therefore, all patients should be assessed for VWD before proceeding with more specific platelet studies.

Bleeding time

Bleeding time measures the time required for bleeding cessation after a standardized superficial skin incision on a patient's forearm. Due to its invasive nature, insensitivity, poor reproducibility, and lack of correlation with bleeding symptoms, it is seldom used nowadays [10,11]. Most mild platelet disorders will not prolong bleeding time but a prolonged bleeding time is always abnormal and must be investigated further.

Platelet function analyzer

The platelet function analyzer (PFA-100) is a simple, rapid test increasingly used to evaluate platelet dysfunction [12]. Citrated whole blood at high shear rate is passed through an aperture coated with collagen and either epinephrine or ADP. As a thrombus occludes the aperture, closure times are reported (CEPI and CADP). Closure times are significantly prolonged in Bernard–Soulier syndrome, Glanzmann's thrombasthenia, and VWD (except type 2N). Aspirin and NSAIDs usually prolong CEPI but not CADP [13].

PFA-100 has its shortcomings. It is insensitive for platelet storage pool defects and false negatives are common. Thrombocytopenia ($<50 \times 10^9$/L) and anemia (hematocrit $<25\%$) prolong closure times [14]. Most severe platelet disorders are detected by PFA-100 but milder ones may be missed. If clinical suspicion is high, further evaluation with more specific tests such as aggregometry or flow cytometry is warranted.

Platelet aggregometry

Arguably, the most important platelet function test is platelet aggregometry. Platelet-rich plasma obtained by centrifugation of whole blood is stirred in a cuvette between a light source and a sensor. Upon adding various agonists, platelets aggregate and turbidity is reduced, allowing more light to be transmitted. For each individual agonist, this increase in light transmission is recorded as a curve against time and compared to normal controls. Commonly used agonists include ADP, epinephrine, collagen, arachidonic acid, thrombin, and ristocetin (an antibiotic that induces platelet aggregation through Gp-Ib/IX/V). The typical curve in response to ADP and epinephrine is biphasic (Figure 16.2). A primary wave of aggregation is followed by a larger secondary wave mediated by the platelet release reaction. The secondary wave is absent in storage pool diseases. Other agonists produce a monophasic response [15].

Drawbacks to platelet aggregation studies include its time-consuming nature and the need for technical expertise. There is significant inter-laboratory variability and efforts to standardize results are ongoing [16]. Aggregometry is sensitive to even mild thrombocytopenia ($<120 \times 10^9$/L) and controls must be diluted to obtain accurate comparisons [17]. In contrast to the turbidometric method detailed above, the electrical impedance method uses whole blood and may overcome some limitations of turbidometric aggregometry [18].

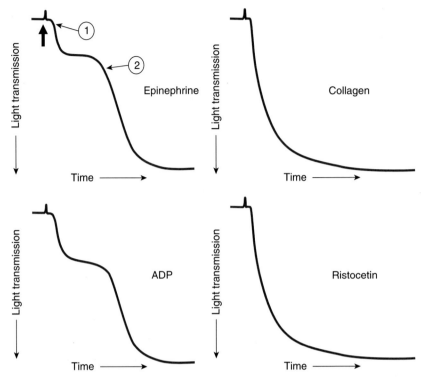

Figure 16.2 Schematic representation of normal platelet aggregometry: Epinephrine and ADP are added (bold arrow) to induce primary (1) and secondary waves (2) of aggregation. Other agonists produce a monophasic curve.

Nucleotide assays

Storage pool and release defects can be diagnosed by measuring platelet ATP/ADP content and release. One-fourth of patients with storage pool defects may have normal platelet aggregometry, so ideally nucleotide content and release assays should both be performed in patients suspected to have platelet dysfunction [19]. These assays are only performed by select specialized centers.

Flow cytometry

Platelet flow cytometry has emerged as a useful tool, particularly for the assessment of inherited surface glycoprotein disorders such as Bernard–Soulier syndrome (Gp-Ib/IX/V) and Glanzmann's thrombasthenia (Gp-IIb/IIIa) [17]. It requires only a small amount of blood and is not limited by thrombocytopenia.

Electron microscopy

Although not widely available, transmission electron microscopy (TEM) is helpful in the evaluation of dense granule defects (e.g., in Hermansky–

Pudlak syndrome; HPS) and ultrastructure abnormalities (e.g., MYH-9 disorders).

As is obvious from the above discussion, no single diagnostic test can identify all platelet disorders. Some tests are indicated in all patients suspected of having a platelet disorder, whereas other tests should be performed selectively based on the suspicion for a particular defect.

Disorders of platelets

Often qualitative and quantitative platelet disorders coexist; however, we will review them separately to improve understanding of their pathophysiologic basis and to differentiate the therapeutic strategies employed. Platelet transfusions are the only effective treatment in severe thrombocytopenia but other options, discussed in their respective sections, are available for disorders of platelet function.

Qualitative platelet disorders

Acquired platelet function disorders are more prevalent than inherited platelet disorders, yet the pathophysiology of congenital platelet disorders is better understood. A detailed discussion of all acquired and inherited qualitative disorders is beyond the scope of this chapter. The more common conditions are discussed below.

Inherited platelet disorders

Congenital platelet disorders are rare. They have been variably classified based on their mode of inheritance, the presence or absence of thrombocytopenia, and the various phases of hemostasis affected. Any step of platelet plug formation can be compromised including adhesion, aggregation, secretion, interaction with the coagulation system, the cytoskeleton or even the second messenger systems involved. Some inherited disorders lead to thrombocytopenia and characteristic morphologic changes on the peripheral smear. Others are associated with phenotypic skeletal and neurologic abnormalities. A discussion of inherited platelet disorders is followed by an overview of their treatment.

Platelet adhesion defects
Bernard–Soulier syndrome
First reported in 1948, Bernard–Soulier syndrome (BSS) is a rare inherited platelet disorder resulting from quantitative or qualitative defects in the

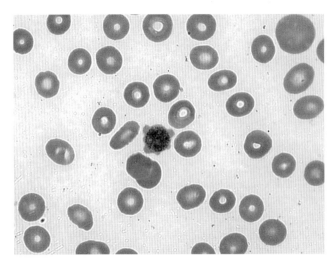

Figure 16.3 Macrothrombocyte: a platelet equal in size to a red blood cell. Image courtesy of Ling Zhang MD, Moffitt Cancer Center, Tampa, FL. (See also Plate 16.3.)

Gp-Ib/IX/V complex [20]. Binding of platelets to VWF and adhesion are impaired. Severity of bleeding is variable. BSS is characterized by a mild to moderate thrombocytopenia and giant platelets on the peripheral smear (Figure 16.3). Macrothrombocytopenia is thought to be a direct result of abnormal Gp-Ib/IX/V [21].

BSS is most commonly inherited in an autosomal recessive pattern, although autosomal dominant inheritance has also been reported [22]. It is more prevalent in areas where consanguinity is common. Gp-Ib/IX/V is encoded by four separate genes and mutations in all genes except Gp-V have been linked to BSS [23].

Most patients present in early childhood with frequent epistaxis, gum bleeds, and easy bruising. Menorrhagia and bleeding during childbirth can be severe in women. Major trauma and surgery can lead to life-threatening hemorrhage. Occasionally, mildly affected patients are not diagnosed until adulthood when they are first faced with a hemostatic challenge. Patients are often misdiagnosed as having ITP which can also present with macro-thrombocytopenia and bleeding.

BSS should be suspected when bleeding is out of proportion to the degree of thrombocytopenia. Platelet counts usually range between $30 \times 10^9/L$ and $200 \times 10^9/L$ [24]. Peripheral film reveals giant platelets. Bleeding time and PFA-100 are invariably prolonged with closure times (CEPI and CADP) often exceeding 300 seconds (300 s) [17]. On aggregometry, platelets fail to aggregate with ristocetin; however, response to other agonists is normal (Figure 16.4). Unlike VWD, addition of normal plasma does not correct response to ristocetin. Diagnosis can be confirmed by

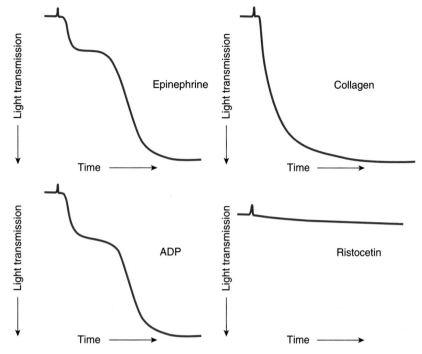

Figure 16.4 Platelet aggregometry in Bernard–Soulier syndrome: there is no response to ristocetin but normal response to other agonists.

platelet flow cytometry for Gp-Ib/IX density [25]. Molecular genetic testing is possible if the particular mutation in the family is known.

Platelet aggregation defects
Glanzmann's thrombasthenia

Glanzmann's thrombasthenia (GT), a relatively severe autosomal recessive congenital bleeding disorder, arises from abnormalities in Gp-IIb/IIIa. Platelets are unable to cross-link fibrinogen or VWF and aggregation is impaired despite a normal count. Based on whether a deficiency or dysfunction of Gp-IIb/IIIa is present, three types of GT have been described: type 1 with <5% expression, type 2 <20% expression, and type 3 with >50% expression but dysfunctional receptors [26].

Similar to BSS, inheritance is autosomal recessive. More than 100 mutations have been reported in the two closely related genes on chromosome 17 encoding for Gp-IIb and Gp-IIIa [27]. Clusters are found in populations where intermarriages are common (e.g., Southern Indians, French gypsies, and Iraqi Jews) [28–30].

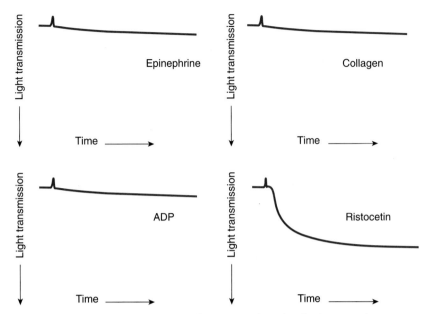

Figure 16.5 Platelet aggregometry in Glanzmann's thrombasthenia: normal response to ristocetin but lack of response to other agonists.

In a review of 177 patients, purpura, epistaxis, gingival bleeding, and menorrhagia were the most common symptoms [26]. Most patients present before 5 years of age, often at birth or in early infancy. Epistaxis and menorrhagia can be severe enough to require blood transfusions. Spontaneous gastrointestinal bleeding and hematuria are less frequent, but prolonged bleeding after trauma or surgery is common.

Patients with GT have normal platelet counts and morphology, a prolonged bleeding time, significantly prolonged closure times on PFA-100, and abnormal aggregation. In contrast to BSS, platelets aggregate normally with ristocetin but fail to aggregate with other agonists (Figure 16.5). Platelet flow cytometry for Gp-IIb (CD41) and Gp-IIIa (CD61) is confirmatory and differentiates it from congenital afibrinogenemia which can also impair aggregation. Normal coagulation studies (PT, aPTT and TT) rule out afibrinogenemia. Genetic testing and prenatal diagnosis is possible in families where the mutation has been identified [31].

Platelet secretion and secondary activation defects

As a group, these disorders are probably the most common inherited platelet disorders. Defective granules, abnormal second messengers, and deficient receptors all lead to impaired platelet secretion and activation.

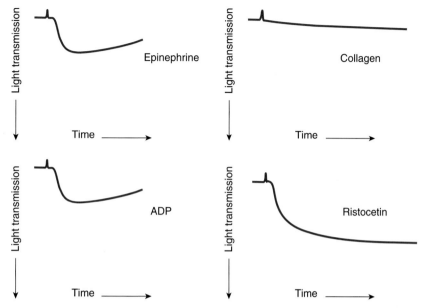

Figure 16.6 Platelet aggregometry in storage pool diseases (SPDs): absent secondary wave of aggregation with epinephrine and ADP.

Characteristically, the addition of ADP or epinephrine to platelet-rich plasma fails to produce a secondary wave of aggregation (Figure 16.6).

Storage pool diseases

Storage pool diseases (SPD) are a heterogeneous group of disorders characterized by abnormal, deficient, or absent α-granules, dense-granules or, less commonly, both α- and δ-granules.

Dense-granule disorders

Isolated δ-SPDs may occur as autosomal dominant disorders, but more commonly they are inherited as part of congenital syndromes. Dense-granules are specialized lysosome-like organelles related to melanosomes and secretory granules of cytotoxic T-lymphocytes. Defects affect all these organelles, resulting in a constellation of oculocutaneous albinism, immune deficiency, and a mild to moderate bleeding diathesis. Bleeding time is often, but not invariably, prolonged. In δ-SPDs, platelet counts and morphology on peripheral smear are normal; however, dense granules are absent on electron microscopy. A secondary wave of aggregation in response to ADP or epinephrine is absent or impaired (Figure 16.6). Diagnosis can be confirmed by direct measurement of nucleotides which shows an increased ratio of ATP to ADP [17].

Hermansky–Pudlak syndrome

Worldwide, Hermansky–Pudlak syndrome (HPS) is rare, but the prevalence in Puerto Rico is as high as 1 in 1,800 [32]. At least eight different gene mutations result in this autosomal recessive disorder. HPS-1 is the most prevalent [33]. Common to all forms of the disease are oculocutaneous albinism and δ-granule defects. Additional manifestations are dictated by the underlying mutation. HPS-1 is associated with pulmonary fibrosis and granulomatous colitis, whereas HPS-2 leads to neutropenia [33]. Like other SPDs, bleeding is mild to moderate.

Chediak–Higashi syndrome

Chediak–Higashi syndrome (CHS) is another rare autosomal recessive disorder resulting from mutations in the gene encoding for the lysosomal trafficking regulator (LYST) on chromosome 1 [34]. In addition to oculocutaneous albinism and dense-granule defects, patients often suffer from recurrent infections, neurologic symptoms, and an accelerated lymphoproliferative phase, leading to multiorgan failure and death by the first decade. All cell lines have cytoplasmic inclusions and the diagnosis is established by finding large peroxidase-positive granules in neutrophils. Similar to other dense-granule disorders, bleeding manifestations are mild to moderate. Hematopoietic stem cell transplantation is the only cure for this otherwise aggressive disease.

Alpha-granule disorders

Alpha-granules are more abundant than dense-granules and contain essential proteins synthesized by platelets as well as those endocytosed from the blood. Disorders of α-granules lack a consistent pattern on aggregometry but often have coexistent thrombocytopenia.

Gray platelet syndrome

Gray platelet syndrome (GPS) is an extremely rare condition characterized by the absence of α-granules on electron microscopy and a variable degree of thrombocytopenia. Platelets appear gray on the peripheral film, hence the name. Normal to elevated levels of PF4 have been noted in the plasma, suggesting that the underlying defect is in the packaging of α-granule contents rather than production [35]. Elevated plasma PDGF may lead to myelofibrosis in patients with GPS [35]. Both autosomal recessive and dominant inheritance are seen. Bleeding symptoms are mild to moderate but platelet counts can be as low as $20 \times 10^9/L$ and severe bleeding can occur. The diagnosis is confirmed by electron microscopy as platelet aggregation studies may be normal.

Quebec platelet syndrome

Quebec platelet syndrome (factor V Quebec) is a rather unique autosomal dominant condition. Alpha-granule contents are produced and packaged appropriately, but undergo premature degradation due to overexpression of urokinase-like plasminogen [36]. In this extremely rare condition, despite normal plasma factor V levels, platelet factor V levels are low. Unlike other platelet disorders, bleeding is delayed and severe, reminiscent of coagulopathies. Transfusing platelets does not improve bleeding but antifibrinolytics are effective. Thromboelastography (TEG) can aid diagnosis [37].

Signal transduction and receptor defects

Inherited platelet disorders can compromise any step of platelet activation. Defects have been identified in agonist receptors, G-proteins coupled to receptors, second messengers, and in the enzymes responsible for synthesizing effectors. Isolated platelet dysfunction without thrombocytopenia is usually seen in these conditions. Patients may be asymptomatic or have mild bleeding. Most remain undiagnosed due to minimal symptoms.

Defects in receptors for thromboxane A2, collagen (Gp-Ia/IIa and Gp-VI), epinephrine, and ADP have all been reported [38,39]. Aggregation is absent or impaired in response to the corresponding agonist but variable with other agonists. Of the three different ADP receptors, abnormalities have only been described in the $P2Y_{12}$ receptor, also the target of thienopyridines (e.g., clopidogrel). Bleeding is generally mild in this autosomal recessive disorder [39]. Platelets fail to aggregate with ADP and sometimes with TXA2.

G-proteins ($G\alpha q$, $G\alpha i_2$, $G\alpha s$) link receptors to effector enzymes in several cell lines. Patients with inherited G-protein disorders often have clinical manifestations in addition to bleeding due to the multitude of cells affected.

Thromboxane A2 is an important in-vivo platelet agonist which acts synergistically with other agonists and induces vasoconstriction at the site of injury. Case reports of patients lacking enzymes necessary for the production of TXA2 from arachidonic acid are present in the literature [40]. An aspirin-like defect is observed.

Cytoskeletal defects
MYH9-related disorders

MYH9-related disorders are autosomal dominant macrothrombocytopenias arising from mutations in the *MYH9* gene and include entities previously classified as May–Hegglin anomaly, Fetchner syndrome, Epstein syndrome, and Sebastian syndrome. It is now known that these disorders

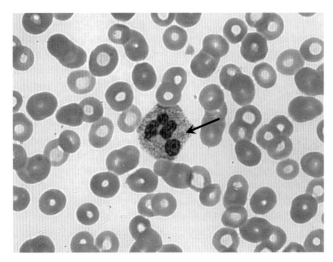

Figure 16.7 Döhle-like body (arrow). Image courtesy of Ling Zhang MD, Moffitt Cancer Center, Tampa, FL. (See also Plate 16.7.)

are not distinct syndromes, rather a spectrum of the same disease with different phenotypes.

The *MYH9* gene encodes for non-muscle myosin II-A heavy chain (NMMHC-IIA) abundant in the kidneys, cochlea, platelets, and neutrophils. Patients present with variable constellations of nephritis, sensorineural hearing loss, bleeding, and cataracts. Bleeding is a result of macrothrombocytopenia and a qualitative platelet dysfunction. NMMHC-IIA is a component of the platelet cytoskeleton and is involved in thrombopoiesis, platelet shape change upon activation, and proper expression of Gp-Ib/IX/V [41].

Albeit variable, bleeding is out of proportion to the degree of thrombocytopenia (platelet counts 20–130 $\times$ 10^9/L). The peripheral smear can be diagnostic. Giant platelets and Döhle-like bodies within neutrophils are seen. Döhle-like bodies are large intracellular myosin aggregates (Figure 16.7). Immunohistochemistry with anti-NMMHC-IIA can aid diagnosis; however, mutation studies are necessary for confirmation [41]. Many patients do not have renal failure, sensorineural hearing loss, or cataracts at presentation, but are at risk for developing them in the future and should be carefully monitored.

Wiskott–Aldrich syndrome

Wiskott–Aldrich syndrome (WAS) is an X-linked recessive disorder resulting from mutations in the WAS gene. Although clinical presentation is variable, a triad of microthrombocytopenia, eczema, and immunodeficiency is classic. The WAS protein responsible for transducing signals from the cell surface to the actin cytoskeleton is either deficient or dysfunctional. Exact phenotype depends on the particular mutation. Some patients may only develop thrombocytopenia (i.e., X-linked thrombocytopenia; XLT).

Most patients present in infancy with significant bleeding after circumcision, bruising, bloody diarrhea, and occasionally intraventricular hemorrhage. Humoral and cellular immune defects are both present, but bacterial sinopulmonary infections are most common. Eczema can be debilitating and predisposes to super-infection. Autoimmune hemolytic anemia, vasculitis, and malignancies are common.

Platelets are characteristically small and thrombocytopenia is present from birth (5–50 × 10^9/L) [17]. WAS should be suspected in any male infant presenting with bleeding and microthrombocytopenia. Genetic testing confirms the diagnosis. Flow cytometry may be helpful in the minority of patients who lack a detectable mutation [42]. Hematopoietic stem cell transplantation remains the only cure, although gene therapy is also being explored [43].

Others
Scott syndrome
In this extremely rare autosomal recessive condition, patients are unable to translocate phosphatidylserine (PS) from the inner to outer membrane leaflet of activated platelets. Since both Xase and prothrombinase require phosphatidylserine to generate thrombin, this results in a serious bleeding disorder. The exact molecular basis of Scott syndrome remains unclear but mutations in the *TMEM16F* gene have been proposed [44]. Platelet transfusions are therapeutic.

Treatment
Bleeding in inherited platelet disorders may vary from mild bruising to life-threatening hemorrhage. No diagnostic test reliably predicts bleeding and treatment has to be individualized. Platelet transfusions are often necessary in severe disorders (e.g., GT and BSS) whereas local measures and alternative therapies such as desmopressin and antifibrinolytics may suffice for milder conditions. Although necessary for life-threatening bleeding, platelet transfusions should be sparingly used due to the risk of alloimmunization and future platelet-refractoriness [45].

Prevention and local measures
Patients and families should be counseled regarding lifestyle issues such as avoidance of contact sports and antiplatelet agents (e.g., NSAIDs and aspirin). Special attention to dental hygiene from childhood can pre-empt future invasive dental procedures. All patients need to be vaccinated

against hepatitis B. Families must be educated about the risk of bleeding during dental and surgical procedures, and a comprehensive plan formulated prior to elective procedures. Prenatal diagnosis is available for some disorders and should be offered to affected families.

Local measures such as compression or application of topical sealants (thrombin or fibrin) remain the mainstay of treatment for mild bleeding and superficial wounds. Epistaxis refractory to compression may be controlled with nasal packing. Antifibrinolytic mouthwashes (e.g., tranexamic acid) can help prevent or control oral mucosal bleeding. Intrauterine devices (IUDs) and endometrial ablation are options for refractory menorrhagia, particularly when fertility is not desired.

Antifibrinolytics
Use of antifibrinolytics (aminocaproic acid and tranexamic acid) for epistaxis, gingival bleeding, or menorrhagia can be platelet-sparing. Available in oral and intravenous forms, these agents are effective alone in mild platelet disorders or as adjuncts to other therapies in more severe disorders.

Desmopressin
Intravenous, subcutaneous, or intranasal desmopressin/DDAVP (1-desamino-8-D-arginine vasopressin) can variably improve bleeding symptoms in patients with platelet disorders. The exact mechanism of action is unknown, but is likely related to release of VWF and factor VIII from endothelial cells [46]. As an off-label use, desmopressin is given intravenously at a dose of 0.3 µg/kg (maximum dose 20 µg) over 30 minutes prior to procedures [47]. Doses may be repeated after 12 hours, although tachyphylaxis occurs. Hyponatremia with seizures is a serious adverse reaction necessitating fluid restriction and careful electrolyte monitoring. Desmopressin must be used cautiously in the elderly. It is most effective in mild platelet disorders. Some patients with BSS and HPS also respond, but desmopressin rarely improves bleeding time in patients with GT [46].

Hormonal therapy
Menorrhagia can be troublesome in young females and most patients require some form of treatment. Antifibrinolytics or intranasal desmopressin at the start of menses may mitigate bleeding. Oral contraceptives or depo-medroxyprogesterone administered subcutaneously are effective alternatives. High-dose intravenous estrogens can be used for more severe bleeding.

Platelet transfusions

Platelet transfusions remain the most effective treatment for bleeding due to platelet dysfunction. Most patients with mild conditions do not require transfusions, but those with severe disorders such as BSS and GT need platelets for trauma, bleeding, and preoperative prophylaxis. In addition to transfusion-associated risks, the most feared complication is alloimmunization and future platelet-refractoriness. Antibodies may form against either HLA alloantigens or missing isoantigens. Unfortunately, the patients most likely to require transfusions are also those most likely to develop antibodies. In one study antibodies were found in 29 of 54 GT (49%) patients evaluated; 16 had anti-Gp-IIb/IIIa, 8 had anti-HLA, and 5 had both [45]. Smaller studies have reported prevalence rates ranging from 25% to 81%, the highest among patients completely lacking Gp-IIb/IIIa (type 1 GT) [48].

Avoiding unnecessary platelet transfusions is crucial to prevent alloimmunization. However, transfusions should not be withheld in life-threatening situations. Use of leuko-reduced blood products and single-donor platelets can minimize the chances of alloimmunization. All patients must be HLA typed at diagnosis and whenever possible HLA-matched platelets transfused. In disorders with concomitant immunodeficiency, irradiated blood products are necessary to prevent transfusion-associated graft-versus-host disease. If stem cell transplantation is being contemplated, blood products from related donors should be avoided. Alternative therapies should be utilized in conjunction with transfusions to minimize platelet use.

Recombinant factor VIIa

Recombinant factor VIIa (rFVIIa), approved in the US for treatment of hemophilia with inhibitors, is approved in Europe for GT with antibodies and platelet-refractoriness. Data for use in inherited platelet disorders is limited. Its approval in Europe was based on an international registry of 59 GT patients and a few case reports. In the registry, rFVIIa was utilized for 34 invasive procedures and 108 bleeding episodes; 29 patients had platelet antibodies and 23 were platelet refractory. Of the evaluable events, rFVIIa was effective for 29/31 (94%) invasive procedures and 69/103 (67%) bleeding events. It was less effective in GI bleeds (9/17; 53%) [45]. For severe bleeds, the authors recommend a regimen of 90 μg/kg every 2 hours until bleeding ceases; lower doses were less effective. Two patients receiving continuous infusion rFVIIa developed thromboembolic complications [45].

Experience in other inherited platelet disorders is even more limited, but rFVIIa appears to be an effective adjunct or alternative to platelet transfusions for both perioperative prophylaxis and treatment of bleeding in severe platelet disorders.

Hematopoietic stem cell transplantation

Hematopoietic stem cell transplantation (HSCT) carries significant morbidity and mortality. It is not usually recommended for bleeding but may be indicated for other reasons in select inherited platelet disorders such as immunodeficiency in WAS, aplasia in CAMT, and multi-organ failure in the accelerated phase of CHS. Transplantation has been performed in a handful of patients with severe refractory GT or BSS with variable results [49].

Future therapeutic approaches

Gene therapy is a promising approach being evaluated in WAS and GT models [43]. With an improved understanding of the underlying genetic defects in inherited platelet disorders and further research, one day we may have curative therapies for these maladies.

Acquired platelet disorders

Acquired disorders of platelet function are far more common than inherited disorders. Mucocutaneous bleeding in the absence of thrombocytopenia or a family history should raise suspicion of an acquired platelet dysfunction. A detailed history of comorbid conditions and medications is often revealing. After ruling out VWD, platelet function tests can aid the diagnosis. In contrast to inherited disorders, the pathophysiology of most acquired conditions is less well understood and usually multifactorial. Coexistent thrombocytopenia often complicates the picture. If possible, treatment should aim at correcting the underlying acquired condition (e.g., removal of the offending drug, or dialysis). General therapies discussed above for inherited disorders are also effective for acquired conditions and, despite normal counts, platelet transfusions may be needed.

Drugs

Drugs are the most common etiology of acquired platelet dysfunction. Numerous medications affect platelet function in vitro but only a few are clinically relevant in otherwise healthy subjects. Most important are the antiplatelet agents, which predictably inhibit platelet function and are used therapeutically to prevent or treat arterial thrombosis. Aspirin is the oldest antithrombotic which inhibits platelet aggregation by irreversibly acetylating cyclooxygenase-1 (COX-1), the enzyme responsible for thromboxane A2 (TXA2) production. Platelet adhesion is not impaired by aspirin.

Risk of bleeding with aspirin alone is low, but its combined use with other antiplatelet agents (e.g., clopidogrel) or with anticoagulants (e.g., warfarin) is associated with increased bleeding [50]. One large meta-analysis reported major bleeds in 0.1% per year in subjects taking low-dose aspirin versus 0.07% in the placebo group [51]. A recent prospective study reported a much higher, almost fivefold incidence [52]. In addition to its antiplatelet effects, aspirin inhibits COX-1-dependent prostaglandin production in the gastric mucosa promoting gastrointestinal bleeding. A single dose of 325 mg or three daily doses of low-dose aspirin (e.g., 81 mg) completely inhibit TXA2 synthesis with effects lasting for the lifespan of platelets (7–10 days). Higher doses of aspirin do not enhance antiplatelet activity; however, risk of gastrointestinal bleeding increases significantly. An analysis of 192,036 patients enrolled in 31 clinical trials reported a statistically significant increased risk of major and minor bleeding in patients receiving high-dose (>200 mg/day) versus low-dose aspirin (<100 mg/day) [53]. A minority of patients have a suboptimal antiplatelet response to aspirin, but the exact mechanism for this "aspirin resistance" is not clearly understood. Increased platelet turnover, genetic polymorphisms, and alternate pathways of platelet activation are all proposed mechanisms.

Other non-steroidal anti-inflammatory drugs (NSAIDs) also inhibit COX-1 and platelet function but their effects are reversible and short-lived. Platelet function assays normalize within 24 hours of taking 600 mg of ibuprofen [54]. Major bleeding due to NSAIDs is uncommon but gastrointestinal bleeding due to prostaglandin inhibition and gastric ulceration is a concern, particularly at high doses. Inhibitors of COX-2 have minimal effects on platelet function.

Thienopyridines are a group of antithrombotics that inhibit platelet aggregation by irreversibly blocking the $P2Y_{12}$ ADP receptor. Three thienopyridines are currently approved by the FDA: ticlopidine, clopidogrel, and prasugrel. Ticlopidine is rarely used nowadays due to concerns for hematologic toxicity and thrombotic thrombocytopenic purpura (TTP). Clopidogrel is used for secondary stroke prevention and in conjunction with aspirin after coronary artery stent placement. Risk of bleeding is much higher when used in combination with aspirin [50]. The recently approved drug ticagrelor also inhibits $P2Y_{12}$ receptors, but unlike thienopyridines it is a reversible inhibitor and does not require biotransformation to become active [55].

Gp-IIb/IIIa antagonists are frequently used during percutaneous coronary interventions in conjunction with heparin and aspirin. Approved agents include the antibody abciximab, and two smaller molecules, eptifibatide and tirofiban. By blocking binding of Gp-IIb/IIIa to fibrinogen, they inhibit aggregation and lead to mucocutaneous bleeding mimicking

Glanzmann's thrombasthenia. Occasionally they induce severe thrombo-cytopenia even after the first exposure. Antiplatelet effects of the antibody abciximab can persist for several days but the half-life of the other agents is much shorter.

Phosphodiesterase inhibitors (e.g., dipyridamole) block degradation of cAMP and act as weak antiplatelet agents. A new class of drugs targeting the thrombin receptor (PAR-1) is currently under development.

Drug-induced platelet dysfunction can also be seen as a side effect of other commonly used agents. It is usually clinically insignificant, unless there is concomitant thrombocytopenia or a preexisting bleeding diathesis. Notable exceptions include the β-lactam antibiotics which inhibit platelet aggrega-tion by interfering with binding of agonists to receptors [56]. Penicillins and less commonly cephalosporins prolong bleeding time and, at high doses, can lead to hemorrhage. Another class of drugs increasingly implicated are the antidepressant selective serotonin reuptake inhibitors (SSRIs). By decreas-ing platelet uptake of serotonin, SSRIs induce a storage pool-like defect and increase the risk of postoperative bleeding [57]. Various food supplements (e.g., omega-3 fatty acids), herbals (e.g., ginkgo), and alcohol also impair platelet function. Given their increasing popularity, supplements are becom-ing an important cause of acquired platelet dysfunction.

Renal failure

Hemorrhage due to platelet dysfunction is common in uremia. Adhesion, aggregation, and secretion are all impaired. The pathophysiology is complex but accumulation of substances normally excreted by the kidneys likely leads to dysfunction. This is supported by the observation that plate-let function improves with dialysis. Furthermore, platelet dysfunction resolves within 8 weeks of renal transplantation. Guanidinosuccinic acid (GSA), a nitric oxide (NO) donor, is found at higher levels in patients with renal failure. Increased NO inhibits platelets through activation of guan-ylate cyclase and elevation of cGMP levels [58].

Patients with chronic kidney disease often have concomitant anemia and thrombocytopenia. Fewer red blood cells in the central bloodstream are unable to displace platelets outwards, resulting in decreased platelet–vessel wall interactions and adhesion. Correction of anemia with blood transfusions or erythropoietin improves bleeding [59]. The most effective treatment for uremic bleeding is aggressive dialysis. Acute life-threatening bleeds warrant platelet transfusions. Desmopressin and high-dose estro-gens are useful adjuncts.

Liver disease

Gastrointestinal bleeding can be challenging in patients with cirrhosis. Although studies have shown functional platelet abnormalities in liver disease, bleeding is usually a result of thrombocytopenia, coagulopathy, and vascular malformations. Platelet dysfunction likely exacerbates bleeding but the underlying mechanisms are unclear.

Paraproteinemia

Bleeding in Waldenström's macroglobulinemia, multiple myeloma, and other plasma cell dyscrasias is multifactorial but paraprotein-induced platelet dysfunction is of particular interest. Paraproteins nonspecifically coat the platelet surface and interfere with adhesion, aggregation, and other platelet–platelet interactions. Platelet transfusions are largely ineffective as transfused platelets quickly become coated and lose function. Removal of the abnormal protein by plasmapheresis remains the single most effective therapy for significant bleeding. Treatment of the underlying clonal disorder results in longer remissions. Acquired VWD frequently complicates plasma cell dyscrasias.

Myeloproliferative disorders

At least partly a result of platelet dysfunction, thrombosis and hemorrhage are both seen in patients with myeloproliferative disorders (MPDs). Arterial thrombosis is more common than hemorrhage and likely a result of increased platelet activation in vivo. Additionally, platelets in MPDs are derived from the abnormal clonal stem cell with aberrant expression of c-MPL, surface glycoproteins, and P-selectin [60]. Reduced incidence of thrombosis with cytoreductive therapy suggests the role of elevated cell counts. Low-dose aspirin can effectively reduce thrombotic complications in patients with MPDs [61].

Bleeding is more frequently seen in MPD patients with extremely high platelet counts. Prolonged bleeding time and closure time on PFA-100, and impaired aggregation studies have all been reported. Although functional platelet abnormalities are contributory, they are not the dominant mechanism. Large numbers of platelets can adsorb and clear high-molecular-weight VWF, inducing a type 2 VWD-like disorder and hemorrhage.

Cardiopulmonary bypass

During cardiopulmonary bypass, exposure to non-physiologic surfaces activates platelets and leads to degranulation ex vivo. Degranulation combined with prolonged hypothermia, exposure to large doses of heparin, and alteration in glycoprotein expression results in platelet dysfunction [62]. Platelet dysfunction after bypass is usually transient; however, platelet transfusions may be required if bleeding is prolonged or persistent. Thrombocytopenia due to adherence to foreign surfaces frequently accompanies dysfunction and promotes bleeding.

Summary

Platelets are anucleate blood cells essential for hemostasis. Through various glycoprotein interactions and a complex series of events, platelets establish primary hemostasis and activate the coagulation system following injury. A number of inherited and acquired conditions can interfere with these steps and result in platelet dysfunction with or without significant bleeding. Inherited disorders are rare, but have been instrumental in enhancing our understanding of normal platelet physiology. Acquired disorders are far more prevalent but less well understood. A detailed personal and family history can help narrow the differential, but diagnostic tests are often required for confirmation. Hence knowledge of the various laboratory tests available is essential for accurate diagnosis and monitoring. Unfortunately, no test can reliably predict bleeding in a particular patient and treatment has to be individualized. Exact therapy depends on the underlying defect and entails general as well as specific measures. Desmopressin, antifibrinolytics, oral contraceptives, and rFVIIa may control mild to moderate bleeding and minimize the need for platelet transfusions. Although necessary for life-threatening hemorrhage, platelet transfusions should be used judiciously. In acquired disorders, efforts should also be directed at controlling the underlying disease or removing the offending drug.

References

1. Chang Y, Bluteau D, Debili N, Vainchenker W. From hematopoietic stem cells to platelets. *J Thromb Haemost* 2007;5:318–27.
2. Dowling MR, Josefsson EC, Henley KJ, et al. Platelet senescence is regulated by an internal timer, not damage inflicted by hits. *Blood* 2010;116:1776–8.
3. Gerrard JM, White JG, Peterson DA. The platelet dense tubular system: its relationship to prostaglandin synthesis and calcium flux. *Thromb Haemost* 1978;40:224–31.
4. Maynard DM, Heijnen HF, Horne MK, et al. Proteomic analysis of platelet alpha-granules using mass spectrometry. *J Thromb Haemost* 2007;5:1945–55.
5. Siess W, Siegel FL, Lapetina EG. Arachidonic acid stimulates the formation of 1,2-diacylglycerol and phosphatidic acid in human platelets. Degree of phospholipase C activation correlates with protein phosphorylation, platelet shape change, serotonin release, and aggregation. *J Biol Chem* 1983;258:11236–42.
6. Peterson P, Hayes TE, Arkin CF, et al. The preoperative bleeding time test lacks clinical benefit: College of American Pathologists' and American Society of Clinical Pathologists' position article. *Arch Surg* 1998;133:134–9.
7. Sadler JE. Von Willebrand disease type 1: a diagnosis in search of a disease. *Blood* 2003;101:2089–93.
8. Sadler JE, Rodeghiero F. Provisional criteria for the diagnosis of VWD type 1. *J Thromb Haemost* 2005;3:775–7.

9. Lombarts AJ, de Kieviet W. Recognition and prevention of pseudothrombocytopenia and concomitant pseudoleukocytosis. *Am J Clin Pathol* 1988;89:634–9.

10. Lind SE. The bleeding time does not predict surgical bleeding. *Blood* 1991;77:2547–52.

11. Rodgers RP, Levin J. A critical reappraisal of the bleeding time. *Semin Thromb Hemost* 1990;16:1–20.

12. Jilma B. Platelet function analyzer (PFA-100): a tool to quantify congenital or acquired platelet dysfunction. *J Lab Clin Med* 2001;138:152–63.

13. Homoncik M, Jilma B, Hergovich N, et al. Monitoring of aspirin (ASA) pharmacodynamics with the platelet function analyzer PFA-100. *Thromb Haemost* 2000;83:316–21.

14. Favaloro EJ. Clinical application of the PFA-100. *Curr Opin Hematol* 2002;9:407–15.

15. Seegmiller A, Sarode R. Laboratory evaluation of platelet function. *Hematol Oncol Clin North Am* 2007;21:731–42,vii.

16. Hayward CP, Moffat KA, Raby A, et al. Development of North American consensus guidelines for medical laboratories that perform and interpret platelet function testing using light transmission aggregometry. *Am J Clin Pathol* 2010;134:955–63.

17. Bolton-Maggs PH, Chalmers EA, Collins PW, et al. A review of inherited platelet disorders with guidelines for their management on behalf of the UKHCDO. *Br J Haematol* 2006;135:603–33.

18. Dyszkiewicz-Korpanty AM, Frenkel EP, Sarode R. Approach to the assessment of platelet function: comparison between optical-based platelet-rich plasma and impedance-based whole blood platelet aggregation methods. *Clin Appl Thromb Hemost* 2005;11:25–35.

19. Nieuwenhuis HK, Akkerman JW, Sixma JJ. Patients with a prolonged bleeding time and normal aggregation tests may have storage pool deficiency: studies on one hundred six patients. *Blood* 1987;70:620–3.

20. Bernard J, Soulier JP. [Not available]. *Bull Mem Soc Med Hop Paris* 1948;64:969–74.

21. Poujol C, Ware J, Nieswandt B, et al. Absence of GPIbalpha is responsible for aberrant membrane development during megakaryocyte maturation: ultrastructural study using a transgenic model. *Exp Hematol* 2002;30:352–60.

22. Savoia A, Balduini CL, Savino M, et al. Autosomal dominant macrothrombocytopenia in Italy is most frequently a type of heterozygous Bernard–Soulier syndrome. *Blood* 2001;97:1330–5.

23. Poujol C, Ramakrishnan V, DeGuzman F, et al. Ultrastructural analysis of megakaryocytes in GPV knockout mice. *Thromb Haemost* 2000;84:312–18.

24. Lopez JA, Andrews RK, Afshar-Kharghan V, Berndt MC. Bernard–Soulier syndrome. *Blood* 1998;91:4397–418.

25. Linden MD, Frelinger AL, 3rd, Barnard MR, et al. Application of flow cytometry to platelet disorders. *Semin Thromb Hemost* 2004;30:501–11.

26. George JN, Caen JP, Nurden AT. Glanzmann's thrombasthenia: the spectrum of clinical disease. *Blood* 1990;75:1383–95.

27. French D. The Samuel Bronfman Department of Medicine: Glanzmann thrombasthenia database. [updated 06/29/2012; cited July 5, 2012]; Available from: http://sinaicentral.mssm.edu/intranet/research/glanzmann/listmutations?mut=all.

28. Khanduri U, Pulimood R, Sudarsanam A, et al. Glanzmann's thrombasthenia. A review and report of 42 cases from South India. *Thromb Haemost* 1981;46:717–21.

29. Schlegel N, Gayet O, Morel-Kopp MC, et al. The molecular genetic basis of Glanzmann's thrombasthenia in a gypsy population in France: identification of a new mutation on the alpha IIb gene. *Blood* 1995;86:977–82.

30. Seligsohn U, Rososhansky S. A Glanzmann's thrombasthenia cluster among Iraqi Jews in Israel. *Thromb Haemost* 1984;52:230–1.
31. Nurden AT, Fiore M, Pillois X, Nurden P. Genetic testing in the diagnostic evaluation of inherited platelet disorders. *Semin Thromb Hemost* 2009;35:204–12.
32. Witkop CJ, Nunez Babcock M, Rao GH, et al. Albinism and Hermansky–Pudlak syndrome in Puerto Rico. *Bol Asoc Med P R* 1990;82:333–9.
33. Wei ML. Hermansky–Pudlak syndrome: a disease of protein trafficking and organelle function. *Pigment Cell Res* 2006;19:19–42.
34. Nagle DL, Karim MA, Woolf EA, et al. Identification and mutation analysis of the complete gene for Chediak–Higashi syndrome. *Nat Genet* 1996;14:307–11.
35. Caen JP, Deschamps JF, Bodevin E, et al. Megakaryocytes and myelofibrosis in gray platelet syndrome. *Nouv Rev Fr Haematol* 1987;29:109–14.
36. Kahr WH, Zheng S, Sheth PM, et al. Platelets from patients with the Quebec platelet disorder contain and secrete abnormal amounts of urokinase-type plasminogen activator. *Blood* 2001;98:257–65.
37. Diamandis M, Adam F, Kahr WH, et al. Insights into abnormal hemostasis in the Quebec platelet disorder from analyses of clot lysis. *J Thromb Haemost* 2006;4: 1086–94.
38. Nurden A, Nurden P. Advances in our understanding of the molecular basis of disorders of platelet function. *J Thromb Haemost* 2011;9:76–91.
39. Cattaneo M. The platelet P2Y(1)(2) receptor for adenosine diphosphate: congenital and drug-induced defects. *Blood* 2011;117:2102–12.
40. Dube JN, Drouin J, Aminian M, et al. Characterization of a partial prostaglandin endoperoxide H synthase-1 deficiency in a patient with a bleeding disorder. *Br J Haematol* 2001;113:878–85.
41. Balduini CL, Pecci A, Savoia A. Recent advances in the understanding and management of MYH9-related inherited thrombocytopenias. *Br J Haematol* 2011;154: 161–74.
42. Ariga T, Nakajima M, Yoshida J, et al. Confirming or excluding the diagnosis of Wiskott–Aldrich syndrome in children with thrombocytopenia of an unknown etiology. *J Pediatr Hematol Oncol* 2004;26:435–40.
43. Boztug K, Schmidt M, Schwarzer A, et al. Stem-cell gene therapy for the Wiskott–Aldrich syndrome. *N Engl J Med* 2010;363:1918–27.
44. Suzuki J, Umeda M, Sims PJ, Nagata S. Calcium-dependent phospholipid scrambling by TMEM16F. *Nature* 2010;468:834–8.
45. Poon MC, D'Oiron R, Von Depka M, et al. Prophylactic and therapeutic recombinant factor VIIa administration to patients with Glanzmann's thrombasthenia: results of an international survey. *J Thromb Haemost* 2004;2:1096–103.
46. Coppola A, Di Minno G. Desmopressin in inherited disorders of platelet function. *Haemophilia* 2008;14:31–9.
47. Seligsohn U. Treatment of inherited platelet disorders. *Haemophilia* 2012;18:161–5.
48. Fiore M, Firah N, Pillois X, et al. Natural history of platelet antibody formation against alpha-IIb/beta3 in a French cohort of Glanzmann thrombasthenia patients. *Haemophilia* 2012;18:e201–9.
49. Alamelu J, Liesner R. Modern management of severe platelet function disorders. *Br J Haematol* 2010;149:813–23.
50. Diener HC, Bogousslavsky J, Brass LM, et al. Aspirin and clopidogrel compared with clopidogrel alone after recent ischaemic stroke or transient ischaemic attack in high-risk patients (MATCH): randomised, double-blind, placebo-controlled trial. *Lancet* 2004;364:331–7.

51. Baigent C, Blackwell L, Collins R, et al. Aspirin in the primary and secondary prevention of vascular disease: collaborative meta-analysis of individual participant data from randomised trials. *Lancet* 2009;373:1849–60.

52. De Berardis G, Lucisano G, D'Ettorre A, et al. Association of aspirin use with major bleeding in patients with and without diabetes. *JAMA* 2012;307:2286–94.

53. Serebruany VL, Steinhubl SR, Berger PB, et al. Analysis of risk of bleeding complications after different doses of aspirin in 192,036 patients enrolled in 31 randomized controlled trials. *Am J Cardiol* 2005;95:1218–22.

54. McIntyre BA, Philp RB, Inwood MJ. Effect of ibuprofen on platelet function in normal subjects and hemophiliac patients. *Clin Pharmacol Ther* 1978;24:616–21.

55. Giannitsis E, Katus HA. Antiplatelet therapy – ticagrelor. *Hamostaseologie* 2012;32:177–85.

56. Shattil SJ, Bennett JS, McDonough M, Turnbull J. Carbenicillin and penicillin G inhibit platelet function in vitro by impairing the interaction of agonists with the platelet surface. *J Clin Invest* 1980;65:329–37.

57. Gartner R, Cronin-Fenton D, Hundborg HH, et al. Use of selective serotonin reuptake inhibitors and risk of re-operation due to post-surgical bleeding in breast cancer patients: a Danish population-based cohort study. *BMC Surg* 2010;10:3.

58. Noris M, Remuzzi G. Uremic bleeding: closing the circle after 30 years of controversies? *Blood* 1999;94:2569–74.

59. Zwaginga JJ, MJ IJ, de Groot PG, et al. Treatment of uremic anemia with recombinant erythropoietin also reduces the defects in platelet adhesion and aggregation caused by uremic plasma. *Thromb Haemost* 1991;66:638–47.

60. Elliott MA, Tefferi A. Thrombosis and haemorrhage in polycythaemia vera and essential thrombocythaemia. *Br J Haematol* 2005;128:275–90.

61. Landolfi R, Marchioli R, Kutti J, et al. Efficacy and safety of low-dose aspirin in polycythemia vera. *N Engl J Med* 2004;350:114–24.

62. Linden MD. The hemostatic defect of cardiopulmonary bypass. *J Thromb Thrombolysis* 2003;16:129–47.

CHAPTER 17

Contributions of Platelet Polyphosphate to Hemostasis and Thrombosis

James H. Morrissey
Biochemistry Department, University of Illinois, Urbana, IL, USA

Introduction

Polyphosphate (polyP) is an inorganic molecule consisting of linear polymers of phosphates linked together via phosphoanhydride bonds – the same kind of high-energy bonds that link the phosphates together in ATP (Figure 17.1). Polyphosphate is present from microbes to humans, with polymer lengths that can vary from just a few phosphates to thousands of phosphates long, depending on the species and cell type [1,2]. Since each internal phosphate carries a charge of −1, polyphosphate is a highly anionic polymer. The biosynthesis of polyP in higher eukaryotes is poorly understood, but in microorganisms it is synthesized enzymatically by transferring the γ phosphate of ATP to the end of the growing polyP chain [3]. PolyP is degraded by both endopolyphosphatases (cleaving phosphoanhydride bonds within the polyP chain) and exopolyphosphatases (sequentially removing terminal phosphates from polyP). Mammalian alkaline phosphatase has potent exopolyphosphatase activity [4]. PolyP decays in human blood or plasma with a half-life of about 90 minutes, apparently due to degradation by phosphatases [5,6].

The biology of polyP has not been studied as extensively in mammals as it has been in microbes [3]. This is now changing, with polyP having been identified in mammals in lysosomes [7], platelet dense granules [8], mast cell granules [9], mitochondria, and nuclei [10]. This chapter focuses on recent studies that have proposed important roles for polyP in hemostasis, thrombosis, and inflammation [5,11–19].

Hemostasis and Thrombosis: Practical Guidelines in Clinical Management, First Edition.
Hussain I. Saba and Harold R. Roberts.
© 2014 John Wiley & Sons, Ltd. Published 2014 by John Wiley & Sons, Ltd.

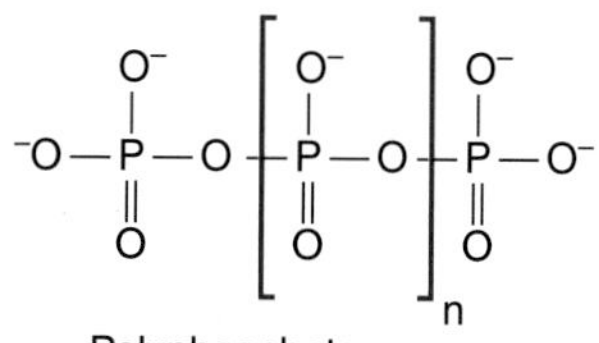

$$^-O-\overset{\displaystyle O^-}{\underset{\displaystyle O}{\overset{\displaystyle |}{\underset{\displaystyle \|}{P}}}}-O\left[\overset{\displaystyle O^-}{\underset{\displaystyle O}{\overset{\displaystyle |}{\underset{\displaystyle \|}{P}}}}-O\right]_n\overset{\displaystyle O^-}{\underset{\displaystyle O}{\overset{\displaystyle |}{\underset{\displaystyle \|}{P}}}}-O^-$$

Polyphosphate

Figure 17.1 PolyP structure. PolyP is a linear polymer of inorganic orthophosphates connected via by high-energy phosphoanhydride bonds. PolyP secreted by activated platelets is approximately 60–100 phosphate units long [8,13,15], while polyP in microbes ranges from dozens to thousands of phosphates long [3,44].

Platelet polyP

In eukaryotes, polyP biology has been studied most extensively in micro-organisms such as trypanosomes and yeast, in which polyP is known to accumulate to high levels in acidocalcisomes and yeast vacuoles [20]. Acidocalcisomes are acidic organelles containing Ca^{2+} and other metal ions, along with abundant levels of phosphates in the form of pyrophosphate (PP_i) and poly P. Acidocalcisomes are thought to function in multiple processes in eukaryotic cells, including: osmoregulation; storage of metal ions and phosphorus; metabolism of PP_i and poly P; calcium homeostasis; and maintenance of intracellular pH. A number of studies have suggested that acidocalcisomes are part of the lysosome-related group of organelles in eukaryotes [20].

In 2004, Ruiz et al. [8] noted that the dense granules of human platelets bear a striking resemblance to acidocalcisomes of trypanosomes and other unicellular organisms. Both acidocalcisomes and platelet dense granules are spherical, acidic [21], electron-dense [22], and contain Na^+, Ca^{2+}, and Mg^{2+} [23]. Platelet dense granules also contain PP_i [23], another hallmark of acidocalcisomes. To test the notion that platelet dense granules may be a type of acidocalcisome, Ruiz et al. [8] isolated dense granules from human platelets and showed that they contained abundant levels of polyP. Furthermore, they found that activated platelets secrete polyP in amounts that could reach about 1–3 µM in whole blood. (Note that polyP concentrations are typically expressed as the concentration of phosphate monomer.) Consistent with this earlier finding, Hernández-Ruiz et al. [24] subsequently reported that patients with hereditary platelet dense granule defects have platelet polyP levels tenfold lower than normal. Microbial polyP is typically very polydisperse, with polymer lengths from hundreds to thousands of phosphate units long [3]. In contrast, polyP in human platelets is shorter and much more uniform in size, with polymer lengths of about 60–100 phosphate units [8,13].

PolyP and the contact pathway of blood clotting

Prompted by the discovery that activated human platelets secrete significant quantities of polyP [8], we began investigating whether polyP could
modulate the blood clotting system. Since polyP and heparin are both
highly anionic, linear polymers, one might expect polyP to be anticoagulant, like heparin. Indeed, back in 1988, Church et al. [25] reported that
polyP (and certain other highly phosphorylated polymers and proteins)
could accelerate the rate inhibition of thrombin by heparin cofactor II,
although polyP had no effect on the inactivation of thrombin by antithrombin. In 2006, we reported that polyP of approximately the size range
secreted by human platelets is strongly procoagulant when added to human
plasma [5]. In particular, we found that polyP initiates the contact (or
intrinsic) pathway of blood clotting. For many years, the contact pathway
has been known to be triggered when plasma comes into contact with a
variety of artificial substances, most of which are anionic surfaces or polymers. Typical contact activators used in such studies include glass, clay
(kaolin), diatomaceous earth, dextran sulfate, ellagic acid, or high concentrations of sulfatides, but the true activators of this pathway in vivo have
been elusive. In recent years, a number of candidates have been identified
as physiologic/pathophysiologic activators of the contact pathway, including extracellular RNA, collagen, misfolded proteins, and certain bacterial
substances (reviewed by Maas and Renné [26]).

PolyP can now be added to the relatively short list of potential pathophysiologic activators of the contact pathway, and subsequent work from
our lab and others has delved into the mechanisms by which polyP modulates blood clotting [5,15,27]. Triggering of clotting by polyP exhibits a
bell-shaped concentration-dependence, consistent with polyP functioning
as a template for assembling the multiple proteins necessary to initiate
clotting via the contact pathway [5,15]. The ability of polyP to trigger the
contact pathway is highly dependent on polyP polymer length, with specific activity increasing dramatically with increasing polymer length [15].
Microbes tend to accumulate long-chain polyP (up to thousands of phosphates long) and, in fact, polyP purified from *Salmonella* is extremely
potent in triggering the contact pathway [15]. Platelet polyP is considerably shorter ($\sim$60 to 100 phosphates long) and, while it can measurably
trigger the contact pathway [5,13], it is thousands of times less potent than
long-chain polyP [15].

The findings that platelets secrete polyP and that polyP can trigger clotting via the contact pathway provide a potential mechanism for reports
dating back to the 1960s that activated human platelets exhibit a weak
but measurable ability to trigger clotting in a factor XII-dependent manner
[28]. On the other hand, the relatively low specific activity of platelet

polyP in triggering the contact pathway is consistent with the concept that platelets are very effective at accelerating blood clotting but are much weaker at initiating clotting. This is also consistent with findings from both humans and animals that the proteins responsible for triggering the contact pathway (factor XII, prekallikrein, and high-molecular-weight kininogen) are all dispensable for normal hemostasis [26]. It seems reasonable to conclude that the ability of polyP to trigger the contact pathway, which requires very long polyP polymers for optimal activity, may function in host responses to pathogens and possibly also thrombotic disease, rather than normal hemostasis [19].

Acceleration of thrombin generation by polyP

Factor Va occupies a central place in blood clotting as the essential protein cofactor for the activation of prothrombin by factor Xa. PolyP accelerates the rate of factor V activation by factor Xa and thrombin, which results in an earlier thrombin burst during the clotting of human plasma [5]. This procoagulant activity of polyP requires much shorter polymers than are required for triggering the contact pathway, and is optimal with polyP polymers of the size secreted by activated platelets, and just a bit longer [15]. PolyP's ability to accelerate the rate of factor V activation during plasma clotting reactions has the interesting consequence of abrogating the anticoagulant function of tissue factor pathway inhibitor (TFPI) [5,15]. Mast and Broze [29] had previously shown that TFPI has little ability to inhibit factor Xa within the prothrombinase complex (i.e., once factor Xa binds to factor Va, and especially in the presence of its substrate, prothrombin). We found that simply adding preactivated factor Va to plasma is as effective in abrogating the anticoagulant activity of TFPI as is adding polyP to plasma [5]. The releasates from activated human platelets also inhibit the anticoagulant function of TFPI, with the majority of this activity being directly attributable to the presence of polyP in the releasates [5,13].

Effects of polyP on fibrin clot structure and fibrinolysis

Adding polyP to clotting reactions consisting of purified fibrinogen and thrombin, in the presence of plasma concentrations of Ca^{2+}, results in fibrin clots that are more turbid than in the absence of polyP. The resulting fibrin fibrils have higher mass/length ratios, and are more resistant to elastic stretching and fibrinolysis than are clots formed in the absence of polyP [12,18]. Such clots stain in a characteristic way with toluidine blue, indicating that polyP may be directly incorporated into fibrin clots [12]. Part of the antifibrinolytic effect of polyP is mediated by thrombin-activatable fibrinolysis inhibitor (TAFI) [5], but much of the effect may be due to direct interactions between polyP and fibrin that decrease the ability of fibrinolytic proteases (in particular, tissue-type plasminogen activator and plasminogen) to associate with fibrin and thus to degrade the fibrin strands [18]. PolyP in the size range secreted by activated human platelets – and just a bit longer – is very effective in enhancing fibrin clot structure and delaying fibrinolysis [15]. This work also showed that PP_i potently blocks the ability of polyP to enhance fibrin clot structure [15]. While activated platelets are known to secrete PP_i, biological roles for this secreted PP_i have been elusive. Platelet PP_i may thus be a regulator of fibrin structure.

Platelet polyP and the role of factor XI in normal hemostasis

In classic models of the blood coagulation cascade, factor XIIa activates factor XI, with the resulting factor XIa activating factor IX. However, severe deficiencies in factor XII do not lead to bleeding problems in either humans or mice, while severe factor XI deficiencies are associated with bleeding diatheses in humans – particularly following surgery or trauma in tissues with a high fibrinolytic potential [30]. Thus, for factor XI to have a role in normal hemostasis, it must be activated by a protease other than factor XIIa. A potential answer to this conundrum was provided in 1991, when two groups reported that factor XI can be back-activated by thrombin, providing a feedback loop that could cause sustained thrombin generation and diminished fibrinolysis TAFI activation [31,32]. On the other hand, the kinetics for back-activation of factor XI by thrombin are very slow unless one adds a nonphysiologic polyanion like dextran sulfate or heparin to the reactions [31–34], leading some to question the physiologic significance of factor XI activation by thrombin in plasma [35]. We recently found that polyP accelerates factor XI activation by thrombin (and factor XI autoactivation) by orders of magnitude [17]. Furthermore, we found that platelet releasates strongly accelerate factor XI activation by thrombin, and that essentially all of this activity is due to polyP. We also found that polyP of the size released by platelets binds to thrombin and factor XI; this finding and others suggest that polyP acts as a template for factor XI/XIa and thrombin, thereby accelerating the rate of factor XI activation [17]. Thus, platelet polyP appears to act as a potent, natural cofactor for factor XI activation, which may now explain how factor XI can function in normal hemostasis in a manner that is independent of factor XII and the rest of the contact pathway.

PolyP in thrombosis and inflammation

In vivo roles for polyP have recently been investigated in mouse models of thrombosis and inflammation [13,36]. High doses of polyP injected intravenously into mice resulted in lethal pulmonary embolism, but mice deficient in factor XII given factor XIIa inhibitors survived the polyP challenge [13]. Factor XII-deficient mice were likewise protected from an otherwise lethal intravenous dose of an agonist peptide that stimulates protease-activated receptors, as were wild-type mice that had been administered high levels of alkaline phosphatase (a potent exopolyphosphatase) [13]. Thus, polyP can be highly thrombogenic in vivo, in a factor XII-dependent manner [13].

A proinflammatory consequence of activating the contact pathway of blood clotting is the proteolytic release of the vasoactive peptide, bradykinin, from high-molecular-weight kininogen. Injecting wild-type mice subcutaneously with polyP provoked localized capillary leak, which was not observed in mice lacking factor XII or bradykinin B_2 receptors [13]. Intraperitoneal injection of bacterial polyP into wild-type mice caused a rapid drop in blood pressure and death of 90% of the mice, but mice without factor XII or bradykinin B_2 receptors survived [13]. PolyP can therefore be proinflammatory in vivo, in a factor XII- and bradykinin-dependent manner.

In another proinflammatory pathway, polyP was recently shown to enhance the ability of extracellular histones to activate platelets and promote thrombin generation [16]. The mechanism for this effect is not known and, surprisingly, appears to be independent of factor XII or tissue factor. In yet another proinflammatory mechanism, cultured endothelial cells have been shown to respond to polyP, in an NF-κB-dependent manner, resulting in enhanced barrier permeability, increased apoptosis, and upregulation of cell adhesion molecules [37].

PolyP as a potential drug target

The contributions of polyP to thrombosis and inflammation make it a potential target for new antithrombotic drugs, possibly with reduced bleeding risk compared with conventional anticoagulant/antithrombotic agents. In one approach to inhibiting the procoagulant activity of polyP, we have used the isolated recombinant polyP-binding domain of *E. coli* exopolyphosphatase to block the ability of polyP in platelet releasates to stimulate factor XI activation by thrombin [17]. Other studies have chosen to degrade polyP with phosphatases, including recombinant yeast exopolyphosphatase [38] and alkaline phosphatase (a highly active exopolyphosphatase, albeit not specific for polyP) [5,13]. Injecting alkaline phosphatase was shown to diminish activation of the contact system, bradykinin generation, and thrombosis in mice [13]. Another approach is to use the isolated polyP-binding domain of *E. coli* exopolyphosphatase (PPXbd) in a manner analogous to using a blocking antibody. PPXbd has previously been used to localize polyP in yeast [39], in mast cell granules [9], and in acidocalcisomes of the eggs of sea urchins [40] and insects [41]. We have employed PPXbd successfully to block polyP procoagulant activity in vitro [17,36].

Most recently, our lab undertook a large-scale, high-throughput screen for polyP inhibitors [36]. The screen was based on blocking the binding of thrombin to immobilized polyP which, in turn, was based on the knowledge that polyP binds with high affinity to exosite II of thrombin [14]. We identified several cationic small molecules, polymers, and proteins (including PPXbd) that potently inhibit polyP procoagulant activity as assessed in a variety of in vitro clotting assays using plasma and whole blood [36]. At the concentrations used in the study, the two inhibitors chosen for intensive study (a generation 1.0 cationic PAMAM dendrimer and the antibiotic, polymyxin B) strongly inhibited clotting triggered by polyP but not by tissue factor. These polyP inhibitors significantly diminished the severity of both arterial and venous thrombosis in mouse models, and the generation 1.0 dendrimer significantly blocked polyP-induced capillary leak in the skin of mice. Another study showed similar efficacy of a generation 3.0 cationic PAMAM dendrimer in attenuating thrombosis in mice, while not promoting bleeding in a mouse surgical model [42]. These studies, therefore, provide proof of principle that polyP represents an attractive target for developing novel antithrombotic and anti-inflammatory drugs with potentially decreased bleeding risk compared to drugs that directly target clotting proteases.

Conclusions and future directions

PolyP of the type secreted by activated human platelets accelerates factor V activation, abrogates the anticoagulant function of TFPI, enhances fibrin clot structure, inhibits fibrinolysis, and very potently promotes the activation of factor XI by thrombin and factor XIa. PolyP can also reverse the activity of several anticoagulant drugs [11]. These findings help to explain how platelets enhance plasma clotting reactions – perhaps surprisingly, by secreting an inorganic compound instead of a protein.

It is likely that polyP has other roles in blood. Recently, polyP was shown to be present in mast cells, co-localizing with serotonin- but not with histamine-containing granules [9]. Activated mast cells secrete polyP, suggesting that polyP could help mediate proinflammatory and procoagulant activities of mast cells.

In another very recent study, polyP was shown to bind to purified von Willebrand factor (VWF); and furthermore, circulating VWF isolated from human platelets and plasma was shown to contain tightly bound polyP [43]. PolyP was shown to enhance VWF ristocetin cofactor activity but not to alter binding of VWF to collagen or VWF multimerization.

Doubtless, there are many more contributions of polyP to platelet function that remain to be elucidated.

Acknowledgments

The author's studies were supported by grant R01 HL047014 from the National Heart, Lung and Blood Institute of the National Institutes of Health. Conflict-of-interest disclosure: the author is a co-inventor on patents and pending patent applications on medical uses of polyP.

References

1. Ault-Riché D, Fraley CD, Tzeng CM, Kornberg A. Novel assay reveals multiple pathways regulating stress-induced accumulations of inorganic polyphosphate in *Escherichia coli*. *J Bacteriol* 1998;180:1841–7.
2. Brown MR, Kornberg A. Inorganic polyphosphate in the origin and survival of species. *Proc Natl Acad Sci USA* 2004;101:16085–7.
3. Kornberg A, Rao NN, Ault-Riché D. Inorganic polyphosphate: a molecule of many functions. *Annu Rev Biochem* 1999;68:89–125.
4. Lorenz B, Schröder HC. Mammalian intestinal alkaline phosphatase acts as highly active exopolyphosphatase. *Biochim Biophys Acta* 2001;1547:254–61.
5. Smith SA, Mutch NJ, Baskar D, et al. Polyphosphate modulates blood coagulation and fibrinolysis. *Proc Natl Acad Sci USA* 2006;103:903–8.
6. Lorenz B, Leuck J, Kohl D, Muller WE, Schröder HC. Anti-HIV-1 activity of inorganic polyphosphates. *J Acquir Immune Defic Syndr Hum Retrovirol* 1997;14:110–18.
7. Pisoni RL, Lindley ER. Incorporation of [^{32}P]orthophosphate into long chains of inorganic polyphosphate within lysosomes of human fibroblasts. *J Biol Chem* 1992; 267:3626–31.
8. Ruiz FA, Lea CR, Oldfield E, Docampo R. Human platelet dense granules contain polyphosphate and are similar to acidocalcisomes of bacteria and unicellular eukaryotes. *J Biol Chem* 2004;279:44250–7.

9. Moreno-Sanchez D, Hernandez-Ruiz L, Ruiz FA, Docampo R. Polyphosphate is a novel pro-inflammatory regulator of mast cells and is located in acidocalcisomes. *J Biol Chem* 2012;287:28435–44.

10. Kornberg A. Inorganic polyphosphate: toward making a forgotten polymer unforgettable. *J Bacteriol* 1995;177:491–6.

11. Smith SA, Morrissey JH. Polyphosphate as a general procoagulant agent. *J Thromb Haemost* 2008;6:1750–6.

12. Smith SA, Morrissey JH. Polyphosphate enhances fibrin clot structure. *Blood* 2008;112:2810–16.

13. Müller F, Mutch NJ, Schenk WA, et al. Platelet polyphosphates are proinflammatory and procoagulant mediators in vivo. *Cell* 2009;139:1143–56.

14. Mutch NJ, Myles T, Leung LL, Morrissey JH. Polyphosphate binds with high affinity to exosite II of thrombin. *J Thromb Haemost* 2010;8:548–55.

15. Smith SA, Choi SH, Davis-Harrison R, et al. Polyphosphate exerts differential effects on blood clotting, depending on polymer size. *Blood* 2010;116:4353–9.

16. Semeraro F, Ammollo CT, Morrissey JH, et al. Extracellular histones promote thrombin generation through platelet-dependent mechanisms: involvement of platelet TLR2 and TLR4. *Blood* 2011;118:1952–61.

17. Choi SH, Smith SA, Morrissey JH. Polyphosphate is a cofactor for the activation of factor XI by thrombin. *Blood* 2011;118:6963–70.

18. Mutch NJ, Engel R, Uitte de Willige S, et al. Polyphosphate modifies the fibrin network and down-regulates fibrinolysis by attenuating binding of tPA and plasminogen to fibrin. *Blood* 2010;115:3980–8.

19. Morrissey JH, Choi SH, Smith SA. Polyphosphate: an ancient molecule that links platelets, coagulation, and inflammation. *Blood* 2012;119:5972–9.

20. Docampo R, Moreno SN. Acidocalcisomes. *Cell Calcium* 2011;50:113–19.

21. Dean GE, Fishkes H, Nelson PJ, Rudnick G. The hydrogen ion-pumping adenosine triphosphatase of platelet dense granule membrane: differences from F_1F_0- and phosphoenzyme-type ATPases. *J Biol Chem* 1984;259:9569–74.

22. White JG. The dense bodies of human platelets: inherent electron opacity of the serotonin storage particles. *Blood* 1969;33:598–606.

23. Fukami MH, Dangelmaier CA, Bauer JS, Holmsen H. Secretion, subcellular localization and metabolic status of inorganic pyrophosphate in human platelets: a major constituent of the amine-storing granules. *Biochem J* 1980;192:99–105.

24. Hernández-Ruiz L, Sáez-Benito A, Pujol-Moix N, et al. Platelet inorganic polyphosphate decreases in patients with delta storage pool disease. *J Thromb Haemost* 2009;7:361–3.

25. Church FC, Pratt CW, Treanor RE, Whinna HC. Antithrombin action of phosvitin and other phosphate-containing polyanions is mediated by heparin cofactor II. *FEBS Lett* 1988;237:26–30.

26. Maas C, Renne T. Regulatory mechanisms of the plasma contact system. *Thromb Res* 2012;129(suppl 2):S73–6.

27. Choi SH, Collins JN, Smith SA, et al. Phosphoramidate end labeling of inorganic polyphosphates: facile manipulation of polyphosphate for investigating and modulating its biological activities. *Biochemistry* 2010;49:9935–41.

28. Caen J, Wu Q. Hageman factor, platelets and polyphosphates: early history and recent connection. *J Thromb Haemost* 2010;8:1670–4.

29. Mast AE, Broze GJ, Jr. Physiological concentrations of tissue factor pathway inhibitor do not inhibit prothrombinase. *Blood* 1996;87:1845–50.

30. Walsh PN, Gailani D, Factor XI. In Colman RW, Marder VJ, Clowes AW, George JN, Goldhaber SZ (eds), *Hemostasis and Thrombosis: Basic Principles and Clinical Practice*, 5th edition. Philadelphia: Lippincott Williams & Wilkins, 2006;221–33.

31. Naito K, Fujikawa K. Activation of human blood coagulation factor XI independent of factor XII. Factor XI is activated by thrombin and factor XIa in the presence of negatively charged surfaces. *J Biol Chem* 1991;266:7353–8.

32. Gailani D, Broze GJ, Jr. Factor XI activation in a revised model of blood coagulation. *Science* 1991;253:909–12.

33. Gailani D, Broze GJ, Jr. Factor XII-independent activation of factor XI in plasma: effects of sulfatides on tissue factor-induced coagulation. *Blood* 1993;82:813–19.

34. Gailani D, Broze GJ, Jr. Effects of glycosaminoglycans on factor XI activation by thrombin. *Blood Coagul Fibrinolysis* 1993;4:15–20.

35. Pedicord DL, Seiffert D, Blat Y. Feedback activation of factor XI by thrombin does not occur in plasma. *Proc Natl Acad Sci USA* 2007;104:12855–60.

36. Smith SA, Choi SH, Collins JN, et al. Inhibition of polyphosphate as a novel strategy for preventing thrombosis and inflammation. *Blood* 2012;120:5103–10.

37. Bae JS, Lee W, Rezaie AR. Polyphosphate elicits pro-inflammatory responses that are counteracted by activated protein C in both cellular and animal models. *J Thromb Haemost* 2012;10:1145–51.

38. Jimenez-Nunez MD, Moreno-Sanchez D, Hernandez-Ruiz L, et al. Myeloma cells contain high levels of inorganic polyphosphate which is associated with nucleolar transcription. *Haematologica* 2012;97:1264–71.

39. Saito K, Ohtomo R, Kuga-Uetake Y, et al. Direct labeling of polyphosphate at the ultrastructural level in *Saccharomyces cerevisiae* by using the affinity of the polyphosphate binding domain of *Escherichia coli* exopolyphosphatase. *Appl Environ Microbiol* 2005;71:5692–701.

40. Ramos IB, Miranda K, Pace DA, et al. Calcium- and polyphosphate-containing acidic granules of sea urchin eggs are similar to acidocalcisomes, but are not the targets for NAADP. *Biochem J* 2010;429:485–95.

41. Ramos I, Gomes F, Koeller CM, et al. Acidocalcisomes as calcium- and polyphosphate-storage compartments during embryogenesis of the insect *Rhodnius prolixus* Stahl. *PloS one* 2011;6:e27276.

42. Jain S, Pitoc GA, Holl EK, et al. Nucleic acid scavengers inhibit thrombosis without increasing bleeding. *Proc Natl Acad Sci USA* 2012;109:12938–43.

43. Montilla M, Hernández-Ruiz L, García-Cozar FJ, et al. Polyphosphate binds to human von Willebrand factor *in vivo* and modulates its interaction with glycoprotein Ib. *J Thromb Haemost* 2012;10:2315–23.

44. Brown MR, Kornberg A. The long and short of it – polyphosphate, PPK and bacterial survival. *Trends Biochem Sci* 2008;33:284–90.

CHAPTER 18

Thrombotic Microangiopathy: Biology, Diagnosis, and Management

Samir Dalia[1] and Hussain I. Saba[2]
[1]H. Lee Moffitt Cancer & Research Center, University of South Florida, Tampa, FL, USA
[2]Hematology and Oncology, University of South Florida, Tampa, FL, USA

History and pathophysiology

Thrombotic microangiopathy refers to a group of disorders in which a microangiopathic hemolytic anemia (MHA), thrombocytopenia, and microvascular thrombosis lead to dysfunction of various organs. Disorders such as thrombotic thrombocytopenic purpura (TTP) and hemolytic uremic syndrome (HUS) are in the spectrum of thrombotic microangiopathy. They differ in pathophysiology, but can be difficult to distinguish by clinical features. Prompt diagnosis and treatment are required to reduce morbidity and mortality, especially in cases of TTP.

History: thrombotic thrombocytopenic purpura

TTP is a form of thrombotic microangiopathy in which there is MHA, thrombocytopenia with neurologic damage, and fever. Renal failure can be present but is usually non-oliguric. TTP was first described by Eli Moschcowitz in 1924 when he reported the case of a 16-year-old girl with fever, severe anemia, leukocytosis, petechiae, and hemiparesis with normal renal function. She became comatose and died 2 weeks after her first symptoms. On autopsy, hyaline thrombi were found diffusely in terminal arterioles and capillaries [1]. In 1966, a review of 272 published cases defined the major clinical features of TTP [2]. They described a classic "pentad" in patients with TTP, including thrombocytopenia, hemolytic anemia with schistocytes, neurologic findings, renal damage, and fever. There was a 90% mortality rate with an average hospital stay of 14 days

Hemostasis and Thrombosis: Practical Guidelines in Clinical Management, First Edition.
Hussain I. Saba and Harold R. Roberts.

prior to death. Splenectomy was shown to provide dramatic recovery in some cases. By 1976, whole blood exchange was used to attempt to treat TTP and resulted in remissions in 8 patients of a case series of 14 patients [3]. By 1991 plasma exchange became the treatment of choice and reduced mortality to less than 20% [4]. Based upon the Oklahoma TTP-HUS registry, which records all TTP or HUS patients who receive plasma exchange in 58 of 77 Oklahoma counties, it is estimated that TTP in the United States occurs at 4.5 per million per year with a peak incidence between ages 30 and 50; 40% of patients present with idiopathic TTP. Risk factors include gender (female), African ancestry, and obesity [5].

Pathophysiology: thrombotic thrombocytopenic purpura

TTP is thought to be secondary to a disintegrin and metalloproteinase with a thrombospondin type 1 motif, member 13 (ADAMTS-13) deficiency that leads to ultra large von Willebrand factor (VWF) which, in turn, leads to platelet thrombosis [6–9]. Large VWF multimers mediate platelet adhesion at areas of vascular injury. When VWF multimers bind to collagen under conditions of high fluid shear stress, the VWF multimer is stretched and is accessible to ADAMTS-13. ADAMTS13 normally cleaves the large VWF multimer but, in TTP, the deficiency leads to platelet aggregation and thrombus formation [5–7, 10, 11].

TTP is usually caused by a IgG autoantibody that inhibit ADAMTS-13 [11]. Thrombi and subendothelial hyaline deposits are found in the small arterioles and capillaries of any organ, with common organs being the myocardium, pancreas, kidney, adrenal, and brain.

History: hemolytic uremic syndrome

HUS refers to thrombotic microangiopathy that mainly affects the kidney and leads to oliguric-anuric renal failure. Typical HUS or diarrhea-associated HUS is caused by enteric infections with Shiga toxin-producing organisms and occurs in patients without any other predisposing conditions. HUS was first proposed in 1995 for thrombotic microangiopathy occurring in children and associated with acute anuric renal failure [10,12–15]. This was preceded by a diarrheal illness and most patients survived and recovered normal renal function with only supportive care.

Pathophysiology: hemolytic uremic syndrome

Diarrhea-associated HUS (typical HUS) usually occurs in patients younger than 10 years of age and arises sporadically. It is associated with the ingestion of foods or other materials contaminated with Shiga toxin-producing bacteria. *Escherichia coli* O157:H7 accounts for 80% of cases [16,17]. It can also be caused by other toxin-bearing *E. coli* or by *Shigella dysenteriae* type 1. ADAMTS-13 levels are normal in patients with typical HUS.

Non-diarrheal HUS (atypical HUS) is much less common and is defined as MHA, thrombocytopenia, and anuric renal failure. Half of the cases are secondary to inherited defects in complement regulatory proteins. Loss of function in factor H, membrane cofactor protein, factor I, factor H-related proteins 1 and 3, and C4 binding protein have all been found in patients with atypical HUS [18].

Congenital thrombotic thrombocytopenic purpura: Upshaw–Schulman syndrome

Congenital TTP refers to TTP that is caused by inherited deficiency of ADAMTS-13 with an inactivation of *ADAMTS-13* gene on chromosome 9q34 [7]. The mutation impairs the synthesis or secretion of ADAMTS-13. Patients usually present in infancy and have neonatal jaundice and hemolysis without any ABO blood group or Rh incompatibility. Half of these patients have a chronic relapsing course from infancy. Acute exacerbations are triggered by infections, pregnancy, stress, or surgery. Most patients have some renal involvement with proteinuria, hematuria, and elevated creatinine. Chronic renal failure can occur. Congenital TTP is treated with periodic fresh frozen plasma infusions. The frequency of relapses varies among individuals and prophylactic plasma may not be needed in all cases [5,19–21].

Diagnosis

Clinical features: thrombotic thrombocytopenic purpura

TTP remains a clinically diagnosed disease. The classic pentad of microangiopathic hemolytic anemia, thrombocytopenia, fever, neurologic dysfunction, and renal failure occurs in less than 20% of cases [15]. Only microangiopathic hemolytic anemia and thrombocytopenia are required to make a diagnosis of TTP today. Microangiopathic hemolytic anemia is established by evaluating a peripheral blood smear for more than two schistocytes per 100× high-power field. There should be an increase in indirect bilirubin, an elevated serum lactate dehydrogenase (LDH), and a negative direct antiglobulin test. Thrombocytopenia can be severe but usually has a mean platelet count of 25,000/μL [15,21]. When fever is present, other entities such as sepsis need to be ruled out. Neurologic symptoms can range from headache to stroke-like symptoms. Renal involvement ranges from mild proteinuria to kidney failure requiring dialysis. Microthrombi may lead to chest pain or myocardial infarction in patients with cardiac involvement. Gastrointestinal symptoms include abdominal pain; nausea and vomiting are common. Infrequent findings

Box 18.1 Secondary causes of TTP

Drugs

Quinine: the most common drug causing TTP

Chemotherapeutic agents (usually dose-dependent)

- Mitomycin C
- Cisplatin
- Oxaliplatin
- Pentostatin
- Bevacizumab
- Bleomycin
- Gemcitabine

Ticlopidine

Clopidogrel

Cyclosporine

Tacrolimus

Valacyclovir

Cancer

Disseminated malignancy, especially mucin-producing adenocarcinomas

Allogenic transplant associated microangiopathy

Pregnancy

HIV infection

Less in post-HAART era

Cardiovascular surgery

Idiopathic

include retinal hemorrhage or detachment, arthralgia, myalgia, or Raynaud phenomenon.

There are multiple secondary causes of TTP. Box 18.1 lists common secondary causes of TTP that should be excluded in all patents with a clinical presentation of TTP.

Laboratory features: thrombotic thrombocytopenic purpura

Review of the peripheral blood smear is required to diagnosis TTP. A marked increase in schistocytes, irregularly shaped fragments of split red cells with two or more sharp projections, should be seen. Hemolysis will be indicated by an elevated LDH, decreased serum haptoglobin, elevated reticulocyte count, and indirect hyperbilirubinemia. Plasma fibrinogen, prothrombin time, and activated partial thromboplastin time are normal. Direct antiglobulin test is almost always negative. Evidence of myocardial

---

damage is commonly seen by elevations of troponin T levels. ADAMTS-13 functional assays can be sent out in order to confirm a deficiency, but results are not usually received in time to aid in a treatment plan [22,23].

Clinical and laboratory features: hemolytic uremic syndrome

Typical HUS is more commonly seen in children younger than the age of 10 years. The disease presents with painful diarrhea without fever that evolves to bloody diarrhea within 3 days of ingestion of the bacteria. MHA, thrombocytopenia, and renal injury follow. Renal signs include proteinuria, hematuria, and elevated creatinine, with anuria and oliguria being common. PT and aPTT are normal and ADAMTS-13 levels are normal. Serologies can be sent for causative organisms [24].

Atypical HUS is much less common and diagnosis and laboratory workup should be similar to that for TTP, with attention to renal involvement.

Differential diagnosis

In addition to the multiple drug-induced causes of TTP there are other disease processes which can have a similar presentation. Disseminated intravascular coagulation (DIC) secondary to infection or other processes should be considered, especially in those with elevated PT and aPTT levels. Vasculitis should be considered in those individuals with peripheral neurologic involvement and rash without a low platelet count. Malignant hypertension should be considered in those with papilledema or a history of hypertension. Aspergillus and cytomegalovirus infections and catastrophic antiphospholipid syndrome should also be considered. In pregnant patients postpartum renal failure and thrombocytopenia along with the HELLP syndrome should be considered [14,15,21]. Box 18.2 summarizes the differential diagnosis in TTP/HUS.

Box 18.2 Differential diagnosis for TTP/HUS

Disseminated intravascular coagulation
Pregnancy-associated
• Preeclampsia
• Eclampsia
• HELLP syndrome
Autoimmmune disorders
• Antiphospholipid syndrome
• Vasculitis include systemic lupus erythematosus
• Evans syndrome
Malignant hypertension
Aspergillus infection
Cytomegalovirus infection

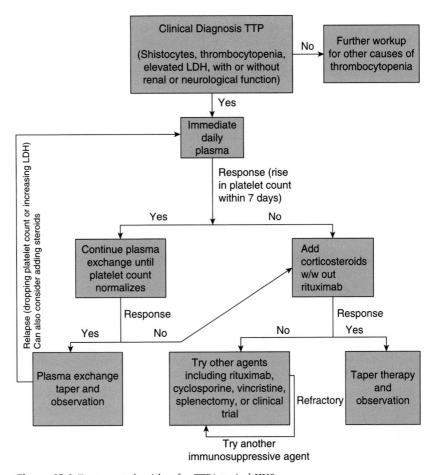

Figure 18.1 Treatment algorithm for TTP/atypical HUS.

Treatment: thrombotic thrombocytopenic purpura

Acute

Figure 18.1 shows a treatment algorithm for TTP/atypical HUS.

Plasma exchange

Initially, plasma infusion was used to treat TTP with variable success. Plasma exchange was tried as well and showed promising results. Neither was ever compared to placebo because both were shown to improve survival in TTP. It was not until 1991 that Rock et al. carried out a randomized trial that proved plasma exchange was superior to plasma infusion to treat. In this trial, plasma exchange at 1–1.5 times plasma volume was randomized against plasma infusion at 30 mL/kg on day 1 followed by 15 mL/kg until platelets returned to normal. At 6 months of follow-up 78% of those in the plasma exchange group survived against 63% in the plasma infusion group. The findings were statistically significant with a *p*-value of 0.04. From this study, plasma exchange became the standard first-line therapy in TTP [4]. Experts and systematic reviews also agree that plasma exchange is the standard of care for patients with TTP [5,25–31].

Plasma exchange should be initiated within 24 hours of a suspected case of TTP. Plasma exchange is administered through an apheresis catheter, which must be placed in order to initiate treatment; 1–1.5 times plasma volume is the normal amount of plasma that is exchanged. Fresh frozen plasma is used most frequently, but other plasma components such as cryoprecipitate have been shown to work just as well. Plasma exchange should be continued daily until the platelet count normalizes and hemolysis stops (LDH normal). The average number of treatment days required is 7–16 [4,5,21,32]. There is no expert consensus on how to taper plasma exchange once the platelet count has normalized, with some experts stopping it completely and watching the platelet count for relapse while others taper therapy over a longer period of time.

The Oklahoma TTP-HUS registry showed that complications of plasma exchange included venous thrombosis, hypotension, systemic infection, catheter insertion complications including pneumothorax, and death from sepsis or hemorrhage from catheter insertion. In the registry of 249 patients, 26% had a major complication with three deaths reported [5,32].

Corticosteroids

There is no randomized clinical trial that compares plasma exchange alone to plasma exchange and corticosteroids as first-line therapy in acute TTP. Most experts agree that, since corticosteroids have shown a response in patients with low levels of ADAMTS-13, they should be added as first-line therapy [5,33,34]. Prednisone at 1 mg/kg/day or methylprednisone (125 mg intravenously twice daily) can be used in conjunction with plasma exchange.

Refractory or relapsed

In 10–20% of patients TTP is refractory to plasma exchange, or relapses after a period of remission. Refractory TTP is defined as TTP in which the platelet count does not improve after 7–10 days of plasma exchange therapy. Plasma exchange should not be stopped in the refractory setting. Other agents should be added to improve outcomes.

Corticosteroids

If corticosteroids were not used in conjunction with plasma exchange as first-line therapy, they should be started in refractory cases. One randomized study compared high-dose to regular-dose corticosteroids in TTP.

This study showed benefit with the addition of corticosteroids, but failed to show a statistical difference between high-dose and regular-dose corticosteroids [33]. If relapse occurs after corticosteroids are tapered, experts agree to increase the dose to high-dose steroids to see if there will be an effect on platelet count. If corticosteroids were not initially used, either prednisone at 1 mg/kg/day or methylprednisone at 125 mg intravenously twice daily are recommended [5,25,34,35].

Rituximab

Rituximab is the most studied agent for refractory and relapsed TTP. Two systematic reviews show that 93% of patients have a clinical benefit with the addition of this monoclonal antibody [36,37]. In one study of 118 patients with TTP between 2002 and 2009, clinical remission was documented in 85% of patients treated with rituximab [36]; 65% of these patients had refractory disease. Complete remission was achieved after between two and eight cycles of therapy [36].

Rituximab was also studied in a phase II clinical trial as first-line therapy in conjunction with corticosteroids and plasma exchange. The number of plasma exchanges was not reduced and there was no difference in survival when compared to historical controls [38]. The STAR study was a phase III clinical trial to assess rituximab use in the front line. This study was terminated due to poor accrual.

While it is unclear if rituximab should be used as a first-line agent, it is the drug of choice for refractory or relapsed disease.

Other agents

There are multiple other agents that have been tested to assess response in refractory or relapsed TTP.

Cyclosporine

Cyclosporine is a promising immunosuppressant with very little current data. One study comparing outcomes at 30 days post treatment showed that a cohort of patients treated with cyclosporine and plasma exchange had fewer relapses than patients treated with corticosteroids and plasma exchange [39]. This was a small study involving only 20 subjects but the results showed that cyclosporine may have activity in TTP. Currently, there is a phase II clinical trial comparing cyclosporine with plasma exchange to prednisone and plasma exchange in patients with TTP. Data collection should be complete by November 2012 [40].

Vincristine

Vincristine has also been shown to be active in relapsed TTP, especially when combined with other agents. Vincristine has only been reported to have efficacy in TTP in small case series and case reports. One case series described 8 patients in which vincristine at 2 mg intravenously weekly was used for relapsed TTP. Four of eight patients responded, with four deaths [41]. It remains a salvage option in TTP.

Danazol
Danazol is currently being tested in a phase II clinical trial to assess its efficacy in TTP. This trial will finish accrual in December 2013 [42].

Splenectomy
Splenectomy has been shown to result in lasting remissions for some patients with TTP who are refractory to plasma exchange or other second-line therapies. The proposed mechanism is that spleen removal eliminates a major site of anti-ADAMTS-13 antibody production. The addition of cyclosporine and splenectomy has been shown to result in remissions in refractory patients. Splenectomy should be used when other treatments fail to result in a remission [43–46].

Platelets
Direct harm from transfusion of platelets is hard to ascertain in the medical literature. Platelet transfusion should only be used in life-threatening cases or if needed with insertion of central venous access for plasma exchange. Ideally, platelets should be given after the start of plasma exchange [12,47].

In cases of chemotherapy-induced TTP or transplant-associated TTP, plasma exchange has not been shown to help the disease course. Supportive care measures are taken and the associated agent is removed [11,15].

Treatment: hemolytic uremic syndrome

Typical HUS may first be treated with plasma exchange because its etiology may initially be unknown. Once typical HUS is confirmed, plasma exchange can be stopped and supportive care should be initiated. Patients will recover on their own as the infection terminates. There is no role for antibiotics to treat the underlying cause. Dialysis may be required and chronic kidney disease may occur.

Atypical HUS, in general, should be treated similarly to TTP with plasma exchange as first-line therapy. New research has recently shown that, in patients with complement H defects, eculizumab (a monoclonal antibody against complement protein C5) has efficacy in treating patients with atypical HUS [48–50]. Further research is needed to confirm these findings.

Thrombotic thrombocytopenic purpura in pregnancy

TTP in pregnancy can be difficult to differentiate from gestational thrombocytopenia and the hemolysis, preeclampsia, eclampsia, acute fatty liver of pregnancy, and elevated liver enzymes, low platelet (HELLP) syndrome. ADAMTS-13 levels can help to differentiate TTP from HELLP syndrome (low in TTP) but can take multiple days for test results to be available. If TTP is suspected, treatment is similar to that used in non-pregnant patients. Plasma exchange should be immediately administered, and the role of corticosteroids is unclear. If the fetus is mature, delivery should be considered since HELLP syndrome and other causes of thrombocytopenia in pregnancy should improve after delivery. Management should involve both obstetric and hematologic teams while the patient is admitted to a hospital [51–54].

References

1. Moschcowitz E. An acute febrile pleiochromic anemia with hyaline thrombosis of the terminal arterioles and capillaries. *Arch Intern Med* 1925;36:89–93.
2. Amorosi EL, Ultmann JE. Thrombotic thrombocytopenic purpura: report of 16 cases and review of the literature. *Medicine* 1966;45:139–60.
3. Bukowski RM, Hewlett JS, Harris JW, et al. Exchange transfusions in the treatment of thrombotic thrombocytopenic purpura. *Sem Hematol* 1976;13:219–32.
4. Rock GA, Shumak KH, Buskard NA, et al. Comparison of plasma exchange with plasma infusion in the treatment of thrombotic thrombocytopenic purpura. Canadian Apheresis Study Group. *N Engl J Med* 1991;325:393–7.
5. George JN. How I treat patients with thrombotic thrombocytopenic purpura: *Blood* 2010;116:4060–9.
6. Zheng X, Majerus EM, Sadler JE. ADAMTS13 and TTP. *Curr Opin Hematol* 2002; 9:389–94.
7. Peyvandi F, Palla R, Lotta LA, et al. ADAMTS-13 assays in thrombotic thrombocytopenic purpura. *J Thromb Hemost* 2010;8:631–40.
8. Tsai HM, Lian EC. Antibodies to von Willebrand factor-cleaving protease in acute thrombotic thrombocytopenic purpura. *N Engl J Med* 1998;339:1585–94.
9. Furlan M, Robles R, Galbusera M, et al. von Willebrand factor-cleaving protease in thrombotic thrombocytopenic purpura and the hemolytic-uremic syndrome. *N Engl J Med* 1998;339:1578–84.
10. Zheng XL, Sadler JE. Pathogenesis of thrombotic microangiopathies. *Annu Rev Pathol* 2008;3:249–77.
11. Tsai HM. Pathophysiology of thrombotic thrombocytopenic purpura. *Int J Hematol* 2010;91:1–19.
12. George JN, Sadler JE, Lammle B. Platelets: thrombotic thrombocytopenic purpura. *Hematology Am Soc Educ Program* 2002:315–34.
13. Sadler JE, Moake JL, Miyata T, George JN. Recent advances in thrombotic thrombocytopenic purpura. *Hematology Am Soc Educ Program* 2004:407–23.
14. Elliott MA, Nichols WL. Thrombotic thrombocytopenic purpura and hemolytic uremic syndrome. *Mayo Clin Proc* 2001;76:1154–62.

15. George JN. The thrombotic thrombocytopenic purpura and hemolytic uremic syndromes: evaluation, management, and long-term outcomes experience of the Oklahoma TTP-HUS Registry, 1989–2007. *Kidney Int Suppl* 2009;112:S52–4.
16. Hosler GA, Cusumano AM, Hutchins GM. Thrombotic thrombocytopenic purpura and hemolytic uremic syndrome are distinct pathologic entities. A review of 56 autopsy cases. *Arch Path Lab Med* 2003;127:834–9.
17. Sadler JE. Thrombotic thrombocytopenic purpura: a moving target. *Hematology Am Soc Educ Program* 2006:415–20.
18. Kavanagh D, Richards A, Atkinson J. Complement regulatory genes and hemolytic uremic syndromes. *Annu Rev Med* 2008;59:293–309.
19. Schulman I, Pierce M, Lukens A, Currimbhoy Z. Studies on thrombopoiesis. I. A factor in normal human plasma required for platelet production; chronic thrombocytopenia due to its deficiency. *Blood* 1960;16:943–57.
20. Upshaw JD, Jr. Congenital deficiency of a factor in normal plasma that reverses microangiopathic hemolysis and thrombocytopenia. *N Engl J Med* 1978;298:1350–2.
21. George JN. Clinical practice. Thrombotic thrombocytopenic purpura. *N Engl J Med* 2006;354:1927–35.
22. Cataland SR, Wu HM. Practical issues in ADAMTS13 testing and emerging therapies in thrombotic thrombocytopenic purpura. *Sem Hematol* 2011;48:242–50.
23. Sadler JE. Von Willebrand factor, ADAMTS13, and thrombotic thrombocytopenic purpura. *Blood* 2008;112:11–18.
24. Michael M, Elliott EJ, Craig JC, et al. Interventions for hemolytic uremic syndrome and thrombotic thrombocytopenic purpura: a systematic review of randomized controlled trials. *Am J Kidney Dis* 2009;53:259–72.
25. George JN. Evaluation and management of patients with thrombotic thrombocytopenic purpura. *J Intens Care Med* 2007;22:82–91.
26. Rock GA. Management of thrombotic thrombocytopenic purpura. *Br J Haematol* 2000;109:496–507.
27. Rock G. Plasma exchange in the management of thrombotic thrombocytopenic purpura. *Vox Sang* 2002;83(S1):141–3.
28. Nguyen TC, Han YY. Plasma exchange therapy for thrombotic microangiopathies. *Organogenesis* 2011;7:28–31.
29. Brunskill SJ, Tusold A, Benjamin S, et al. A systematic review of randomized controlled trials for plasma exchange in the treatment of thrombotic thrombocytopenic purpura. *Trans Med* 2007;17:17–35.
30. Altuntas F, Aydogdu I, Kabukcu S, et al. Therapeutic plasma exchange for the treatment of thrombotic thrombocytopenic purpura: a retrospective multicenter study. *Transfus Apher Sci* 2007;36:57–67.
31. Bandarenko N, Brecher ME. United States Thrombotic Thrombocytopenic Purpura Apheresis Study Group (US TTP ASG): multicenter survey and retrospective analysis of current efficacy of therapeutic plasma exchange. *J Clin Apheresis* 1998;13:133–41.
32. George JN, Kremer Hovinga JA, Terrell DR, et al. The Oklahoma Thrombotic Thrombocytopenic Purpura-Hemolytic Uremic Syndrome Registry: the Swiss connection. *Euro J Haematol* 2008;80:277–86.
33. Balduini CL, Gugliotta L, Luppi M, et al. High versus standard dose methylprednisolone in the acute phase of idiopathic thrombotic thrombocytopenic purpura: a randomized study. *Ann Hematol* 2010;89:591–6.

34. Michael M, Elliott EJ, Ridley GF, et al. Interventions for haemolytic uraemic syndrome and thrombotic thrombocytopenic purpura. *Cochrane Database Syst Rev* 2009;21(1), CD003595.

35. Rock G, Porta C, Bobbio-Pallavicini E. Thrombotic thrombocytopenic purpura treatment in year 2000. *Haematologica* 2000;85:410–19.

36. Caramazza D, Quintini G, Abbene I, et al. Relapsing or refractory idiopathic thrombotic thrombocytopenic purpura-hemolytic uremic syndrome: the role of rituximab. *Transfusion* 2010;50:2753–60.

37. George JN, Woodson RD, Kiss JE, et al. Rituximab therapy for thrombotic thrombocytopenic purpura: a proposed study of the Transfusion Medicine/Hemostasis Clinical Trials Network with a systematic review of rituximab therapy for immune-mediated disorders. *J Clin Apheresis* 2006;21:49–56.

38. Scully M, McDonald V, Cavenagh J, et al. A phase 2 study of the safety and efficacy of rituximab with plasma exchange in acute acquired thrombotic thrombocytopenic purpura. *Blood* 2011;118:1746–53.

39. Cataland SR, Jin M, Ferketich AK, et al. An evaluation of cyclosporin and corticosteroids individually as adjuncts to plasma exchange in the treatment of thrombotic thrombocytopenic purpura. *Br J Haematol* 2007;136:146–9.

40. NCT00713193. Study of Cyclosporine or Corticosteroids as an Adjunct to Plasma Exchange in Thrombotic Thrombocytopenic Purpura (TTP). Clinical Trials.gov; 2012 [cited 2012 05/03]; Available from: http://clinicaltrials.gov/ct2/show/NCT00713193?term=thrombotic+thrombocytopenic&recr=Open&rank=3.

41. Bobbio-Pallavicini E, Porta C, Centurioni R, et al. Vincristine sulfate for the treatment of thrombotic thrombocytopenic purpura refractory to plasma-exchange. The Italian Cooperative Group for TTP. *Euro J Haematol* 1994;52:222–6.

42. NCT00953771. Safety Study of Danazol With Plasma Exchange and Steroids for the Treatment of Thrombotic Thrombocytopenic Purpura (TTP). 2012 [cited 2012 05/03]; Available from: http://clinicaltrials.gov/ct2/show/NCT00953771?term=danazol&rank=2.

43. Veltman GA, Brand A, Leeksma OC, et al. The role of splenectomy in the treatment of relapsing thrombotic thrombocytopenic purpura. *Ann Hematol* 1995;70:231–6.

44. Beloncle F, Buffet M, Coindre JP, et al. Splenectomy and/or cyclophosphamide as salvage therapies in thrombotic thrombocytopenic purpura: the French TMA Reference Center experience. *Transfusion* 2012;52:2436–44.

45. Kappers-Klunne MC, Wijermans P, Fijnheer R, et al. Splenectomy for the treatment of thrombotic thrombocytopenic purpura. *Br J Haematol* 2005;130:768–76.

46. Jhaveri KD, Scheuer A, Cohen J, Gordon B. Treatment of refractory thrombotic thrombocytopenic purpura using multimodality therapy including splenectomy and cyclosporine. *Trans Apher Sci* 2009;41:19–22.

47. Swisher KK, Terrell DR, Vesely SK, et al. Clinical outcomes after platelet transfusions in patients with thrombotic thrombocytopenic purpura. *Transfusion* 2009;49:873–87.

48. Nurnberger J, Philipp T, Witzke O, et al. Eculizumab for atypical hemolytic-uremic syndrome. *N Engl J Med* 2009;360:542–4.

49. Al-Akash SI, Almond PS, Savell VH, Jr., et al. Eculizumab induces long-term remission in recurrent post-transplant HUS associated with C3 gene mutation. *Pediatr Nephrol* 2011;26:613–19.

50. Kose O, Zimmerhackl LB, Jungraithmayr T, et al. New treatment options for atypical hemolytic uremic syndrome with the complement inhibitor eculizumab. *Sem Thromb Hemostas* 2010;36:669–72.

51. Baron JM, Baron BW. Thrombotic thrombocytopenic purpura and its look-alikes. *Clin Adv Hematol Oncol* 2005;3:868–74.

52. Pels SG, Paidas MJ. Microangiopathic disorders in pregnancy. *Hematol Oncol Clin North Am* 2011;25:311–22,viii.

53. McCrae KR. Thrombocytopenia in pregnancy. *Hematology Am Soc Hematol Educ Program* 2010;397–402.

54. Martin JN, Jr., Bailey AP, Rehberg JF, et al. Thrombotic thrombocytopenic purpura in 166 pregnancies: 1955–2006. *Am J Obstet Gynecol* 2008;199:98–104.

CHAPTER 19

Hemostasis and Aging

Lodovico Balducci
H. Lee Moffitt Cancer Center & Research Institute, Tampa, FL, USA

Introduction

This chapter explores the role of hemostasis in the aging process and in the diseases associated with aging. The goal is to achieve a better insight into the biology of aging which may help preventing its medical and social complications.

The world population is aging [1,2]. This phenomenon entails increased incidence and prevalence of chronic diseases [3,4] and of functional dependence [5] which lead to increased medical and social costs [2], and to a decline in the quality of life of older individuals [6]. Aging involves a number of systemic changes that conspire together to reduce a person's functional reserve and life expectancy, and result from the combination of genetic and environmental effects that are different for each individual. As it is highly individualized in terms of causes, mechanisms, and rate of development, aging is poorly reflected in chronologic age. Better than in demographic terms, aging is defined by physiologic outcomes. At most, chronologic age may be considered a landmark, generally established around age 70, beyond which the majority of individuals who are physiologically aged are found.

After providing an operational definition of aging, we will review clotting-related abnormalities in the aged person, the incidence and prevalence of clotting-related disease in the aged, and the related research opportunities.

Clinical definition of aging

Though a standard definition of aging is wanted, general agreement exists on these points:

Hemostasis and Thrombosis: Practical Guidelines in Clinical Management, First Edition.
Hussain I. Saba and Harold R. Roberts.
© 2014 John Wiley & Sons, Ltd. Published 2014 by John Wiley & Sons, Ltd.

- Aging implies a progressive reduction of a person's ability to withstand stress due to a progressive loss of the functional reserve of multiple organ systems [7].
- Aging is associated with polymorbidity [3] and may be associated with a decline in social resources [8]. Anemia represents a crossroads of multiple aging-related events [9]; as such, it may have a central role in aging. Chronic anemia, even mild anemia, is predictive of functional dependence, geriatric syndromes, and mortality [9].
- Aging implies allostasis, a progressive failure of homeostatic regulation [10], which is the ability of an organism to return to basic physiologic condition after stress. Inflammation has been the most studied of various manifestations of allostasis [11]. A chronic and progressive inflammation leads to activation of intravascular coagulation and of fibrinolysis in the aged.
- Aging is associated with increased risk of mortality that may be estimated from the extent of comorbidity and of functional decline [12].
- Aging is associated with a shortening of leukocyte telomeres [13,14].

Assessment of physiologic age

The physiologic age of a person may be expressed as the risk of unfavorable outcomes, especially mortality, functional dependence, and vulnerability to stress [12]. It may be assessed by clinical evaluation, laboratory parameters, functional tests, or a combination of these. A comprehensive geriatric assessment (CGA) (Table 19.1) provides the best validated estimate of physiologic age.

The basic activities of daily living (ADLs) are essential to support basic living and include continence, transferring, grooming, ability to go to the bathroom, to dress, and to eat without assistance. The IADLs are activities necessary for independent living, and include ability to use transportation, ability to take medications, to prepare one's own meal, to use the telephone, and to manage money.

Comorbidity may be associated with a reduction both in life expectancy and tolerance of stress [12,15–17]. Comorbidity may be assessed as number of comorbid conditions or as a comorbidity index reflecting the severity of each condition [18]. At the Moffitt Cancer Center, the Cumulative Index Rating Scale–Geriatric (CIRS-G) is commonly used [19]. In addition to being very comprehensive, the CIRS-G has the advantage that it may be converted into the Charlson's index, another comorbidity index in widespread use [19]. Two forms of comorbidity have special interest for the older cancer patient: depression and anemia [10,20]. Both conditions may be reversible and may compromise patients' function and treatment tolerance. In addition, chronic renal insufficiency, cancer, chronic pulmonary disease, and congestive heart failure are associated with increased

Table 19.1 Elements of a comprehensive geriatric assessment and potential clinical applications.

CGA element	Application
Functional status	
Activities of Daily Living (ADL) and Instrumental Activities of Daily Living (IADL)	Relation to life expectancy, functional dependence, and tolerance of stress
Comorbidity	
Number of comorbid conditions and comorbidity indices	Relation to life expectancy and tolerance of stress
Mental status	
Folstein Mini Mental Status	Relation to life expectancy and dependence
Emotional conditions	
Geriatric Depression Scale (GDS)	Relation to survival; may indicate motivation to receive treatment
Nutritional status	
Mini Nutritional Assessment (MNA)	Reversible condition; possible relationship to survival
Polypharmacy	
	Risk of drug interactions
Geriatric syndromes	
Delirium, dementia, depression, falls, incontinence, spontaneous bone fractures; neglect and abuse, failure to thrive	Relationship to survival; functional dependence

mortality risk [12,21]. The Geriatric Depression Scale is a simple 30-item, self-administered questionnaire very sensitive to subclinical depression, and is a practical instrument to screen older individuals [20]. The optimal level of hemoglobin is controversial [10], but it is clear that even mild anemia is associated with increased risk of mortality and of functional decline [10].

Geriatric syndromes include a number of conditions, from different causes, that are typical of, though not exclusive to, advanced age, and are associated with decreased survival and increased risk of functional dependence [22]. The early recognition of geriatric syndromes is important because some of them (such as depression) may be reversed and others (dementia, failure to thrive, falls, neglect and abuse, severe osteoporosis) may be arrested and managed. The Holstein Mini Mental Status (MMS) is a short instrument that may detect mild as well as advanced dementia, and is administered by an expert interviewer in approximately 15 minutes. Because of its practicality, the MMS is utilized in different institutions to screen older individuals for dementia [23]. The MMS is not sensitive to progressive cognitive changes that may lead to dementia, though they do not represent dementia yet. The presence of one or more geriatric syndromes generally suggests the need for at least a part-time caregiver, and for special precautions aimed to manage the specific conditions. In addition to shortening life expectancy and increasing the risk of treatment-related toxicity, comorbidity represents a cause of polypharmacy which may be associated with complications including increased risk of mortality and functional dependence.

The causes of polypharmacy [24] are multiple and include comorbidity, the consultation of several different healthcare specialists, and the use of multiple over-the-counter preparations. Polypharmacy is a major cause of adverse drug reactions and interactions, as well as of health-related costs.

The risk of malnutrition increases with age, and malnutrition is an independent risk factor for the toxicity of chemotherapy [25]. Causes of malnutrition are multiple, and include reduced food intake due to isolation, depression, poverty, and anorexia from polypharmacy, reduced threshold for bitter and increased threshold for sweet flavor, gastric atrophy and hypomobility, and reduced splanchnic circulation. The Mini Nutritional Assessment (MNA) identifies patients who are malnourished and those at risk of malnutrition [26], and is widely used because it is at the same time comprehensive and user-friendly.

Laboratory tests for the determination of physiologic age should be considered investigative, and include measurement of inflammatory markers in the circulation [11] and leukocyte telomere length [13,14]. Among the inflammatory markers, the fibrin split products and, in particular, the concentrations of D-dimer are particularly relevant to this review [27]. The concentration of this substance increases in the circulation of older individuals and is predictive of mortality and functional dependence [27,28]. Currently, both the sensitivity and the specificity of these tests are inadequate for useful clinical purposes. More studies are necessary to establish whether the concentration of inflammatory cytokines (especially interleukin 6, C-reactive protein, and D-dimer) in conjunction with other clinical parameters may be predictive of outcome for individual patients. At present, the main use of this determination is to conduct two types of clinical studies. These include population studies looking at an interaction between inflammation and geriatric syndromes, and clinical trials to establish whether reversal of inflammation may prevent or delay the complications of aging.

A clear correlation has been established between the length of leukocyte telomeres and the risk of cancer, geriatric syndromes, and death [13,14,29,30]. The individual variation in the telomere length, however, makes this test inadequate for the determination of individual physiologic age. Current investigations are aimed to establish whether the individual rate of telomere shortening over time may be used for this purpose.

The allostatic load [7] and the frailty index [31] involve the assessment of clinical, laboratory, and functional parameters. They are very useful in clinical research but they are too cumbersome to be used in clinical practice at present.

A taxonomy of aging

Aging is multidimensional and occurs at a different rate for different individuals, and for different functions within the same individual. For this reason it has been difficult to identify specific biologic landmarks of aging, as one has established for growth (puberty; epiphyseal ossification). Virtually all students of aging agree on a condition called "frailty" that is a situation of critically increased vulnerability to stress. The frail person is one that is still capable of independent living, but may become dependent following a minor stress that would not affect the function of a more fit subject [32,33]. There is general agreement that the construct of frailty is real, but a clinical definition of this condition is still wanted. In 2001, the investigators of the Cardiovascular Health Study established a definition of frailty based on five parameters (Box 19.1) [34]. They followed more than 8,500 subjects 65 and older for an average of 11 years, and were able to identify three groups of individuals with different life expectancy and risk of functional dependence based on the number of abnormalities present. Currently, this definition is utilized in most studies as the gold standard of frailty against which new definitions are compared.

Controversy exists over whether the terms "frailty" and "vulnerability" indicate different phenotypes [35,36]. For some students, vulnerability is a condition that precedes frailty and is reversible, whereas frailty is irreversible. We will not refer to vulnerability in the following discussion, but the reader should be aware of the controversy.

Box 19.1 Conclusions of the Cardiovascular Health Study [34]

A. Variables of interest
- Involuntary weight loss of ≥10% of the original body weight over 1 year or less
- Decreased grip strength
- Early exhaustion
- Slow walk
- Difficulty in starting movements

B. Clinical groups
- Fit: negative assessment
- Pre-frail: 1 or 2 abnormal parameters
- Frail: 3 or more abnormal parameters

Interactions of aging and hemostasis

We will explore these interactions at three levels: hemostatic manifestations of aging, thrombotic disorders in the elderly, and bleeding disorders.

Hemostatic manifestations of aging

As already mentioned, aging involves a chronic and progressive inflammation that leads to chronic intravascular coagulation and chronic fibrinolysis. Of the markers of fibrinolysis, the D-dimer has been the most extensively studied [37]. As the circulating levels of this substance may increase with age, the specificity of circulating D-dimer levels for the diagnosis of pulmonary embolism and deep vein thrombosis is reduced [37,38]. Almost ten years ago, Duke's investigators established that in otherwise healthy persons aged 70 and older, increased levels of D-dimer in the circulation were associated with a fourfold increased risk of death or functional dependence over the following 2 years [28]. The Baltimore Longitudinal Study investigators [27] studied cross-sectionally the levels of D-dimer in 776 individuals aged 65 and older. They found that levels above normal (100 ng/mL) were associated with increased erythrocyte sedimentation rate and levels above 200 ng/mL were associated with age, increased levels of triglycerides, creatinine, lower hemoglobin, and higher body mass index. The investigators of the BARI 2D study (a study that explored the risk of cardiovascular disease in patients with type 2 diabetes) found that the level of circulating D-dimer increased and that of plasminogen activator inhibitor 1 (PAI-1) decreased with aging [39]. According to these investigators, the activation of fibrinolysis may represent a compensatory mechanism that prevents coronary occlusion in older patients at risk. This view seems at odds with most other studies that saw increased circulating levels of D-dimer as a poor prognostic factor for the aged. In reality, the conclusions of the BARI investigators are not necessarily incongruent with those of others. It is reasonable to assume that the D-dimer levels reflect a condition of chronic inflammation that implies poor prognosis. At the same time the activation of the fibrinolytic system may be beneficial for patients at risk of arterial obstruction. Germane to this discussion is the finding of recent studies that increased circulating levels of D-dimer are associated with three genes (F3, F5, and FGA) in healthy adults of European ancestry [40]. It is possible that these genes may be associated with longevity, which may explain the association of increased circulating levels of D-dimer and aging, at least in part.

In a recent review, PAI-1 levels were also proposed as a marker of aging, though this substance has not been as extensively studied as the D-dimer

[41]. In addition to coagulation abnormalities, aging seems to be associated with vascular endothelial activation [42]. In the Established Population for Epidemiologist Studies in the Elderly (EPESE) study, increased circulating concentration of the marker of endothelial activation s-VCAM predicted increased risk of functional dependence and death, independently from the circulating values of D-dimer and interleukin 6.

While chronic intravascular coagulation and fibrinolysis are hallmarks of aging, it is important to underline that aging may also be associated with increased concentration of clotting factors including fibrinogen, factor VIII, and von Willebrand factor (VWF) [43]. In the meantime, the concentrations of VWF-cleaving proteases decline with aging. Of special interest, these clotting factors are generally increased in the centenarian, who also has higher frequency of thrombophilic mutations. These include the 4G allele of the PAI-1-675 polymorphism, mutant factor V, and prothrombin gene *G20210A*. This finding is referred to as the "centenarian paradox" [44]. While the increased concentration of these substances generally purports increased risk of thromboembolic manifestations, subjects of advanced age, and especially centenarians, seem immune to this risk.

In conclusion, aging is associated with increased incidence of intravascular coagulation and fibrinolysis and increased activation of vascular endothelium, seemingly as a result of chronic and progressive inflammation. The circulating levels of D-dimer, VCAM, and possibly PAI-1 predict the risk of poor outcome, especially of death and functional dependence. The predictive value of each of these substances alone is inadequate to assess a person's physiologic age. Future studies should explore the predictive value of these substances in combination with markers of inflammations (C-reactive protein, interleukin 6) and the role of these abnormalities in the pathogenesis of geriatric syndromes and other conditions that become more common with age (e.g., cerebrovascular and cardiovascular disease, renal insufficiency, and sarcopenia).

Aging is also associated with increased concentration of a number of thrombophilic substances, whose role in the pathogenesis of arterial thromboembolic disease is controversial (the aging or centenarian paradox).

Aging and thromboembolic diseases

The risk of deep vein thrombosis and pulmonary embolism increases steeply after age 55 [45–49]. It is tempting to hypothesize that intravascular coagulation may be responsible for venous thrombosis, and increased concentration of clotting factors, especially VWF, responsible for arterial thrombosis. The evidence supporting this association is inconclusive, however. The following points are emphasized:

- In patients of advanced age, and especially in centenarians, increased concentration of clotting factors and D-dimer and decreased concentrations of PAI-1 do not seem to be associated with increased risk of thrombosis.
- Age is definitely a risk factor for venous thrombosis [49]. The age-related factors that increase the risk of venous thrombosis include malignancies and comorbidities. In addition, factor V Leiden and prothrombin mutations may be responsible for 7–22% of the cases of venous thrombosis in the elderly.
- The role of circulating anticoagulants in the thromboembolic diseases of aging is poorly understood. A recent study showed that increased circulating levels of beta2-glycoprotein I were protective from myocardial infarction for men 60 and older, but not for younger men [50]. This observation suggests that the levels of circulating anticoagulant may be critical to prevent arterial thrombosis in some older individuals with a thrombophilic status.
- The treatment of thromboembolic conditions in older individuals is not different from that of younger patients. In older individuals the risk of drug interactions with oral anticoagulants, however, is increased due to polypharmacy [51]. Currently, there is no indication for prophylactic anticoagulant treatment in patients with evidence of intravascular coagulation in the absence of thrombosis or embolism.

Bleeding disorders in the elderly

The information about this topic is very limited. I will limit my comments to two subjects: the aging of patients with hemophilia, and diagnosis of hemophilia in older individuals.

The survival of patients with hemophilia has progressively improved between 1970 and 1979 thanks to the introduction of factor replacement therapy [52,53]. The median life expectancy of patients with hemophilia dropped from 57 to 40 years between 1979 and 1994, due to the AIDS epidemics, and started increasing again thereafter. Currently, the average life expectancy of patients with hemophilia and without AIDS is 64 years and a substantial portion of the population is aged 70 and older. Thus, it is important to define the medical profile and the medical need of aging patients with hemophilia. A review of 404 hemophilic individuals registered in the Gulf State Hemophilia and Thrombophilia Center (GBHTC) was published [54]. Of 404 patients 45 were over 40 and 14 over 60. Unlike the US population of the same age, 100% of the adults with hemophilia had at least one comorbid condition and 12% had seven or more comorbidities. In addition to HIV infections, present in 25% of patients, hepatitis C was present in approximately 80%, obesity in 65%, cardiovascular disease in 47%, hypertension in 46%, and chronic arthropathy in

52%. Cancer was present in 15.9% of patients and was mainly related to hepatitis C and HIV infections. While one may expect that the prevalence of serum-transmitted infections will decrease in the next cohorts of hemophilic individuals, the other comorbidities appear more difficult to eliminate and will represent a significant disease burden for aging patients with hemophilia. A review of the literature [55] indicates that chronic arthropathy, pain, and the need for joint replacement represent the major source of morbidity in the aged with hemophilia. While the overall prevalence of cardiovascular disease may be lower among aged patients with hemophilia than in the general population, the risk of non-valvular atrial fibrillation increases among the former. This condition represents a special problem due to the need for oral anticoagulation.

In 1992, our group reported three cases diagnosed with hemophilia A after age 70 [56]. All three were veterans; two had participated in war actions, and all three had undergone some type of trauma, including elective surgery in their past life, without excessive bleeding. None of them had family history of hemophilia or other bleeding disorders. No factor VIII inhibitor was present. These findings were puzzling and a satisfactory explanation was not found. It is possible that these individuals had a very mild form of hemophilia A or, alternatively, that age-related hypogonadism led to decreased release of VWF from the endothelium into the circulation. To our knowledge, these are the only cases ever reported of acquired hemophilia in the absence of an inhibitor. The incidence, prevalence, and mechanisms of this condition are unknown.

Conclusions

Age is a physiologic event that involves a progressive reduction in the functional reserve of multiple organ systems as well as increased prevalence of comorbidity and geriatric syndromes. The outcomes of aging include functional dependence and death.

Aging is associated with increased incidence and prevalence of chronic intravascular anticoagulation, due to chronic and progressive inflammation. In the aged, increased concentration of circulating D-dimer, factor VIII fibrinogen, and VWF and decreased concentration of PAI-1 are harbingers of increased mortality and increased risk of functional dependence and geriatric syndromes.

Aging is associated with increased risk of thromboembolic disorders that is only in part related to the clotting abnormalities of aging. The centenarian paradox implies that centenarians are at decreased risk of thromboembolic events despite increased concentration of clotting factors in the circulation. The explanation of this paradox is unknown.

With the advent of replacement therapy, patients with hemophilia have achieved an almost normal life expectancy (despite a drop in life expectancy between 1979 and 1989 due to HIV). Elderly patients with hemophilia appear to have increased prevalence of comorbid conditions. In addition to those due to HIV and hepatitis C, these include those related to chronic arthropathy and joint replacement.

References

1. Kapteyn A. What can we learn from (and about) global aging? *Demography* 2010;47(suppl):191–209.
2. Alamayehu B, Warner KE. The lifetime distribution of health care costs. *Health Serv Rev* 2004;39:627–42.
3. Boyd CM, Ritchie CS, Tipton EF, et al. From Bedside to Bench: Summary from the American Geriatric Society/National Institute of Aging Research Conference on Comorbidity and Multiple morbidities in Older Adults. *Aging Clin Exper Res* 2008;20:181–8.
4. Yancik R, Ershler W, Satariano W, et al. Report of the national Institute of Aging Task Force on Comorbidity. *J Gerontol A Biol Sci Med Sci* 2007;62:275–80.
5. Moreh E, Jacobs JM, Stessman J. Fatigue, function, and mortality in older adults. *J Gerontol A Biol Sci Med Sci* 2010;65:887–95.
6. Motl RW, McAuley E. Physical activity, disability, and quality of life in older adults. *Phys Med Rehabil Clin N Am* 2010;21:299–308.
7. Mariano J, Min LC. Assessment. In Naeim A, Reuben DB, Ganz PA (eds), *Management of Cancer in the Older Patient*. St Louis, MO: Elsevier Saunders, 2012;39–50.
8. Murumatsu N, Yin H, Hedeker D. Functional decline, social support, and mental health in the elderly: Does living in a state supportive of home and community-based services make a difference? *Social Sci Med* 2010;70:1050–8.
9. Balducci L. Anemia, fatigue, and aging. *Transfus Clin Biol* 2010;17:375–81.
10. Grunewald TM, Seeman TE, Karlamangla AS, et al. Allostatic load and frailty in Older Adults. *J Am Geriatr Soc* 2009;57:1525–31.
11. Ferrucci L, Corsi A, Lauretani F et al. The origin of age-related pro-inflammatory state. *Blood* 2005;105:2294–9.
12. Yourman LC, Lee SJ, Schonberg MA, et al. Prognostic indices for older adults: A systematic review. *JAMA* 2012;307:182–92.
13. Willeit P, Willeit J, Kloss-Blandstätter A, et al. Fifteen year follow-up of the association between telomere length and incident cancer and cancer mortality. *JAMA* 2011;306:42–4.
14. Ma H, Zou Z, Wei S, et al. Shortened telomere length is associated with increased risk of cancer: A meta-analysis. *PLoS One* 2011;6:e20466.
15. Hurria A, Togawa K, Mohile SG, et al. Predicting chemotherapy toxicity in older adults with cancer. *J Clin Oncol* 2011;29:3457–65.
16. Extermann M, Boler I, Reich RR, et al. Predicting the risk of chemotherapy toxicity in older patients: The Chemotherapy Toxicity Assessment Scale in High Age patients (CRASH) score. *Cancer* 2012;118:3377–86.
17. Kristjansson SR, Nesbakken A, Jordy MS, et al. Comprehensive Geriatric Assessment can predict complications in elderly patients after elective surgery for colorectal

cancer: A prospective observation cohort study. *Crit Rev Oncol Hematol* 2010; 76:208–17.

18. de Groot V, Beckerman H, Lankhorst GJ, et al. How to measure comorbidity. A critical review of available methods. *J Clin Epidemiol* 2003;56:221–9.

19. Extermann M. Measurement and impact of comorbidity in older cancer patients. *Crit Rev Oncol Hematol* 2000;35:181–200.

20. Covinsky KE, Kahana E, Chin MH. et al. Depressive symptoms and three year mortality in older hospitalized medical patients. *Ann Intern Med* 1999;130:563–9.

21. Lee SJ, Lindquist K, Segal MR, et al. Development and validation of a prognostic index for 4 year mortality in older adults. *JAMA* 2006;295:801–8.

22. Mohile SG, Fan L, Reeve E, et al. Association of cancer with geriatric syndromes in older Medicare beneficiaries. *J Clin Oncol* 2011;29:1458–64.

23. Folstein ME, Folstein SE, McHugh PR. A Mini Mental State: A practical method for grading the cognitive status of patients for the clinician. *J Psychiatr Res* 1975;12: 189–98.

24. Hamilton H, Gallagher P, Ryan C, et al. Potentially inappropriate medications defined by STOPP criteria and the risk of adverse drug events in older hospitalized patients. *Arch Intern Med* 2011;171:1013–19.

25. Hughes VA, Roubenoff R, Wood M, et al. Anthropometric assessment of 10 yr changes in body composition in the elderly. *Am J Clin Nutr* 2004;80:475–82.

26. Guigoz Y, Vellas B, Garry PJ. *Mininutritional assessment: A practical assessment tool for grading the nutritional state of elderly patients*. In *Facts, Research, Interventions in Geriatrics*. New York: Serdi, 1997;15–60.

27. Tita-Nwa F, Bos A, Adiel A, et al. Correlates of D-Dimer in older persons. *Aging Clin Exp Res* 2010;22:20–3.

28. Cohen HJ, Harris T, Pieper CF. Coagulation and activation of inflammatory pathways in the development of functional decline and mortality in the elderly. *Am J Med* 2003;114:180–7.

29. Zhu H, Belcher M, Van der Harst P. Healthy aging and disease: Role for telomere biology. *Clin Sci Lond* 2011;120:427–40.

30. Mather KA, Jorm AF, Parslow RA, et al. Is telomere length a biomarker of aging? A review. *J Gerontol A Biol Sci Med Sci* 2011;66:202–13.

31. Searle SD, Mitnitski A, Gahbauer EA, et al. A standard procedure for creating a frailty index. *BMC Geriatr* 2008;30:8–24.

32. Ferrucci L, Giallauria F, Sclessinger D. Mapping the road to resilience: Novel math for the study of frailty. *Mech Ageing Dev* 2008;129:677–9.

33. Karunananthan S, Wolfson C, Bergman H, et al. A multidisciplinary systematic literature review on frailty: overview of the methodology used by the Canadian Initiative on Frailty and Aging. *BMC Med Res Methodol* 2009;12:9–68.

34. Fried LP, Tangen CM, Walston J, et al. Frailty in older adults: evidence for a phenotype. *J Gerontol A Biol Sci Med Sci* 2001;56:146–56.

35. Quinlan N, Marcantonio NR, Inoyou SK, et al. Vulnerability: the crossroads of frailty and delirium. *J Am Geriatr Soc* 2011;59(suppl 2):S262–268.

36. Mohile SG. Xian W, Dale W, et al. Association of a cancer diagnosis with vulnerability and frailty in older Medicare beneficiaries. *J Natl Cancer Inst* 2009;101:1206–15.

37. van Es J, Mos I, Douma R, et al. The combination of four different decision rules and an age-adjusted D-Dimer cut-off increases the number of patients in whom pulmonary embolism can be safely excluded. *Thromb Haemost* 2012;107:167–71.

38. Legnani C, Cini M, Cosmi B, et al. Age and gender specific cut-off values to improve the performance of D-dimer assays to predict the risk of of venous thromboembolism recurrence. *Intern Emerg Med* 2013;8:229–36.

39. McBane RD, Hardison AM, Sobel BE, et al. Comparison of levels of plasminogen activator inhibitor 1, tissue type plasminogen activator antigen, fibrinogen and d-dimer in various age decades in patients with type 2 diabetes mellitus and stable coronary artery disease. *Am J Cardiol* 2010;105:17–24.

40. Smith NL, Huffman JE, Strachan DP, et al. Genetic predictors of Fibrin D-Dimer levels in healthy adults. *Circulation* 2011;123:1864–72.

41. Cesari M, Pahor M, Incalzi RA. Plasminogen activator inhibitor-1 (PAI-1): A key factor linking fibrinolysis and age-related subclinical and clinical conditions. *Cardiovascul Ther* 2010;28:e72–e91.

42. Huffman KM, Pieper CF, Kraus VB, et al. Relation of a marker of endothelial activation (s-VCAM) to function and mortality in community-dwelling older adults. *J Gerontol A Biol Sci Med Sci* 2011;66:1369–75.

43. Mari D, Coppola R, Provenzano R. Hemostasis factors and aging. *Exp Gerontol* 2008;43:66–73.

44. Mari D, Mannucci PM, Coppola R, et al. Hypercoagulability in centenarians: the paradox of successful aging. *Blood* 1995;85:3144–9.

45. Silverstein M, Helt J, Mohr D, et al. Trends in the incidence of deep vein thrombosis and pulmonary embolism: a 25-year population based study. *Arch Intern Med* 1998;158:585–93.

46. Wilkerson WR, Sane DC. Aging and thrombosis. *Semin Thromb Hemost* 2002; 28:555–68.

47. Silverstein RL, Bauer KA, Cushman M, et al. Venous thrombosis in the elderly: more questions than answers. *Blood* 2007;110:3097–101.

48. Kirson NY, Bimbaum HG, Ivanova JL, et al. Prevalence of pulmonary arterial hypertension and chronic thrombo-embolic pulmonary hypertension in the United States. *Curr Med Res Opin* 2011;27:1763–8.

49. Engbers MJ, van Hilckama Vileg A, Rosendaal FR. Venous thrombosis in the elderly: Incidence, risk factors, and risk groups. *J Thromb Hemost* 2010;10:2105–12.

50. De Laat B, de Groot PG, Derksen RHWM, et al. Association between beta2glycoprotein I plasma levels and the risk of myocardial infarction in older men. *Blood* 2009;114:3656–61.

51. Gallagher P, Ryan C, Byrne S, et al. STOPP (Screening tool of older person's prescriptions) and START (Screening tool to alert doctors to right treatment). Consensus validation. *Int J Clin Pharmacol Ther* 2008;46:72–83.

52. Soucie SM, Nuss R, Evatt B, et al. Mortality among males with hemophilia: relation with source of medical care. The Hemophilia Surveillance System project Investigation. *Blood* 2000;96:437–42.

53. Konkle BA. Clinical challenges with the aging hemophilia population. *Thromb Res* 2011;127(suppl 1):S10–13.

54. Khleif AA, Rodriguez N, Brown D, et al. Multiple comorbid conditions among middle aged and elderly hemophilia patients: prevalence estimates and implications for future care. *J Aging Res* 2011; ID 985703.

55. Mannucci PM, Schutgens REG, Santagostino E, et al. How I treat age-related morbidities in elderly persons with hemophilia. *Blood* 2009;114:5256–63.

56. Ballester OG, Wang T, Saba HI, et al. Classic hemophilia in elderly patients. *J Am Geriatr Soc* 1992;40:824–6.

CHAPTER 20

Hemostatic Problems in Chronic and Acute Liver Disease

Ton Lisman and Robert J. Porte

Section of Hepatobiliary Surgery and Liver Transplantation, Department of Surgery, University of Groningen, University Medical Center Groningen, Groningen, The Netherlands

Introduction

The liver has a central role in the hemostatic system as it synthesizes many of the proteins involved in coagulation and fibrinolysis. Moreover, the liver synthesizes thrombopoietin and is, therefore, involved in the production of platelets. Patients with chronic or acute liver failure acquire complex alterations in their hemostatic system, which may be a result of decreased synthesis, but may also in part be explained by consumption due to disseminated or local activation of coagulation [1,2]. Specifically, patients with liver failure may be thrombocytopenic and have reduced plasma levels of coagulation factors, inhibitors of coagulation, and fibrinolytic proteins. Plasma levels of von Willebrand factor (VWF) and factor VIII (FVIII), however, are frequently elevated, as are levels of tissue-type plasminogen activator (tPA) and plasminogen activator inhibitor type 1 (PAI-1). As VWF, tPA, and PAI-1 are synthesized by endothelial cells, the elevated levels of these proteins are explained by chronic endothelial cell activation. Elevated levels of factor VIII may be explained by the elevated levels of its carrier protein, VWF. In addition, although FVIII is synthesized in the liver, the synthesis primarily takes place in sinusoidal endothelial cells, whose function is much better preserved in liver disease in comparison to hepatocyte function, which synthesize all other liver-derived coagulation factors.

The effects of liver failure on hemostasis are similar, but not identical, between different etiologies of liver disease [3–5]. Patients with chronic liver failure more frequently experience thrombocytopenia compared to patients with acute liver failure. Conversely, the levels of coagulation factors and inhibitors are decreased to a larger extent in patients with

---

Hemostasis and Thrombosis: Practical Guidelines in Clinical Management, First Edition.
Hussain I. Saba and Harold R. Roberts.

acute liver failure in comparison to patients with chronic disease. Fibri-nolytic proteins are also lower in patients with acute liver failure, but levels of PAI-1 are much more increased in acute liver failure. The hemo-static changes in cholestatic liver disease are less pronounced as com-pared to the changes observed in non-cholestatic liver disease, and platelet function is better preserved in cholestatic disease. The hemostatic changes in patients with non-alcoholic fatty liver disease (NAFLD), the hepatic manifestation of the metabolic syndrome, are initially prothrom-botic with platelet hyperfunction, elevated levels of coagulation factors, and elevated levels of PAI-1. Studies on the hemostatic system in patients with NAFLD who have progressed to liver failure have not yet been performed.

The net effect of the hemostatic changes in liver disease has long been thought to be a hypocoagulable state as evidenced by thrombocytopenia and prolonged clotting times in tests such as the prothrombin time (PT) and activated partial thromboplastin time (aPTT). However, recent clinical and laboratory studies have shown that this interpretation was too simplified [6]. Rather, a commensurate decline in both pro- and antihe-mostatic pathways results in a reset of the hemostatic balance, which will be discussed below.

This chapter will discuss interpretation of routine and advanced labora-tory tests of hemostasis in patients with liver disease. Furthermore, the concept of a "rebalanced" hemostatic status in liver disease will be intro-duced. Finally, the etiology, prevention, and treatment of bleeding com-plications and thrombotic events in patients with liver disease will be discussed.

Laboratory tests of hemostasis in patients with liver disease

The interpretation of routine diagnostic tests of hemostasis is a particular challenge in patients with liver disease due to the multiple alterations that occur simultaneously. Routine tests of hemostasis in general are suitable to diagnose isolated defects or to monitor antihemostatic therapy. In patients without a diagnosed hemostatic defect, laboratory test results are a poor predictor of (procedure-related) bleeding, but are still frequently used for that purpose [7]. Also, in patients with liver disease, routine hemostasis tests are still frequently used to estimate bleeding risk, but these tests have little or no predictive value [8].

The platelet count is frequently reduced in patients with liver disease, but the thrombocytopenia is usually mild to moderate. However, patients with liver disease have complex alterations in their primary hemostatic system including platelet function abnormalities and alterations in VWF and the VWF-cleaving protease, "a disintegrin and metalloproteinase with a thrombospondin type 1 motif, member 13" (ADAMTS-13) [9,10]. The substantially elevated levels of VWF and decreased levels of ADAMTS-13 may compensate for the low platelet count, which complicates the interpretation of the thrombocytopenia and platelet function defects in relation to bleeding risk. One recent study found that thrombocytopenia (and not abnormal coagulation tests) was a predictor of procedural bleeding [11], but these results require confirmation. Functional tests of primary hemostasis such as the skin bleeding time and suspension aggregometry are also frequently abnormal in patients with liver disease, but also for these tests the predictive value is, if any, limited.

The PT and aPTT are frequently prolonged in liver disease, but these abnormal test results have little or no predictive value in terms of bleeding risk. A plausible reason for the poor performance of these tests in predicting bleeding is the fact that these tests are insensitive to levels of natural anticoagulants. Since both pro- and anticoagulant proteins (with the exception of tissue factor pathway inhibitor; TFPI, and factor VIII) are decreased in patients with liver disease, the PT and aPTT do not adequately reflect the balance in the coagulation system. This has been elegantly shown in studies assessing the endogenous thrombin potential (ETP) in samples taken from patients with cirrhosis and an elevated PT. In these patients, the ETP was indistinguishable from that of healthy volunteers, provided thrombomodulin, the natural activator of protein C, was added to the test mixture [12]. Interestingly, when the thrombomodulin-modified ETP was performed in platelet-rich plasma, it was demonstrated that a minimal platelet count of ~50–60 G/L was required for normal thrombin generation, which may suggest that thrombocytopenia may indeed be a risk factor for bleeding [13]. It has not yet been examined whether the thrombomodulin-modified ETP has any predictive value. Regardless, the complexity of the test will probably limit its use in routine diagnostics.

The interpretation of circulating markers of hemostasis activation such as, for example, prothrombin fragment 1 + 2, D-dimer, or platelet factor 4/β-thromboglobulin is a challenge as these markers are primarily cleared by the liver. Elevated levels of these markers may indicate hemostasis activation, but may also be explained by accumulation due to defective clearance. D-dimers are important in the workup of patients with suspected venous thrombosis, but this test is probably of little use in patients with liver disease as 100% of patients with severe cirrhosis have elevated D-dimer levels in the absence of a venous thrombosis [14].

The concept of rebalanced hemostasis in liver disease

Laboratory studies have shown a reset in the balance of primary hemostasis, secondary hemostasis, and the fibrinolytic system in patients with chronic liver disease [9,12,14]. Hemostatic changes that lead to a diminished hemostatic potential are compensated by hemostatic changes leading to enhanced hemostatic potential. Specifically, thrombocytopenia and platelet function defects are balanced by elevated VWF and decreased ADAMTS-13 levels. Decreased levels of procoagulant proteins are balanced by decreased levels of anticoagulant proteins, and decreased levels of the profibrinolytic plasminogen are balanced by decreased levels of antifibrinolytic proteins. A similar reset in the hemostatic balance is probably also present in patients with acute liver failure although data are scarce [15]. Table 20.1 shows an overview of the hemostatic changes in patients with liver disease.

Clinical evidence for a rebalanced hemostatic system in patients with liver disease primarily originates from studies on transfusion requirements during liver transplantation. Although liver transplantation was accompanied by extreme blood loss and transfusion requirements frequently exceeding multiple circulating volumes in the past, developments in the last 15–20 years have resulted in a steady decline in blood loss and transfusion requirements [16]. Nowadays, many centers report transfusion-free liver transplantation even in the absence of attempts to correct the coagulopathy prior to surgery [17]. The absence of significant bleeding in patients with end-stage liver disease undergoing transplant surgery argues

Table 20.1 Alterations in the hemostatic system in patients with liver disease that contribute to bleeding (middle column) or counteract bleeding (right-hand column). Source: Adapted from Lisman et al. 2002 [1]. With permission of Elsevier.

	Changes that impair hemostasis	Changes that promote hemostasis
Primary hemostasis	Thrombocytopenia Platelet function defects Enhanced production of nitric oxide and prostacyclin	Elevated levels of von Willebrand factor (VWF) Decreased levels of ADAMTS-13
Secondary hemostasis	Low levels of factors II, V, VII, IX, X, and XI Vitamin K deficiency Dysfibrinogenemia	Elevated levels of factor VIII Decreased levels of protein C, protein S, antithrombin, α_2-macroglobulin, and heparin cofactor II
Fibrinolysis	Low levels of α_2-antiplasmin, factor XIII, and TAFI Elevated levels of tPA	Low levels of plasminogen

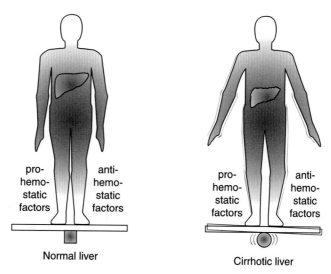

Figure 20.1 The hemostatic balance in patients with liver disease as compared to that of healthy individuals. This cartoon depicts the stable hemostatic balance in healthy individuals and shows that, although the hemostatic system in patients with liver disease is (re)balanced, the balance is fragile and may easily tip to either a hypo- or a hypercoagulable status.

against a profound hemostatic defect as suggested by the abnormal routine hemostasis tests including platelet count, PT, and aPTT. In patients with acute liver failure, who frequently present with extreme abnormalities in particular in levels of coagulation factors and inhibitors, the absence of spontaneously clinically relevant bleeding in the majority of patients also argues in favor of a rebalanced hemostatic system in these patients [3,15].

Although the hemostatic system in patients with liver disease appears relatively balanced, the balance is much more unstable as compared to healthy individuals (Figure 20.1).

Indeed, both bleeding and thrombosis may complicate liver disease, and these events are likely triggered (in part) by acquired factors or comorbidities such as renal failure, bacterial infection, alterations in blood flow including the hemodynamic changes related to portal hypertension, endothelial cell activation, and changes in vasoreactivity. Unfortunately, currently available hemostasis tests do not appear to discriminate between patients in hemostatic balance and patients at risk for either bleeding or thrombosis.

Bleeding in liver disease

Bleeding complications in patients with liver disease occur frequently, but are not necessarily related to alterations in hemostasis. The most frequent and clinically relevant bleeding complication in patients with cirrhosis is bleeding from ruptured gastroesophageal varices [18]. This life-threatening complication is related to local vascular abnormalities and portal hypertension. The role of hemostatic abnormalities is limited and therefore procoagulant treatment is not indicated. This section will focus on bleeding complications that are (in part) related to hemostatic failure.

Etiology

Spontaneous bleeding complications associated with hemostatic failure in patients with cirrhosis include bruising, purpura, epistaxis, gingival bleeding, and menorrhagia. The etiology of these complications is likely multifactorial, but since most of these complications do not require prohemostatic treatment, the mechanisms behind these complications are clinically irrelevant. Spontaneous bleeding that is clinically relevant is uncommon in patients with acute liver failure. In contrast, bleeding may complicate invasive procedures in both chronic and acute liver failure [5]. In general, bleeding may be related to thrombocytopenia or coagulation defects. One study has shown that thrombocytopenia, but not laboratory evidence of coagulation abnormalities, is related to an increased risk of procedural bleeding [11]. Also, anemia may contribute to procedural bleeding risks due to the stimulating effects of erythrocytes on platelet–vessel wall interactions. In patients with cirrhosis, hyperfibrinolysis may contribute to procedural bleeding, and in particular during liver transplantation a temporary hyperfibrinolytic state may develop, most commonly after graft reperfusion [19]. Patients with acute liver failure have laboratory evidence of severe hypofibrinolysis [20], so the role for fibrinolysis in bleeding in these patients is presumably absent. Heparin-like substances have been shown to circulate in patients with chronic and acute liver failure [21]; these molecules may have relevant anticoagulant activity and thereby contribute to bleeding. Bacterial infections, which are common in patients with cirrhosis, result in a hypocoagulable status and an increased bleeding risk which is in part related to elevated levels of heparin-like substances [22,23]. Finally, renal failure impairs hemostasis by multiple mechanisms and has been shown to contribute to procedural bleeding [24].

Treatment

It has long been common practice to correct the coagulopathy of liver failure prior to invasive procedures by administration of blood component transfusion. An increasing proportion of centers are switching from this prophylactic transfusion approach to a "wait-and-see" policy in which blood components are only transfused in patients with active bleeding which does not have a surgical origin. Accumulating clinical evidence suggest that a more restrictive transfusion policy is safe and has numerous advantages over a prophylactic transfusion strategy. First, prophylactic blood component transfusion is associated with an increase in central venous and portal pressure, which may in fact promote bleeding when surgical damage is inflicted. Indeed, maintenance of a low central venous pressure by conservative fluid and transfusion management or even by preoperative phlebotomy results in a reduction in intraoperative blood loss and transfusion requirements [17]. Second, transfusion of blood product components is associated with increased morbidity and mortality [25]. Besides recognized transfusion reactions, more recently recognized complications such as transfusion-related acute lung injury (TRALI) contribute to transfusion-associated morbidity and mortality. Importantly, the risk of TRALI appears to be increased in patients with liver disease compared to the general population [26,27]. Finally, avoidance of blood component transfusion results in a decrease in health-care costs.

Besides red cell concentrates, fresh frozen plasma, and platelet concentrates, other pharmacologic strategies to prevent or treat bleeding are frequently used, although randomized clinical studies to examine efficacy and safety of the various strategies are still lacking. Advantages and disadvantages of the various prohemostatic strategies are summarized in Table 20.2.

Thrombosis in liver disease

It has long been assumed that patients with liver disease were protected against thrombotic disease as a result of the prohemostatic defects. Recent epidemiologic research and clinical observations have unequivocally demonstrated that patients with liver disease may experience a number of thrombotic complications. Treatment or prevention of thrombosis in patients with liver failure is a particular challenge due to the fragile hemostatic system.

Etiology

Systemic venous as well as arterial thrombotic events may occur in patients with liver disease. Venous thrombosis occurs in patients with liver failure, even in those patients that receive mechanical or pharmacologic thromboprophylactic treatment [33]. Studies on the risk of venous thrombosis in patients with liver disease compared to patients without liver disease are conflicting; some studies report liver disease to be an independent risk factor for venous thrombosis whereas other studies report patients with liver disease to be protected [34,35]. The possibly increased risk for venous

Table 20.2 The advantages and disadvantages of various strategies available to prevent or treat bleeding in patients with liver disease. Source: Adapted from Lisman et al. 2010 [5]. With permission of Elsevier.

Product	Advantage	Disadvantage
Red cell concentrate	Life-saving in cases of severe anemia, improvement of platelet function	Transfusion-related side effects, adversely affects outcome of liver transplantation [25]
Fresh frozen plasma	Repletes both pro- and anticoagulants	Transfusion-related side effects, fluid overload, exacerbation of portal hypertension. Complete normalization is often not achieved [31]
Platelet concentrate	Improves primary hemostasis. Recent data showed adequate thrombin production with levels exceeding 50–60 G/L [13]	Transfusion-related side effects, adversely affects outcome of liver transplantation [25]
Recombinant factor VIIa	Small volume product, encouraging data from uncontrolled studies and case reports	Cost, no proven effect in randomized trials in patients with liver disease, theoretical risk of thrombosis [32]
DDAVP	Laboratory improvement of primary hemostasis, relative lack of side effects, easy administration	Efficacy in patients with liver disease is not proven
Factor concentrates	Small volume product	Only repletes part of the coagulation factors (some products only replete procoagulants), no data from controlled studies yet, theoretical risk of thrombosis
Thrombopoietin receptor agonists	Effectively increases endogenous platelet count, no transfusion-related side effects	No data from controlled studies on efficacy, theoretical risk of thrombosis
Antibiotics	Reduces variceal bleeding, and improves coagulation status in patients with active infection, improvement of systemic hemodynamics [28–60]	Bacterial resistance or overgrowth

thrombosis in patients with liver disease may be explained by low levels of the natural anticoagulants protein C, protein S, and antithrombin, elevated levels of FVIII, and a resistance against the anticoagulant action of thrombomodulin [36]. Also, studies on the occurrence of arterial thrombosis, including coronary artery disease, are conflicting, except in patients with NAFLD, who have a clearly increased risk for coronary artery disease possibly related to the hypercoagulable state associated with the metabolic syndrome [5,37].

Liver-related thrombotic events include portal vein thrombosis (PVT) and intrahepatic microthrombosis. The risk of PVT increases with the severity of the disease, is associated with profound complications, and may even result in a reduced prognosis after liver transplantation [38,39]. Risk factors for PVT include the prothrombin 20210A mutation and decreased portal flow. Microthrombi have been demonstrated in human biopsies from patients with both chronic and acute liver failure [40,41]. Studies in animal models have shown that prevention of clot formation reduces disease progression by mechanisms that may involve prevention of micro-ischemia or reduction of cellular activation by coagulation proteases such as thrombin or factor Xa [42,43].

Treatment

Treatment or prevention of venous thrombosis in patients with liver disease is challenging for a number of reasons. Anticoagulation in these patients may be associated with a high bleeding risk as a consequence of the altered hemostatic status. Furthermore, dosing of vitamin K antagonists is a particular challenge, as many patients with liver failure have a prolonged INR as a result of the decreased levels of procoagulants, and the target INRs for patients with liver failure have not been established. Also, dosing of heparins is difficult as patients with liver disease frequently have strongly decreased circulating levels of antithrombin. Furthermore, anti-Xa measurements in patients with liver disease receiving a standard dose of low-molecular-weight heparin (LMWH) suggest that these patients are under-anticoagulated. This is likely due to an inherent flaw in the anti-Xa test, since thrombin generation tests suggest that plasma from patients with cirrhosis is more susceptible to LMWH as compared to plasma from healthy volunteers [44,45].

Aspirin has been successfully used to prevent hepatic artery thrombosis following liver transplantation [46]. Patients with NAFLD have a clearly increased risk of arterial events, and prophylactic administration of antiplatelet drugs may be indicated. Also, patients with NAFLD or non-alcoholic steatohepatitis may need to undergo vascular stenting which may require antiplatelet treatment to avoid restenosis. These patients pose a particular challenge, as the bleeding risk in patients with liver disease-associated hemostatic disorders is substantial. Furthermore, the use of antiplatelet agents that require metabolizing in the liver forms a particular challenge.

Clinical experience with antihemostatic therapy to treat liver micro-thrombosis with the aim of slowing down progression of disease is scarce, although one randomised study showed long-term LMWH to reduce morbidity and mortality in patients with cirrhosis [47].

Conclusion

Patients with chronic and acute liver disease have complex alterations in their hemostatic system. However, the net effect of these changes is a hemostatic system that is in balance as a result of changes in both pro- and antihemostatic pathways. Routine diagnostic tests of hemostasis, however, fail to capture this hemostatic rebalance, and may lead to prophylactic correction of the abnormal test results by administration of blood products or pharmacologic prohemostatic agents. This approach is without a scientific basis, and may in fact pose unwarranted risks with little or no benefit. Accumulating evidence from the liver transplantation community suggest that a restricted transfusion policy directed at treating bleeding complications when they occur is safe and effective. Nevertheless, both bleeding and thrombotic episodes may complicate the treatment of patients with liver disease and, unfortunately, current laboratory tests are not able to predict which patients are at risk for bleeding or thrombosis. The optimal management of bleeding and thrombosis in patients with liver disease is complex and clinical studies to define the risk/benefit of possible therapeutic approaches are required. Until these data become available, clinicians need to be aware of the limitations of currently available laboratory tests of hemostasis.

References

1. Lisman T, Leebeek FW, de Groot PG. Haemostatic abnormalities in patients with liver disease. *J Hepatol* 2002;37:280–7.
2. Lisman T, Porte RJ. Activation and regulation of hemostasis in acute liver failure and acute pancreatitis. *Semin Thromb Hemost* 2010;36:437–43.
3. Munoz SJ, Stravitz RT, Gabriel DA. Coagulopathy of acute liver failure. *Clin Liver Dis* 2009;13:95–107.
4. Ben-Ari Z, Panagou M, Patch D, et al. Hypercoagulability in patients with primary biliary cirrhosis and primary sclerosing cholangitis evaluated by thrombelastography. *J Hepatol* 1997;26:554–9.
5. Lisman T, Caldwell SH, Burroughs AK, et al. Hemostasis and thrombosis in patients with liver disease: the ups and downs. *J Hepatol* 2010;53:362–71.
6. Lisman T, Porte RJ. Rebalanced hemostasis in patients with liver disease: evidence and clinical consequences. *Blood* 2010;116:878–85.

7. Segal JB, Dzik WH. Transfusion Medicine/Hemostasis Clinical Trials Network. Paucity of studies to support that abnormal coagulation test results predict bleeding in the setting of invasive procedures: an evidence-based review. *Transfusion* 2005;45:1413–25.

8. McVay PA, Toy PT. Lack of increased bleeding after liver biopsy in patients with mild hemostatic abnormalities. *Am J Clin Pathol* 1990;94:747–53.

9. Lisman T, Bongers TN, Adelmeijer J, et al. Elevated levels of von Willebrand Factor in cirrhosis support platelet adhesion despite reduced functional capacity. *Hepatology* 2006;44:53–61.

10. Uemura M, Fujimura Y, Matsumoto M, et al. Comprehensive analysis of ADAMTS13 in patients with liver cirrhosis. *Thromb Haemost* 2008;99:1019–29.

11. Giannini EG, Greco A, Marenco S, et al. Incidence of bleeding following invasive procedures in patients with thrombocytopenia and advanced liver disease. *Clin Gastroenterol Hepatol* 2010;8:899–902; quiz e109.

12. Tripodi A, Salerno F, Chantarangkul V, et al. Evidence of normal thrombin generation in cirrhosis despite abnormal conventional coagulation tests. *Hepatology* 2005;41:553–8.

13. Tripodi A, Primignani M, Chantarangkul V, et al. Thrombin generation in patients with cirrhosis: the role of platelets. *Hepatology* 2006;44:440–5.

14. Lisman T, Leebeek FW, Mosnier LO, et al. Thrombin-activatable fibrinolysis inhibitor deficiency in cirrhosis is not associated with increased plasma fibrinolysis. *Gastroenterology* 2001;121:131–39.

15. Stravitz RT, Lisman T, Luketic VA, et al. Minimal effects of acute liver injury/acute liver failure on hemostasis as assessed by thromboelastography. *J Hepatol* 2012; 56:129–36.

16. de Boer MT, Molenaar IQ, Hendriks HG, et al. Minimizing blood loss in liver transplantation: progress through research and evolution of techniques. *Dig Surg* 2005;22:265–275.

17. Massicotte L, Lenis S, Thibeault L, et al. Effect of low central venous pressure and phlebotomy on blood product transfusion requirements during liver transplantations. *Liver Transpl* 2006;12:117–23.

18. Garcia-Tsao G, Bosch J. Management of varices and variceal hemorrhage in cirrhosis. *N Engl J Med* 2010;62:823–32.

19. Porte RJ, Bontempo FA, Knot EA, et al. Systemic effects of tissue plasminogen activator-associated fibrinolysis and its relation to thrombin generation in orthotopic liver transplantation. *Transplantation* 1989;47:978–84.

20. Pernambuco JR, Langley PG, Hughes RD, et al. Activation of the fibrinolytic system in patients with fulminant liver failure. *Hepatology* 1993;18:1350–6.

21. Senzolo M, Cholongitas E, Thalheimer U, et al. Heparin-like effect in liver disease and liver transplantation. *Clin Liver Dis* 2009;13:43–53.

22. Goulis J, Armonis A, Patch D, et al. Bacterial infection is independently associated with failure to control bleeding in cirrhotic patients with gastrointestinal hemorrhage. *Hepatology* 1998;27:1207–12.

23. Montalto P, Vlachogiannakos J, Cox DJ, et al. Bacterial infection in cirrhosis impairs coagulation by a heparin effect: a prospective study. *J Hepatol* 2002;37: 463–70.

24. Hendriks HG, van der Meer J, Klompmaker IJ, et al. Blood loss in orthotopic liver transplantation: a retrospective analysis of transfusion requirements and the effects of autotransfusion of cell saver blood in 164 consecutive patients. *Blood Coagul Fibrinolysis* 2000;11(suppl 1):S87–93.

25. de Boer MT, Christensen MC, Asmussen M, et al. The impact of intraoperative transfusion of platelets and red blood cells on survival after liver transplantation. *Anesth Analg* 2008;106:32–44.

26. Benson AB, Austin GL, Berg M, et al. Transfusion-related acute lung injury in ICU patients admitted with gastrointestinal bleeding. *Intens Care Med* 2010;36: 1710–17.

27. Toy P, Gajic O, Bacchetti P, et al. Transfusion related acute lung injury: incidence and risk factors. *Blood* 2011;119:1757–67.

28. Jun CH, Park CH, Lee WS, et al. Antibiotic prophylaxis using third generation cephalosporins can reduce the risk of early rebleeding in the first acute gastro-esophageal variceal hemorrhage: a prospective randomized study. *J Korean Med Sci* 2006;21:883–90.

29. Hou MC, Lin HC, Liu TT, et al. Antibiotic prophylaxis after endoscopic therapy prevents rebleeding in acute variceal hemorrhage: a randomized trial. *Hepatology* 2004;39:746–53.

30. Rasaratnam B, Kaye D, Jennings G, et al. The effect of selective intestinal decon-tamination on the hyperdynamic circulatory state in cirrhosis: a randomized trial. *Ann Intern Med* 2003;139:186–93.

31. Youssef WI, Salazar F, Dasarathy S, et al. Role of fresh frozen plasma infusion in correction of coagulopathy of chronic liver disease: a dual phase study. *Am J Gastro-enterol* 2003;98:1391–4.

32. Franchini M, Montagnana M, Targher G, et al. The use of recombinant factor VIIa in liver diseases. *Blood Coagul Fibrinolysis* 2008;19:341–8.

33. Tripodi A, Anstee QM, Sogaard KK, et al. Hypercoagulability in cirrhosis: causes and consequences (1). *J Thromb Haemost* 2011;9:1713–23.

34. Sogaard KK, Horvath-Puho E, Gronbaek H, et al. Risk of venous thromboembolism in patients with liver disease: a nationwide population-based case-control study. *Am J Gastroenterol* 2009;104:96–101.

35. Heit JA, Silverstein MD, Mohr DN, et al. Risk factors for deep vein thrombosis and pulmonary embolism: a population-based case-control study. *Arch Intern Med* 2000;160:809–15.

36. Tripodi A, Primignani M, Chantarangkul V, et al. An imbalance of pro- vs. anti-coagulation factors in plasma from patients with cirrhosis. *Gastroenterology* 2009; 137:2105–11.

37. Argo CK, Caldwell SH. Epidemiology and natural history of non-alcoholic steato-hepatitis. *Clin Liver Dis* 2009;13:511–31.

38. Tsochatzis EA, Senzolo M, Germani G, et al. Systematic review: portal vein throm-bosis in cirrhosis. *Aliment Pharmacol Ther* 2010;31:366–74.

39. Francoz C, Belghiti J, Vilgrain V, et al. Splanchnic vein thrombosis in candidates for liver transplantation: usefulness of screening and anticoagulation. *Gut* 2005;54: 691–7.

40. Wanless IR, Liu JJ, Butany J. Role of thrombosis in the pathogenesis of congestive hepatic fibrosis (cardiac cirrhosis). *Hepatology* 1995;21:1232–7.

41. Hillenbrand P, Parbhoo SP, Jedrychowski A, et al. Significance of intravascular coagulation and fibrinolysis in acute hepatic failure. *Gut* 1974;15:83–8.

42. Anstee QM, Goldin RD, Wright M, et al. Coagulation status modulates murine hepatic fibrogenesis: implications for the development of novel therapies. *J Thromb Haemost* 2008;6:1336–43.

43. Ganey PE, Luyendyk JP, Newport SW, et al. Role of the coagulation system in acetaminophen-induced hepatotoxicity in mice. *Hepatology* 2007;46:1177–86.

44. Rodriguez KI, Rossetto V, Dabrili P, et al. Effect of low molecular weight heparin (LMWH) on thrombin generation in cirrhotic patients at different stages of liver disease. *J Hepatol* 2011;54(suppl 1):s79–s80.

45. Lisman T, Porte RJ. Towards a rational use of low-molecular-weight heparin in patients with cirrhosis. *Liver Int* 2011;31:1063.

46. Vivarelli M, La Barba G, Cucchetti A, et al. Can antiplatelet prophylaxis reduce the incidence of hepatic artery thrombosis after liver transplantation? *Liver Transpl* 2007;13:651–4.

47. Villa E, Cammà C, Marietta M, et al. Enoxaparin prevents portal vein thrombosis and liver decompensation in patients with advanced cirrhosis. *Gastroenterology* 2012;143:1253–60.

CHAPTER 21

Cancer and Thrombosis

Erica A. Peterson and Agnes Y. Y. Lee

Division of Hematology, University of British Columbia and Vancouver Coastal Health, Vancouver, BC, Canada

Introduction

The association between cancer and thrombosis is well established. Deep vein thrombosis (DVT) and pulmonary embolism (PE), collectively referred to as venous thromboembolism (VTE), are the most commonly observed thrombotic complaints in cancer patients; however, arterial thromboses and clots within other venous systems are also encountered.

The etiology of cancer-associated VTE is complex and multifactorial due to systemic activation of the coagulation system directly or indirectly by tumor cells, medical comorbidities, and poor functional status, as well as therapeutic interventions such as chemotherapy, catheterization, and surgery. The cancer-mediated prothrombotic state is believed to result from alterations in the hemostatic system and activation of coagulation in response to release of proinflammatory effectors and oncogenic events in tumor cells. This prothrombotic state is also a key feature of cancer progression as activation of the coagulation system has many pleotropic effects including downstream regulation of angiogenesis.

Venous thromboembolism is a frequent complication of cancer and may be the first clinical sign of an occult malignant state [1]. The occurrence of VTE in patients with malignancies can result in long-term respiratory and post-phlebitic symptoms, negatively affecting the clinical course and overall quality of life. Additionally, the use of anticoagulant therapy in malignancy is associated with increased bleeding complications [2]. The occurrence of VTE or its complications may force treatment changes or delays in administering therapy, which may alter patient outcome. Irrespective of cancer stage, development of VTE has been shown to be an independent risk factor for mortality [2]. In outpatients receiving chemotherapy, mortality rates over a 75-day period of 9.2% have been observed,

Hemostasis and Thrombosis: Practical Guidelines in Clinical Management, First Edition.
Hussain I. Saba and Harold R. Roberts.
© 2014 John Wiley & Sons, Ltd. Published 2014 by John Wiley & Sons, Ltd.

making VTE the second leading cause of death in this cohort [3]. VTE also places a significant burden on the community with increased hospitalization, resource utilization, and healthcare costs.

Prevention of venous thromboembolism in cancer patients

Anticoagulant prophylaxis has proven efficacy in preventing VTE in multiple medical and surgical settings. In patients with cancer, however, it remains uncertain whether the benefit of prophylaxis outweighs the burden and potential harm of anticoagulants in the majority of patients. Physicians are particularly concerned with the risk of bleeding, the cost and inconvenience of available anticoagulant options, and the lack of evidence on quality of life and mortality benefits. Consequently, risk assessment models are needed to help target prophylaxis at patients with higher risks of VTE and minimize exposure to those at high risk of bleeding.

Risk factors for cancer-associated venous thromboembolism

Numerous risk factors have been identified for cancer-associated thrombosis. They can be subdivided into broad categories such as cancer-related, treatment-related, and patient-related factors (Box 21.1). It is important to also bear in mind that VTE risk does not remain static over time due to acquisition of new risk factors, changes in cancer therapy, or progression of the underlying malignancy.

Tumor biology and behavior strongly influence the risk of VTE. The highest rates of VTE are consistently reported in patients with cancer of the pancreas, brain, and stomach, whereas the lowest incidence rates are seen in patients with tumors of the head and neck (Table 21.1) [4–6]. As discussed earlier, advanced stage and metastatic disease are also associated with increased VTE incidence across all types of tumors, likely reflecting the underlying tumor burden.

Treatment modalities also contribute to the thrombotic risk. Cytotoxic chemotherapy, immunomodulatory agents, anti-angiogenic agents, hormonal treatments, and supportive medications have all been associated with an increased thrombotic risk. Certain chemotherapeutic agents, such as cisplatin, 5-flurouracil, and L-asparaginase, are highly thrombogenic [7]. In multiple myeloma, thalidomide and lenalidomide dramatically raise the incidence of thrombotic complications when combined with steroids or chemotherapy. Other anti-angiogenic agents targeting vascular endothelial growth factor (VEGF), such as bevacizumab, also increase VTE risk [8].

Box 21.1 Risk factors for venous thromboembolism in cancer patients

Patient-related risk factors
Older age
Race
Prior venous thromboembolism
Platelet count
Co-morbid conditions

Cancer-related risk factors
Primary tumor site
Histology
Metastatic disease
Length of time since diagnosis

Treatment-related risk factors
Surgery
Chemotherapy
Hormonal therapy
Antiangiogenic therapy
Erythropoiesis-stimulating agents
Hospitalization
Indwelling vascular access devices

Table 21.1 Incidence of cancer-associated thrombosis according to tumor site.

Tumor site	VTE/100 pt-yrs during 1st yr (N = 235,149) [4]	VTE/100 hospitalizations (N = 40,487,000) [5]	VTE/100 neutropenic hospitalized pts (N = 66,106) [6]
Pancreas	20	4.3	12.10
Brain	—	3.5	9.50
Stomach	10.7	2.7	7.41
Bladder	7	1.0	6.60
Uterine	6.4	2.2	—
Kidney	6	2.0	7.55
Lung	5	2.1	7.00
Colon	4.3	1.0	6.75
Ovary	3.6	1.9	6.50
Breast	2.8	1.7	3.93
Lymphoma	2.5	—	5.01
Prostate	0.9	2.0	7.29

VTE, venous thromboembolism.

Tamoxifen and other hormonal agents increase rates of VTE, particularly when used in combination with conventional chemotherapy [9]. Even supportive care modalities, such as erythropoiesis-stimulating agents, can increase the risk of venous thrombosis [10].

Patient factors such as age, ethnicity, and medical comorbidities also influence VTE risk. Specifically, increasing age, having two or more serious medical conditions, and black race are associated with a higher risk [1]. In contrast, Asian ethnicity appears to confer protection against VTE.

Risk stratification of cancer-associated thrombosis

The first validated risk assessment model for chemotherapy-associated thrombosis was developed using data from the Awareness of Neutropenia in Chemotherapy (ANC) Study Group Registry, where patients were followed for adverse outcomes after starting a new chemotherapeutic regimen [11]. Five independent risk factors for cancer-associated VTE were identified: the site of malignancy, body mass index >35, pre-chemotherapy platelet count $\geq 350 \times 10^9/L$, white blood cell count $>11 \times 10^9/L$, and anemia (hemoglobin <100 g/L) or the use of erythropoiesis-stimulating agents. By assigning a score of 1 or 2 to the presence of these risk factors, the risk of a symptomatic episode of VTE could be estimated based on the total score (Table 21.2). The Khorana score has been validated in other outpatient settings. In the Vienna CAT registry, a prospective cohort of 819 patients with newly diagnosed or progressive cancer who were followed primarily for symptomatic VTE, the 6-month incidence rates of VTE for those with a score of 3 or higher was 17.7%, while those with a score of 0 had a low risk of 1.5% (Table 21.2) [12]. In a randomized controlled study (SAVE-ONCO trial), in which an ultra-low-molecular-weight heparin, semuloparin, was evaluated for primary prophylaxis in patients with a variety of solid tumors [13], the VTE incidence rates in the placebo-controlled group over a median follow-up of 3.5 months were 1.3% in those with a score of 0–1, 3.5% with a score of 2, and 5.4% with a score of 3 [14]. Overall, the evidence supports the Khorana score's ability to stratify VTE risk in ambulatory cancer patients, but the absolute risk of VTE varies in different settings. It is possible that the addition of biomarkers such as D-dimer or soluble P-selectin will further improve the accuracy of the Khorana score, but the lack of assay standardization and increased complexity of the model are potential limitations.

Prevention of venous thromboembolism in cancer patients undergoing surgery

Consensus guidelines recommend the use of low-molecular-weight heparin (LMWH) or unfractionated heparin (UFH) prophylaxis in non-orthopedic surgical patients at moderate to high risk of VTE [15] and in

Table 21.2 Khorana score risk assessment model for venous thromboembolism in outpatient cancer patients receiving chemotherapy [11]. (A) Clinical and laboratory variables used in Khorana score calculation. (B) Venous thromboembolism risk according to risk category.

A	
Patient characteristic	Score
Site of cancer	
Very high risk (stomach, pancreas)	2
High risk (lung, lymphoma, gynecologic, genitourinary excluding prostate)	1
Pre-chemotherapy platelet count $\geq$350,000/mm^3	1
Hemoglobin <10 g/dL or use of Erythropoiesis-stimulating agents	1
Pre-chemotherapy leukocyte count >11,000/mm^3	1
BMI $\geq$35	1

B				
	Total score	ANC study[11]*	Vienna CAT Registry[12]	SAVE-ONCO study[13]†
Follow-up		2.5 months	6 months	3.5 months
Low risk	0	0.3%	1.5%	1.3%
Moderate risk	1–2	2.0%	3.8–9.6%	3.5%
High risk	3 or higher	6.7%	17.7%	5.4%

*Khorana score derivation cohort.
†Low-risk group 0–1 points; moderate-risk group 2 points; high-risk group $\geq$3points.

cancer patients undergoing surgical procedures [16]. Trials that have directly compared the efficacy of short-term LMWH and UFH for post-surgical thromboprophylaxis in cancer patients undergoing elective major abdominal or pelvic surgery have reported no significant difference between these agents [17]. The two largest studies demonstrated VTE rates of approximately 15% using screening venography. Rates of major bleeding were also similar. Data on fondaparinux in the oncology surgical setting is very limited and comes from a subgroup analysis of a single study [18]. Fondaparinux showed a relative risk reduction of 38.6% compared with dalteparin (4.7% vs 7.7%) but these results have not been confirmed.

Extended prophylaxis up to 4 weeks after abdominal or pelvic surgery for cancer has also been studied. In the ENOXICAN II study, the group that received 4 weeks of enoxaparin had a relative risk reduction in veno-graphically detected VTE of 60% (12% vs 4.8%) compared with 6–10 days of prophylaxis [19]. This statistically significant difference was maintained at 3 months. Similar results were observed with extended prophylaxis using dalteparin in the FAME trial, in which over half of included patients underwent surgery for malignancy [20]. The CANBESURE trial found that 28 days of bemiparin significantly reduced the risk of major VTE to 0.8% from 4.6% in the 1-week bemiparin group ($p = 0.010$). Overall, available evidence shows that extended prophylaxis can reduce the incidence of VTE and may reduce fatal VTE. The ASCO guidelines recommend a minimum of 7–10 days of postoperative thromboprophylaxis, with consideration of extending prophylaxis to 4 weeks in patients with high-risk features such as obesity, residual malignancy, and prior VTE [16].

Two observational studies provide further evidence that the risk of symptomatic VTE after cancer surgery is sufficiently high and delayed in some patients to warrant extended prophylaxis. The @RISTOS project followed symptomatic VTE events in cancer patients undergoing general, urologic, or gynecologic surgery [21]. The incidence of VTE in the entire cohort was 2.1% and fatal PE was the cause of death in 46.3%. In 40% of patients thrombotic events occurred over 21 days after surgical intervention. In the Million Women study, 947,454 women in the United Kingdom were tracked for symptomatic VTE using the National Health Service hospital admission database [22]. The peak incidence of PE was at 3 weeks after surgery. During the first 6 weeks, the risk of VTE was increased 91.6-fold compared with those who did not have surgery. Even at 12 weeks post-surgery, this risk remained elevated at 53.4-fold. Further studies are required to determine the optimal duration of postoperative thromboprophylaxis in cancer patients.

Prevention of venous thromboembolism in hospitalized cancer patients

Data regarding thromboprophylaxis in hospitalized, medically ill cancer patients is limited as no trials have been completed in this population. Only 5–15% of patients in clinical trials studying inpatient pharmacologic prophylaxis had cancer. Consequently, it is difficult to determine the relative risk/benefit of anticoagulant prophylaxis in oncology patients admitted to hospital. A post-hoc analysis of the MEDENOX study reported that enoxaparin demonstrated a non-significant relative reduction in VTE of 50% in the cancer patient subgroup [23]. However, because cancer and hospitalization are known independent risk factors for the development of VTE, this subgroup of patients is likely at sufficiently high risk of thrombosis to warrant prophylaxis. Based on this consensus, all major guidelines recommend the use of thromboprophylaxis with UFH, LWMH, or fondaparinux in acutely ill, hospitalized cancer patients with no contraindications to anticoagulation [16,24].

Prevention of venous thromboembolism in cancer outpatients

The risks and benefits of pharmacologic thromboprophylaxis in outpatients receiving chemotherapy have been studied in randomized controlled trials in different tumor types. Warfarin was shown to be effective in reducing symptomatic VTE in women receiving chemotherapy for metastatic breast cancer but it has never been used in practice because of its inconvenience [25]. In contrast, early trials evaluating the benefit of LMWH thromboprophylaxis in patients with advanced stage breast cancer, non-small-cell lung cancer, and high-grade gliomas did not demonstrate a statistically significant reduction in VTE rates [26,27]. But in more recent trials that were adequately powered, LMWH appears effective and safe. The PROTECHT study examined the use of nadroparin in patients with advanced lung, gastrointestinal, pancreatic, breast, ovarian, or head and neck cancers for the duration of their chemotherapy treatment up to a maximum duration of 4 months [28]. A combined endpoint of arterial and venous thrombotic complications was significantly reduced with the use of nadroparin (2.0% vs. 3.9%; $p = 0.02$). More dramatic results with LMWH were reported in two open-label trials in advanced pancreatic cancer that used higher doses of LMWH. The CONKO-004 trial examined the use of enoxaparin 1 mg/kg daily for 3 months, followed by 40 mg daily in patients with advanced pancreatic cancer receiving palliative chemotherapy [29]. A significant decrease in VTE rates were observed with enoxaparin at 3 (1.25% vs 9.9%) and 12 months (5.0% vs 13.0%). In the FRAGEM study, therapeutic doses of dalteparin (200 U/kg/day for 4 weeks, followed by 150 U/kg/day for 12 weeks) were used as primary prophylaxis in patients with advanced pancreatic cancer [30]. Dalteparin was associated with statistically significant 85% risk reduction in VTE (3.4% vs 23%; $p = 0.002$) during the treatment period with no increase in bleeding. Finally, in the SAVE-ONCO trial that included patients with advanced lung, colorectal, stomach, ovarian, pancreatic, or bladder cancer, the use of semuloparin over a median duration of 3.5 months was associated with a 64% relative risk reduction of VTE, with observed VTE rates of 1.2% in the semuloparin group and 3.4% in the placebo group [13]. There was no associated increase in rates of major bleeding (1.2% vs 1.1%).

Primary prophylaxis with ASA, warfarin, and LMWH has been studied in patients with multiple myeloma treated with lenalidomide or thalidomide in combination with steroids or chemotherapy. However, appropriate control groups were not included in the majority of these studies. Hence, although the International Myeloma Working Group recommends using low-dose ASA in low-risk patients and LMWH or warfarin adjusted to an INR of 2.0–3.0 in higher-risk patients, the evidence supporting these recommendations is weak [31–33].

Studies of novel oral anticoagulants for primary prophylaxis have not been performed in cancer patients, with the exception of a single phase II trial of apixaban, an oral direct Xa inhibitor. This small study tested 5, 10, and 20 mg doses of apixaban in 125 patients with metastatic cancer and found that the drug was well tolerated over a 12-week period [34]. Although novel oral agents offer the convenience of oral dosing, stable anticoagulation, and do not requiring laboratory monitoring, interaction with chemotherapeutic agents, inability to rapidly reverse the anticoagulant effect, the higher prevalence of bleeding complications, and liver and renal dysfunction in cancer patients make their use potentially problematic. Therefore, further trials on the efficacy and safety of novel anticoagulants in cancer patients are needed.

Treatment of cancer-associated thrombosis

Initial treatment of VTE in patients with cancer involves the use of parenteral anticoagulants in order to rapidly achieve anticoagulation. Studies specifically comparing UFH, LMWH, and fondaparinux are lacking but data from subgroup analysis of published trials suggests these agents are comparable in efficacy. The same set of data also demonstrates a short-term survival advantage with LMWH, with a statistically significant reduction in 3-month mortality of 29% compared with UFH (RR 0.71; 95% CI 0.52–0.98) [35]. Given that LMWH allows patients to receive therapy on an outpatient basis and reduces the cost associated with hospitalization, LMWH is preferred over UFH for initial therapy of VTE in patients with cancer.

Oral vitamin K antagonists (VKAs) are highly effective in the general population, but their drug and diet interactions, need for frequent laboratory monitoring, dependence on reliable oral intake and normal liver function, and sensitivity to vitamin K stores all contribute to unpredictable anticoagulant responses, leading to difficulties maintaining a therapeutic INR in patients with cancer. Also, cancer patients have higher rates of recurrent VTE and major bleeding when compared to patients without cancer, even while INRs are within therapeutic targets [36,37]. LMWH overcomes many of these problems because of its pharmacokinetic profile. The use of LMWH versus oral VKAs for the long-term treatment of cancer-associated VTE has been studied in several randomized clinical trials (RCTs) [38–41]. The largest trial of these studies, the CLOT trial, demonstrated that dalteparin at a dose of 200 U/kg for the first month followed by a 20–25% dose reduction over the next 5 months was associated with a statistically significant reduction in recurrent VTE compared to oral VKAs (17% vs 9%; RR 0.48; $p = 0.002$). Bleeding and overall mortality were similar between both groups. A meta-analysis of similarly designed trials confirmed these findings [42].

In non-cancer patients with VTE, novel oral anticoagulants directly targeting Xa and thrombin have been evaluated for upfront and long-term therapy. Dabigatran and rivaroxaban have been proven effective in the long-term treatment of VTE and prevention of recurrent thrombotic events (RE-COVER trial, EINSTEIN trial) and other agents are still in phase III testing. Data for the approximate 5% of cancer patients included in these trials has not been published. Given the small numbers and that these cancer patients were highly selected for study inclusion, it is premature to use these agents for treatment of cancer-associated thrombosis. Randomized trials are needed to determine if these new oral anticoagulants are effective and safe in oncology patients.

Consequently, LMWH remains the recommended treatment for both initial and long-term anticoagulation in patients with cancer [16,43]. The optimal duration of anticoagulant therapy has not been determined. However, due to the underlying thrombotic risk associated with cancer and cancer therapy, experts recommend continuing anticoagulation while active disease is present or patients are undergoing cancer treatment [43].

Limited data exist to guide therapy in patients who experience recurrent VTE while on anticoagulation with VKAs or LMWH. In patients treated with VKAs who develop recurrent thrombosis, switching to LMWH is recommended. In patients who develop recurrent events while on standard doses of LMWH, increasing the intensity of anticoagulation with higher doses of LMWH appears to be effective. A small retrospective cohort study of 70 patients with cancer and recurrent VTE found that a 20–25% dose escalation of LMWH was successful at preventing further recurrence in 91% of patients over a follow-up period of 1.9 months [44]. Bleeding complications occurred in 3 patients (4.8%), with only one episode of major bleeding.

References

1. Wun T, White RH. Venous thromboembolism (VTE) in patients with cancer: epidemiology and risk factors. *Cancer Invest* 2009;27:63–74.
2. Kuderer NM, Ortel TL, Francis CW. Impact of venous thromboembolism and anticoagulation on cancer and cancer survival. *J Clin Oncol* 2009;27:4902–11.
3. Khorana AA, Francis CW, Culakova E, et al. Thromboembolism is a leading cause of death in cancer patients receiving outpatient chemotherapy. *J Thromb Haemost* 2007;5:632–4.
4. Chew HK, Wun T, Harvey D, et al. Incidence of venous thromboembolism and its effect on survival among patients with common cancers. *Arch Intern Med* 2006;166: 458–64.

5. Stein PD, Beemath A, Meyers FA, et al. Incidence of venous thromboembolism in patients hospitalized with cancer. *Am J Med* 2006;119:60–8.

6. Khorana AA, Francis CW, Culakova E, et al. Thromboembolism in hospitalized neutropenic cancer patients. *J Clin Oncol* 2006;24:484–90.

7. Haddad TC, Greeno EW. Chemotherapy-induced thrombosis. *Thromb Res* 2006; 118:555–68.

8. Zangari M, Fink LM, Elice F, et al. Thrombotic events in patients with cancer receiving antiangiogenesis agents. *J Clin Oncol* 2009;27:4865–73.

9. Pritchard KI, Paterson AH, Paul NA, et al. Increased thromboembolic complications with concurrent tamoxifen and chemotherapy in a randomized trial of adjuvant therapy for women with breast cancer. National Cancer Institute of Canada Clinical Trials Group Breast Cancer Site Group. *J Clin Oncol* 1996;14:2731–37.

10. Bennett CL, Silver SM, Djulbegovic B, et al. Venous thromboembolism and mortality associated with recombinant erythropoietin and darbepoetin administration for the treatment of cancer-associated anemia. *JAMA* 2008;299:914–24.

11. Khorana AA, Kuderer NM, Culakova E, et al. Development and validation of a predictive model for chemotherapy-associated thrombosis. *Blood* 2008;111:4902–7.

12. Ay C, Dunkler D, Marosi C, et al. Prediction of venous thromboembolism in cancer patients. *Blood* 2010;116:5377–82.

13. Agnelli G, George DJ, Kakkar AK, et al. Semuloparin for thromboprophylaxis in patients receiving chemotherapy for cancer. *N Engl J Med* 2012;366:601–9.

14. George D, Agnelli G, Fisher W, et al. Venous Thromboembolism (VTE) Prevention with Semuloparin in Cancer Patients Initiating Chemotherapy: Benefit-Risk Assessment by VTE Risk in SAVE-ONCO. *Blood* 2011;118:206.

15. Gould MK, Garcia DA, Wren SM, et al. Prevention of VTE in nonorthopedic surgical patients: Antithrombotic Therapy and Prevention of Thrombosis, 9th ed: American College of Chest Physicians Evidence-Based Clinical Practice Guidelines. *Chest* 2012;141:e227S–77S.

16. Lyman GH, Khorana AA, Falanga A, et al. American Society of Clinical Oncology guideline: recommendations for venous thromboembolism prophylaxis and treatment in patients with cancer. *J Clin Oncol* 2007;25:5490–505.

17. ENOXACAN Study Group. Efficacy and safety of enoxaparin versus unfractionated heparin for prevention of deep vein thrombosis in elective cancer surgery: a double-blind randomized multicentre trial with venographic assessment. *Br J Surg* 1997; 84:1099–103.

18. Agnelli G, Bergqvist D, Cohen AT, et al. Randomized clinical trial of postoperative fondaparinux versus perioperative dalteparin for prevention of venous thromboembolism in high-risk abdominal surgery. *Br J Surg* 2005;92:1212–20.

19. Bergqvist D, Agnelli G, Cohen AT, et al. Duration of prophylaxis against venous thromboembolism with enoxaparin after surgery for cancer. *N Engl J Med* 2002; 346:975–80.

20. Rasmussen MS, Jorgensen LN, Wille-Jorgensen P, et al. Prolonged prophylaxis with dalteparin to prevent late thromboembolic complications in patients undergoing major abdominal surgery: a multicenter randomized open-label study. *J Thromb Haemost* 2006;4:2384–90.

21. Agnelli G, Bolis G, Capussotti L, et al. A clinical outcome-based prospective study on venous thromboembolism after cancer surgery: the @RISTOS project. *Ann Surg* 2006;243:89–95.

22. Sweetland S, Green J, Liu B, et al. Duration and magnitude of the postoperative risk of venous thromboembolism in middle aged women: prospective cohort study. *Br Med J* 2009;339:b4583.

23. Alikhan R, Cohen AT, Combe S, et al. Prevention of venous thromboembolism in medical patients with enoxaparin: a subgroup analysis of the MEDENOX study. *Blood Coagul Fibrinolysis* 2003;14:341–6.

24. Khorana AA. The NCCN Clinical Practice Guidelines on Venous Thromboembolic Disease: strategies for improving VTE prophylaxis in hospitalized cancer patients. *Oncologist* 2007;12:1361–70.

25. Levine M, Hirsh J, Gent M, et al. Double-blind randomized trial of a very-low-dose warfarin for prevention of thromboembolism in stage IV breast cancer. *Lancet* 1994;343:886–9.

26. Haas SK, Freund M, Heigener D, et al. Low-molecular-weight heparin versus placebo for the prevention of venous thromboembolism in metastatic breast cancer or stage III/IV lung cancer. *Clin Appl Thromb Hemost* 2012;18:159–65.

27. Perry JR, Julian JA, Laperriere NJ, et al. PRODIGE: a randomized placebo-controlled trial of dalteparin low-molecular-weight heparin thromboprophylaxis in patients with newly diagnosed malignant glioma. *J Thromb Haemost* 2010;8:1959–65.

28. Agnelli G, Gussoni G, Bianchini C, et al. Nadroparin for the prevention of thromboembolic events in ambulatory patients with metastatic or locally advanced solid cancer receiving chemotherapy: a randomized, placebo-controlled, double-blind study. *Lancet Oncol* 2009;10:943–9.

29. Riess H, Pelzer U, Opitz B, et al. A prospective, randomized trial of simultaneous pancreatic cancer treatment with enoxaparin and chemotherapy: Final results of the CONKO-004 trial. *J Clin Oncol* 2010;28:15(suppl) abstr 4033.

30. Maraveyas A, Waters J, Roy R, et al. Gemcitabine versus gemcitabine plus dalteparin thromboprophylaxis in pancreatic cancer. *Eur J Cancer* 2012;48:1283–92.

31. Larocca A, Cavallo F, Bringhen S, et al. Aspirin or enoxaparin thromboprophylaxis for patients with newly diagnosed multiple myeloma treated with lenalidomide. *Blood* 2012;119:933–9.

32. Palumbo A, Cavo M, Bringhen S, et al. Aspirin, warfarin, or enoxaparin thromboprophylaxis in patients with multiple myeloma treated with thalidomide: a phase III, open-label, randomized trial. *J Clin Oncol* 2011;29:986–93.

33. Palumbo A, Rajkumar SV, Dimopoulos MA, et al. Prevention of thalidomide- and lenalidomide-associated thrombosis in myeloma. *Leukemia* 2008;22:414–23.

34. Levine MN, Gu C, Liebman HA, et al. A randomized phase II trial of apixaban for the prevention of thromboembolism in patients with metastatic cancer. *J Thromb Haemost* 2012;10:807–14.

35. Akl EA, Vasireddi SR, Gunukula S, et al. Anticoagulation for the initial treatment of venous thromboembolism in patients with cancer. *Cochrane Database Syst Rev* 2011;6: CD006649.

36. Prandoni P, Trujillo-Santos J, Sanchez-Cantalejo E, et al. Major bleeding as a predictor of mortality in patients with venous thromboembolism: findings from the RIETE Registry. *J Thromb Haemost* 2010;8:2575–7.

37. Hutten BA, Prins MH, Gent M, et al. Incidence of recurrent thromboembolic and bleeding complications among patients with venous thromboembolism in relation to both malignancy and achieved international normalized ratio: a retrospective analysis. *J Clin Oncol* 2000;18:3078–83.

38. Hull RD, Pineo GF, Brant RF, et al. Self-managed long-term low-molecular-weight heparin therapy: the balance of benefits and harms. *Am J Med* 2007;120:72–82.

39. Lee AY, Levine MN, Baker RI, et al. Low-molecular-weight heparin versus a coumarin for the prevention of recurrent venous thromboembolism in patients with cancer. *N Engl J Med* 2003;349:146–53.

40. Meyer G, Marjanovic Z, Valcke J, et al. Comparison of low-molecular-weight heparin and warfarin for the secondary prevention of venous thromboembolism in patients with cancer: a randomized controlled study. *Arch Intern Med* 2002;162: 1729–35.
41. Deitcher SR, Kessler CM, Merli G, et al. Secondary prevention of venous thromboembolic events in patients with active cancer: enoxaparin alone versus initial enoxaparin followed by warfarin for a 180-day period. *Clin Appl Thromb Hemost* 2006;12:389–96.
42. Akl EA, Labedi N, Barba M, et al. Anticoagulation for the long-term treatment of venous thromboembolism in patients with cancer. *Cochrane Database Syst Rev* 2011;6: CD006650.
43. Kearon C, Akl EA, Comerota AJ, et al. Antithrombotic therapy for VTE disease: Antithrombotic Therapy and Prevention of Thrombosis, 9th ed: American College of Chest Physicians Evidence-Based Clinical Practice Guidelines. *Chest* 2012;141: e419S–94S.
44. Carrier M, Le Gal G, Cho R, et al. Dose escalation of low molecular weight heparin to manage recurrent venous thromboembolic events despite systemic anticoagulation in cancer patients. *J Thromb Haemost* 2009;7:760–5.

CHAPTER 22

An Update on Low-Molecular-Weight Heparins

Jawed Fareed,[1] Debra Hoppensteadt, and Walter P. Jeske
[1]Department of Pathology & Pharmacology, Hemostasis & Thrombosis Research Laboratories, Loyola University Chicago, 2160 S. First Avenue, Maywood, IL, USA

Introduction

The low-molecular-weight heparins (LMWHs) represent an important class of anticoagulant drug used for the management of thrombotic and cardiovascular disorders [1,2]. The LMWHs have added a new dimension to heparin therapy. Prior to the introduction of LMWHs, unfractionated heparin was primarily administered to hospitalized patients. Following the introduction of LMWHs, patients could be treated for thrombotic and cardiovascular disorders on an outpatient basis for extended periods of time. Subsequent studies have produced further indications for LMWH including cancer-associated thrombosis, additional cardiovascular indications, and pregnancy-associated thrombosis.

In addition to the antithrombotic properties of LMWHs, these agents exhibit anti-inflammatory effects. The anti-inflammatory properties are mediated by the release of endogenous tissue factor pathway inhibitor. Therefore, the LMWHs demonstrate pleotropic effects and mediate their therapeutic actions by multiple processes.

LMWHs provide a safer alternative to unfractionated heparin. Bleeding and heparin-induced thrombocytopenia (HIT) complications are significantly less across the different indications. Currently, lower-molecular-weight heparins known as ultra-LMWHs and synthetic heparins are in various stages of development.

Available low-molecular-weight heparins

At present, three branded LMWHs, namely enoxaparin, dalteparin, and tinzaparin, are available in the United States. In Europe, several additional

---

Hemostasis and Thrombosis: Practical Guidelines in Clinical Management, First Edition.
Hussain I. Saba and Harold R. Roberts.

Table 22.1 Profiles of low-molecular-weight heparins. Data generated in the Hemostasis and Thrombosis Research Laboratories of the Loyola University Medical Center.

LMWH	Average MW (daltons)	AXa U/mg	AntiIIa U/mg	AXa/AIIa ratio
Ardeparin	5200	90	18	4.8
Bemiparin	3600	85	9	9.7
Certoparin	5400	95	54	2.4
Dalteparin	6000	135	40	2.5
Enoxaparin	4500	100	26	3.9
Fraxiparine	4300	100	23	4.4
Nadroparin	4300	100	30	3.3
Panaparin	5000	90	40	2.3
Reviparin	4400	90	22	4.2
Tinzaparin	6500	98	62	1.6

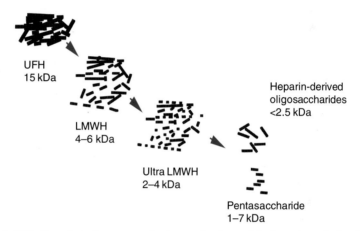

Figure 22.1 Manufacturing process for low-molecular-weight heparin and ultra-low-molecular-weight heparin. UFH, unfractionated heparin.

LMWHs are available, including reviparin, certoparin, parnaparin, and fraxiparine (Table 22.1).

All of the LMWHs are prepared either by chemical or by enzymatic depolymerization of unfractionated heparin (Figure 22.1). The depolymerization processes differ from one LMWH to another, which may result in microchemical changes in the structure of the oligosaccharides. The processes for the production of LMWH are listed below [3].

- Oxidative depolymerization with hydrogen peroxide is used for the manufacture of ardeparin.
- Deaminative cleavage with isoamyl nitrate is used for the manufacture of certoparin.

- β-Elimination (chemical): enoxaparin

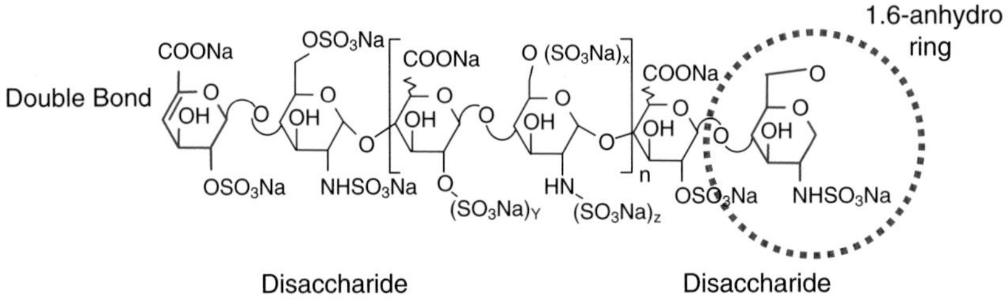

- β-Elimination (enzymatic): tinzaparin

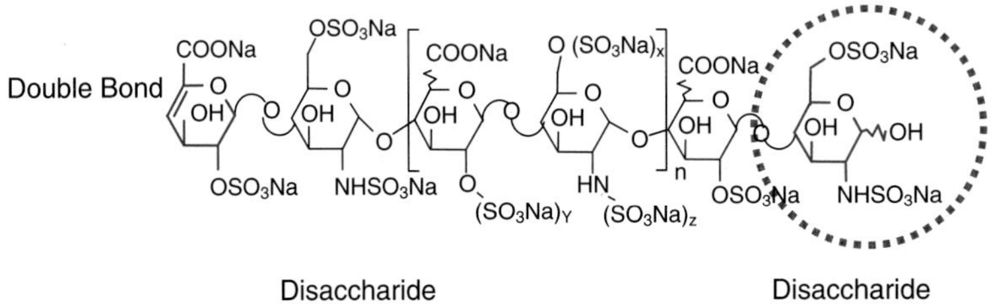

Fareed J, et al. Hematol Oncol Clin North Am. 2005;19:53-68. Linhardt RJ, Gunay NS. Semin Thromb Hemost. 1999;25 suppl 3:5-16.

Figure 22.2 Chemical fingerprint of enoxaparin and tinzaparin [4,47].

- Alkaline beta eliminative cleavage of the benzyl ester of heparin is used for the manufacture of enoxaparin and bemiparin.
- Enzymatic beta eliminative cleavage is used for the manufacture of tinzaparin.
- Deaminative cleavage with nitrous acid is used for the manufacture of dalteparin, reviparin and fraxiparine.

The different depolymerization processes result in certain changes in the heparin molecule and the resulting shorter chains exhibit specific structural differences. A comparison of the differences between enoxaparin (which is prepared by beta elimination using a chemical method) and tinzaparin (which is prepared by digesting heparin by beta elimination with enzyme heparinase) is shown in Figure 22.2. While both methods result in the generation of double bonds, the chemical method results in the formation of anhydro-manno groups. This grouping is considered to be characteristic of enoxaparin. Deaminative cleavage with nitrous acid results in the formation of a novel 2,5-anhydromannose residue at the reducing terminal of the oligosaccharide. This is subsequently transformed into anhydromannitol using a reducing agent.

Since LMWHs are prepared by different methods and exhibit distinct molecular and biologic properties, minor changes in the manufacturing process may result in major variations in biologic properties [4]. Therefore, the US Food and Drug Administration (FDA) requires extensive information on the structure of each LMWH. Stringent biologic specifications along with clinical information are required to assure product identity and safety. It is, therefore, of crucial importance to characterize each product in terms of its biologic and structural properties. Because their molecular, structural, biochemical, and pharmacologic properties differ, each drug is expected to have its own clinical profile in terms of the safety and efficacy in a given indication [5–7].

Despite similar molecular weights and comparable potencies in pharmacologic assays, LMWHs exhibit different pharmacologic properties [8–10]. Each LMWH is considered to be a distinct drug by the FDA, the European Medicines Agency, and the World Health Organization. Each LMWH possesses specific indications for appropriate use.

Enoxaparin is the most widely used LMWH and is indicated for the management of deep vein thrombosis (DVT) and acute coronary syndrome. Recently, generic versions of enoxaparin have become available in certain parts of the world, and are considered comparable to the branded enoxaparin. In the United States, two generic versions of enoxaparin are available. In addition, an authorized generic product from Winthrop has also become available.

Porcine mucosal heparin is used for the manufacture of various LMWHs. The purity and biologic profile of the starting material is important in obtaining a consistent product. Strict quality control measures are in place in the manufacture of LMWH. These specifications are reported in the United States Pharmacopeia (USP) monograph [5]. LMWHs can also be differentiated from unfractionated heparin. Table 22.2 lists some of the differences between unfractionated heparin and LMWH.

Table 22.2 Comparison of heparin and low-molecular-weight heparin.

Parameter	Heparin	LMWH
Origin	Bovine or porcine mucosa, bovine lung	Porcine mucosa
Molecular weight	15–17 kDa	4–6 kDa
USP potency	150–200 U/mg	20–50 U/mg
AXA U/mg	150–200 U/mg	80–130 U/mg
Monitoring	APTT	AXa (amidolytic methods)
Bioavailability	30–40%	100%
Bleeding complications	Moderate	Relatively low
Reversible	Protamine sulfate	No antagonist (high-dose protamine)
Incidence of heparin-induced thrombocytopenia	1–5%	<1%
Osteoporosis	High risk	Low risk
Drug interactions	Rare	Rare

Approved clinical use of low-molecular-weight heparins

The three approved LMWHs in the US (enoxaparin, tinzaparin, and dalta-parin) are marketed for specific indications. These approved indications are based on the clinical data each supplier has provided to the FDA. Enoxaparin possesses the greatest number of indications, reflecting the broadest clinical research profile. Indications for enoxaparin include the following:
- Treatment of unstable angina and non-Q-wave myocardial infarction;
- Prophylaxis of DVT following total hip and knee replacement;
- Prophylaxis of DVT in medical conditions;
- Prophylaxis of DVT following abdominal surgery;
- Treatment of DVT with, or without, pulmonary embolism.

Enoxaparin is classified by the FDA as a Category B drug for pregnancy. It is not expected to harm the fetus and, similar to other LMWHs, it does not cross the placental barrier. Enoxaparin can be used during all stages of pregnancy; however, close monitoring is recommended.

Tinzaparin is approved in the United States for the following indications:
- Prophylaxis of DVT in medically ill and elderly patients;
- Prophylaxis of DVT following total hip and knee replacement;
- Prophylaxis of DVT following abdominal surgery;
- Treatment of DVT with or without pulmonary embolism;
- Prophylaxis and treatment of DVT in pregnant women.
- Tinzaparin is also licensed for the management of gestational hy-percoagulability and is often preferred over other LMWHs in pregnant women.

Like other LMWHs, daltaparin is used for the following indications:
- Prophylaxis of DVT following total hip and knee surgery;
- Treatment of DVT and pulmonary embolism;
- Treatment of unstable angina and non-Q-wave myocardial infarction;
- Treatment of DVT in patients with cancer.

Generic low-molecular-weight heparins

Several generic versions of enoxaparin have been approved in the US and other countries. In the US, there are two approved generic versions of enoxaparin. One version is supplied by Sandoz and the other is supplied

Table 22.3 Generic low-molecular-weight heparins.

Generic LMWH	Country
Cutenoc	India
Markaparin	India
Clenox	India
Lomoparin	India
Lupenox	India
Lomorin-NX	India
Lomoh	India
Troynoxa-40	India
Daltehep	India
Enoxalow	South America
Versa	South America
Heptron	South America
Endocris	South America
Fibrinox	South America
Enoxaparin-Sandoz	United States
Enoxaparin-Amphastar	United States
Enoxparin-Winthrop	United States

All of the above are generic versions of enoxaparin except daltehep which is the generic form of dalteparin.

by Watson Pharmaceuticals. Several additional generic versions of enoxaparin are marketed in Asia and South America. Some of the generic versions of enoxaparin are listed in Table 22.3. The FDA has developed specific guidelines that the manufacturers of generic enoxaparin must follow to prove that their drug is similar to the branded enoxaparin. These guidelines include the following:

1. Origin of the starting material (unfractionated heparin or crude heparin) – species specifications;
2. Manufacturing process – patent adherence;
3. Molecular and structural characterization;
4. Biophysical and biochemical profile;
5. Pharmacologic profile including animal models and pharmacokinetic and pharmacodynamic (PK/PD) testing in humans.

The FDA approval process for enoxaparin does not require any clinical validation of the generic products for any of the approved indications. The generic enoxaparins carry all the indications of the branded enoxaparin. Several other generic versions of enoxaparin and dalteparin are being developed.

Ultra-low-molecular-weight heparins

The ultra-low-molecular-weight heparins have been developed for various indications. They include bemiparin (Rovi, Madrid, Spain) and semuloparin (Sanofi, Paris, France). These drugs show a relatively lower molecular weight profile and a higher anti-Xa and anti-IIa ratio. These agents are not available in the US at this time. Semuloparin has been extensively studied for DVT prophylaxis in post-surgical protocols. Moreover, it has also been studied in the cancer population for the prevention of cancer-associated thrombosis. These drugs have been investigated for their potential value in specific indications such as stroke and atrial fibrillation. Moreover, because of their structural and molecular profile, these drugs may be safer than enoxaparin.

In June 2012, an FDA advisory committee voted against the approval of semuloparin for the prophylaxis of venous thromboembolism (VTE) in cancer patients undergoing chemotherapy. Despite the positive results of the clinical trials, further development of this drug was halted.

Synthetic heparin derivatives

The chemically synthetic pentasaccharide, fondaparinux, has been used in the management of post-surgical DVT. The relative safety of this drug is considered to be better than that of both heparin and the LMWHs. It is chemically synthesized and is, therefore, free of any viral or biologic contaminants. This agent has been found to produce no HIT responses. Various derivatives of this pentasaccharide have been developed for the management of thrombosis, but have met with limited success. A generic version of pentasaccharide has also recently become available. Unlike the LMWHs, pentasaccharide does not have any antithrombin activity and mediates its biologic effects mainly through the inhibition of factor Xa. It also has a long biologic half-life. Fondaparinux has been used in additional indications, including the management of acute coronary syndrome and other anticoagulant management of heparin-compromised patients, such as those with HIT. There have been reports that fondaparinux is used to treat patients with established HIT as it has no affinity with platelet factor 4; however, because of renal excretion it is not recommended for patients with impaired renal function. Fondaparinux is administered subcutaneously and its clinical use includes prevention of DVT in patients after orthopedic surgery as well as for the treatment of DVT and pulmonary embolism.

Other related agents

Danaparoid was a low-molecular-weight glycosaminoglycan mixture containing dermatan, heparan, and LMWH. This agent was used in the anticoagulant management of heparin-compromised patients such as those with HIT, but it has been withdrawn from the market. Additional LMWH-related drugs have also been developed; however, none of these are in clinical use.

Neutralization of low-molecular-weight heparin and fondaparinux

Unlike heparin, the effects of LMWH are only partially neutralized by protamine sulfate. Symptomatic bleeding can be reduced by protamine sulfate; however, the pharmacokinetics of LMWHs and protamine sulfate differ considerably. Protamine sulfate can only be administered intravenously and exhibits a short half-life. The LMWHs have a relatively longer half-life after intravenous and subcutaneous administration. Therefore, rebound responses in both administration modalities may be observed. Protamine neutralizes the anti-IIa effects of LMWH and only partially neutralizes anti-Xa effects. A suitable neutralizing agent for LMWH is yet to be developed.

Fondaparinux is a potent anti-Xa agent which is not reversible by protamine sulfate or fresh frozen plasma. Prothrombin complex concentrates and factor VIIa have been considered in reversal of the anticoagulant effects of fondaparinux [11]. Supportive data on the use of factor VIIa as a reversal agent is available. The role of platelet concentrates and antifibrinolytic agents such as ε-aminocaproic acid (EACA) is not clear.

Contamination of low-molecular-weight heparin

In late 2007 and in 2008, the FDA recalled several batches of heparin due to reports of severe adverse reactions. It was determined that several batches of heparin were adulterated with oversulfated chondroitin sulfate. This contaminant was also found in several batches of various LMWHs. Many of the LMWH products were recalled from the market. The regulatory agencies alerted clinicians and strict quality control methods were instituted. These included stringent analytic requirements to establish the absence of the contaminant from LMWH.

Additional methods to characterize the contaminants were developed and included isolation of the non-heparin contaminant and its characterization by sophisticated methods [12]. The contaminants isolated from heparin and from enoxaparin were comparable to reference semisynthetic oversulfated chondroitin sulfates prepared from chondroitin sulfate obtained from mammalian and marine sources [13]. Beside the main contaminant, several other non-heparin glycosaminoglycans were reportedly present in the contaminated batches of heparin. Some of these contaminants are yet to be characterized.

Additional clinical investigation of low-molecular-weight heparin

LMWHs have been studied in additional indications such as pregnancy-associated thrombosis, cancer-associated thrombosis, pediatrics, kidney disease, and patients with cirrhosis of the liver.

LMWHs have come to play a significant role in the treatment of pregnancy-related thrombosis which has been identified to be one of the leading causes of maternal mortality during pregnancy [14]. Although the use of anticoagulant therapy in pregnancy is challenging due to the potential complications for both the fetus and the mother, LMWH is recommended over unfractionated heparin for the prevention and treatment of VTE [15].

The two most common causes of thrombosis in pregnancy are a previous history of VTE and thrombophilia [16]. There has been an increase in the number of women who are at high risk for thrombosis whom are being treated with LMWH during pregnancy and the puerperium [17]. In one study, women were treated with both therapeutic and prophylactic dosages of LMWH. In this study, the live birth rate was 97% with minimal complications, which included bleeding and decreased bone density [18]. Another study suggested that frequent monitoring of anti-Xa levels may assist in the dose adjustments which may be required throughout pregnancy due to the changes in the weight of the individual patient [19]. LMWHs have also been used to treat pulmonary embolism in pregnant patients [16].

No large trials have been performed in this patient group, most likely due to the fear of adverse outcomes such as bleeding complications to the mother or fetus. Nor have there been any studies to determine the optimal duration of treatment for pregnancy-related thrombosis. However, the current Chest guidelines recommend the use of LMWH for prevention and treatment of venous thrombosis in this patient population [15].

LMWHs have also been shown to reduce the risk of venous thrombosis in patients with cancer [20,21]. In several studies, LMWHs have also been shown to prolong survival in cancer patients [22–24]. In addition to their antithrombotic effects, LMWHs may have antitumor effects by interfering with angiogenesis, tumor growth, and metastasis [22–24].

Although thrombosis is the second most common cause of death in patients with cancer, prophylaxis is underused in this patient group. Recent studies have shown that LMWHs are effective at reducing VTE in patients with breast cancer and ovarian cancer [25–27]. Another study demonstrated that LMWHs are safe and effective for VTE treatment and prevention in cancer patients with renal disease [28]. The ultra-LMWH semuloparin was shown to reduce the incidence of VTE in patients receiving chemotherapy, with no reported increase in major bleeding. In this study, the median treatment duration was 3.5 months [29].

Despite the huge impact of LMWHs on the treatment and prevention of VTE in cancer patients, there are several unanswered questions which emphasize a need for additional clinical trials in this area [23,24].

While the incidence of thrombosis in children is low, treatment in this population has been understudied. Most recommendations for treatment of pediatric patients are extrapolated from adult clinical trials. However, the physiology of children is much different than that of adults. The hemostatic system is not fully developed in young children and, therefore, the dosing regimens and responses vary from adults [30]. Regulatory agencies have released initiatives for the use of LMWHs in children. Despite the lack of clinical trials, LMWHs remain the treatment of choice in the pediatric population for both the treatment and prophylaxis of thrombosis [31].

In addition, there has recently been an increased usage of LMWHs in the trauma setting in children [32,33]. Some publications suggest that, in children and neonates, anti-Xa levels should be monitored by using the anti-Xa method [31]. The Chest guidelines provide weak recommendations for target ranges in the pediatric group. It is clear that additional studies need to be performed in this patient group to provide clear guidelines [31].

Low-molecular-weight heparin in special patient populations

Certain subpopulations, including patients with renal insufficiency, liver disease, and obese patients, have not been extensively studied in pivotal clinical trials. LMWHs have been studied in patients with chronic kidney disease in order to answer the question of whether the dosage needs to be adjusted in these patients [34,35]. In one study, 3 of 61 patients suffered major bleeding and 2 had supratherapeutic anti-Xa levels [35]. The Chest guidelines recommend several possible approaches to the correct dosing of LMWHs in patients with severe chronic kidney disease.

The approved dosages of the different LMWHs may not be optimal for certain patient populations [36]. More importantly, the data on safety and efficacy is limited since it is usually based on pharmacokinetic studies performed in healthy subjects or a small cohort of patient groups.

LMWHs have recently been used in patients with liver cirrhosis. One recent study demonstrates that enoxaparin given over 12 months not only prevented portal vein thrombosis but also delayed hepatic decompensation [36]. Although LMWHs are not cleared by the liver, most liver disease patients have compromised hemostatic systems and may respond differentially to various LMWHs. In obese patients, the dosing of LMWHs has not been optimized. Concerns regarding the possible overdosing of the therapeutic dosage and underdosing of the prophylactic dose are valid. Therefore, LMWHs should be used with caution in special populations, where monitoring may be needed.

Low-molecular-weight heparins in elderly patients

Elderly patients are at high risk for VTE and acute coronary syndrome; however, these patients are also at high risk of bleeding. Most of the clinical trials have excluded this group of patients in studies for various indications. Clinical evidence suggests that when treated with full-dose enoxaparin, dalteparin, and pentasaccharide, elderly patients may exhibit different safety and efficacy profiles. This may be due to pharmacokinetic and pharmacodynamic differences in these patients that put them at high risk of accumulating LMWHs. Dosage adjustments have been proposed to optimize the use of these agents in elderly patients [37].

Low-molecular-weight heparins in patients with inflammatory bowel disease

Patients with ulcerative colitis are at an increased risk of thrombosis [38,39]. Both heparin and LMWH have been used in the management of this disorder. Prophylactic dosage of LMWHs did not show any benefit over placebo for any outcome including clinical remission and endoscopic and histologic improvements. High dosage of LMWH administered via alternate routes and orally administered colonic release tablets demonstrated limited benefit. The use of these agents may be associated with rectal bleeding and, therefore, caution should be exercised in dosing these agents.

Monitoring of low-molecular-weight heparins: prophylactic and therapeutic dosages

The current recommendation is that most patients receiving prophylactic and therapeutic LMWH do not require monitoring [40–42]. This includes patients who are clinically stable and receiving prophylaxis for postoperative VTE. Uncomplicated patients under treatment with higher doses of LMWH for established VTE by a weight-adjusted, fixed dose do not require monitoring. There is little to no risk of having circulating drug concentrations outside the target range in these patients due to the pharmacokinetic behavior of LMWH.

Patients receiving LMWH who do require monitoring include those who are obese, have renal insufficiency, or are pediatric patients or newborns [40,41]. Women should be monitored periodically throughout pregnancy due to changing physiologic requirements as the pregnancy proceeds. Patients receiving LMWH for long-term therapeutic treatment, such as for malignancy, and those receiving LMWH if refractory to warfarin (antiphospholipid, myeloproliferative disorders) or if warfarin derivatives are contraindicated, should be monitored.

LMWH and unfractionated heparin can be assayed by clot or chromogenic-based anti-FXa assays [40–43]. It should be appreciated that monitoring LMWHs by an anti-FXa assay will not always give a complete measure of the drug effect because these drugs have antithrombotic activities other than factor Xa inhibition.

The half-life of LMWH measured by different assays can be different. It has been observed that the anti-FXa activity is longer than the half-life of the anticoagulant effect measured by activated clotting time after protamine neutralization. Similar discrepancies are observed for heparin between these assays where, for example, results from the aPTT do not necessarily reflect the same results from the chromogenic anti-FXa assay.

When LMWH is needed, the chromogenic anti-FXa assay is the currently recommended assay [40,42]. The clot-based aPTT is only sensitive to very high levels of LMWH. The chromogenic anti-FXa assay has sensitivity to LMWH and is a specific assay for LMWH; however, accuracy and reproducibility of results can vary between laboratories.

Blood samples for LMWH monitoring should be obtained 3–4 hours after a subcutaneous injection to obtain the peak circulating concentration. Target peak level for treatment of VTE is 0.5–1.1 anti-FXa U/mL.

Newborns may need a higher dose (1.6 mg/kg) than older pediatric or adult patients (1.0 mg/kg) to reach the target range [29]. If the patient is receiving the drug intravenously, the blood specimen is to be drawn from a different extremity than the one used for drug infusion.

Newer anticoagulants and low-molecular-weight heparin

Over the past decade, several newer anticoagulant drugs have been developed for both parenteral and oral usage. These agents included parenteral anticoagulants such as argatroban, bivalirudin, and hirudin. These drugs are intended as alternative anticoagulation for heparin-compromised patients who developed HIT syndrome. However, unlike LMWH, none of these agents can be administered via the subcutaneous route. Moreover, these agents do not have any neutralizing agent at this time. Furthermore, these agents can only be administered for short-term use.

More recently, newer oral anticoagulants have been developed for the management of post-surgical deep vein thrombosis (DVT) and atrial fibrillation [44,45]. The newer oral anticoagulants target either thrombin or factor Xa. Currently, an oral thrombin inhibitor, dabigatran (Pradaxa), is available for stroke prevention in patients with atrial fibrillation. A factor Xa inhibitor, rivaroxaban (Xarelto), is available for multiple indications including stroke prevention in atrial fibrillation, post-orthopedic surgical prophylaxis of DVT, and the treatment of DVT and pulmonary embolism. Several other agents, such as apixaban and edoxaban, are being developed for similar indications.

While the new oral anticoagulants may offer certain advantages over warfarin, such as rapid onset of action, limited monitoring requirements, decreased population-based variation, and single dosing indications, there are disadvantages. These agents do not have an available antidote, and are not without adverse bleeding events. There are also drug interactions and variations in response. These agents also cross the placental barrier and may not be useful in pregnant patients.

The new oral anticoagulant drugs were initially developed for the prophylaxis of DVT in orthopedic surgical patients and were compared with enoxaparin in various clinical trials. However, their main indication is in stroke prevention in atrial fibrillation. Although in the initial clinical trials many of the newer oral anticoagulants such as apixaban, dabigatran, and rivaroxaban were comparable to enoxaparin, these agents are monotherapeutic agents with certain limitations. In controlled clinical trials, these agents were effective; however, bleeding complications and cardiovascular events occurred with some of these agents. In contrast to the

LMWHs such as enoxaparin, these drugs do not release tissue factor pathway inhibitor. None of these agents exhibit anti-inflammatory effects, which are important in the management of DVT. Currently there is only limited knowledge of population-based variations in response, drug and food interaction, and some of the other biologic effects. The LMWHs offer a predictable and optimal therapeutic and safety profile and many advantages in the management of thrombosis at present. Additional clinical trials are needed to further compare these newer oral anticoagulants with LMWH. Perhaps the post-marketing surveillance data will be helpful in comparing the two classes of these drugs in the management of thromboembolism. The use of new oral anticoagulant drugs in elderly, pediatric, and pregnant patients is also associated with risks and LMWHs should be considered in these populations.

Some of the currently approved or developed oral anticoagulants can be used for the anticoagulant management of heparin-compromised patients. Similar to the parenteral anticoagulant agents, dabigatran and rivaroxaban are synthetic products which do not interact with platelet factor 4. Therefore, none of these agents is expected to produce HIT responses. In-vitro studies on the screening of these agents in HIT studies have demonstrated that dabigatran and rivaroxaban do not mediate HIT antibody aggregation [46]. Furthermore, there have been no reports from the clinical trials and post-marketing surveillance data on the incidence of HIT in patients treated with these agents. However, there are no clinical trials or any other dedicated studies which have provided any clinical evidence on this subject at this time.

Conclusion

As a class of anticoagulants, the LMWHs have added a new dimension in the management of thrombotic and cardiovascular disorders. Not only have these drugs become the standard of care in the approved indications such as the management of venous thrombosis, but these agents are used in indications including adjunct therapy for cancer, autoimmune diseases, neurologic disorders, and inflammatory disorders. Each of the individual LMWHs is considered to be a distinct entity and, as such, is only approved for specific clinical indications where the efficacy is established in clinical trials.

Enoxaparin represents the most widely used LMWH with multiple indications. More recently, generic versions of enoxaparin have become approved by the FDA for all approved indications for which the branded product is approved. Since the initial approval of the first generic LMWH in July 2010, the generic enoxaparin is now widely used. Concerns over the quality of the generic enoxaparin have been expressed; however, no adverse reports have been received.

Until 2007, the regulatory guidelines for the production and approval for LMWHs were vague; however, the contaminant crisis prompted the regulatory bodies to require specific structural and biologic information on LMWHs. The FDA now requires specific data on the manufacturing and biologic profile of each agent prior to its approval. Moreover, specific measures to assess the quality of heparin and LMWHs have been implemented. Thus, the currently available LMWHs are safer and are manufactured to specifications.

The labeled use of each of these LMWHs for specific indications has provided consistent clinical results. In most patients monitoring is not required; however, in certain populations dosage adjustment requires monitoring. In patients that are weight compromised, elderly, or with renal impairment, monitoring may be required to avoid bleeding complications. Unlike with heparin, the prevalence of HIT associated with LMWH is extremely rare. However, these agents should not be used in patients with a history of HIT. Other adverse effects observed with heparin such as osteoporosis, alopecia, and allergic manifestations are also relatively decreased with the use of LMWH.

Ever since their introduction, LMWHs have continued to provide a class of drug for the management of thrombotic disorders in both medical and surgical patients. Newer indications for these agents are continually being explored. The safety and efficacy profile of these agents is predictable. The availability of generic versions of LMWHs has facilitated the use of these drugs by a broader group of patients at an affordable cost. Despite the development of newer anticoagulants, the LMWHs will remain the drugs of choice for many indications for years to come.

References

1. Fareed J, Hoppensteadt DA, Fareed D, et al. Survival of heparins, oral anticoagulants, and aspirin after the year 2010. *Semin Thromb Hemost* 2008;34:58–73.
2. Haas S, Breyer HG, Bacher HO, et al. Prevention of major venous thromboembolism following total hip or knee replacement: a randomized comparison of low-molecular-weight heparin with unfractionated heparin (ECHOS Trial). *Int Angiol* 2006;25: 335–42.
3. Weitz JI. Low-molecular-weight heparins. *N Engl J Med* 1997;337;688–98.
4. Linhardt R, Gunay NS. Production and chemical processing of low molecular weight heparins. *Semin Thromb Hemost* 1999;25:5–16.
5. *US Pharmacopeial Forum* 2011;37(1). www.usp.org. accessed Oct 4, 2012.
6. Garcia DA, Baglin TP, Weitz JI. Parenteral anticoagulants: antithrombotic therapy and prevention of thrombosis. *Chest* 2012;141(2 suppl):e24S–43S.

7. Jeske W, Walenga J, Fareed J. Differentiating between the low-molecular-weight heparin used for VTE treatment and prophylaxis. *Thromb Clin* 2008;2:23–8.

8. Maddineni J, Walenga JM, Jeske WP, et al. Product individuality of commercially available low-molecular-weight heparins and their generic versions: therapeutic implications. *Clin Appl Thromb Hemost* 2006;12:267–76.

9. Jeske WP, Walenga JM, Hoppensteadt DA, et al. Differentiating low-molecular-weight heparins based on chemical, biological, and pharmacologic properties: implications for the development of generic versions of low-molecular-weight heparins. *Semin Thromb Hemost* 2008;34:74–85.

10. Fareed J, Jeske W, Fareed J, et al. Are all low molecular weight heparins equivalent in the management of venous thromboembolism? *Clin Appl Thromb Hemost* 2008; 14:385–92.

11. Elmer J, Wittels KA. Emergent reversal of pentasaccharide anticoagulants: a systematic review of the literature. *Transfus Med* 2012;22(2):108–15.

12. Bienkowski MJ, Conrad HE. Structural characterization of the oligosaccharides formed by depolymerization of heparin with nitrous acid. *J Biol Chem* 1985; 260:356–65.

13. Viskov C, Bouley E, Hubert P, et al. Isolation and characterization of contaminants in recalled unfractionated heparin and low-molecular-weight heparin. *Clin Appl Thromb Hemost* 2009;15:395–401.

14. Hayes-Ryan D, Byrne BM. Prevention of thrombosis in pregnancy: how practical are consensus derived clinical practice guidelines. *J Obstet Gynaecol* 2012;32: 740–2.

15. Bates SM, Greer IA, Middeldorp S, et al. VTE, thromboprophylaxis, antithrombotic therapy and pregnancy. *Chest* 2012;141:691S–736S.

16. Benson MD. Pulmonary embolism in pregnancy: consensus and controversies. *Minerva Ginecol* 2012;64:387–98.

17. Patel J, Auyeung V, Patel R, et al. Women's views and adherence to low molecular weight heparin therapy during pregnancy and the puerperium. *J Thromb Haemost* 2012;10:2526–34.

18. De Sancho MT, Khalid S, Christos PJ. Outcomes in women receiving low-molecular weight heparin during pregnancy. *Blood Coagul Fibrinolysis* 2012;23:751–5.

19. Shapiro NL, Kominiarek MA, Nutescu EA, Chevalier AB, Hibbard JU. Dosing and monitoring of low-molecular-weight heparin in high-risk pregnancy: single-center experience. *Pharmacotherapy* 2011;31:678–85.

20. Lyman GH, Khorana AA, Falanga A, et al. American Society of Clinical Oncology guidelines: recommendations for venous thromboembolism prophylaxis and treatment in patients with cancer. *J Clin Oncol* 2007;25:5490–505.

21. Gould MK, Garcia DA, Wren SM, et al. Prevention of VTE in nonorthopedic surgical patients: antithrombotic therapy and prevention of thrombosis, 9th ed: American College of Chest Physicians Evidence-Based Clinical Practice Guidelines. *Chest* 2012;141(2 Suppl):e227S–77S.

22. Noble S. Low-molecular-weight heparin and survival in lung cancer. *Thromb Res* 2012;129(suppl 1):S114–18.

23. Platek C, O'Connell CL, Liebman HA. Treating venous thromboembolism in patients with cancer. *Expert Rev Hematol* 2012;5:201–9.

24. Lee AY. Treatment of established thrombotic events in patients with cancer. *Thromb Res* 2012;129(suppl 1):S146–53.

25. Medioni J, Guastalla JP, Drouet L. Thrombosis and breast cancer: incidence, risk factors, physiology and treatment. *Bull Cancer* 2012;99:199–210.

26. Kyriazi V. Breast cancer is an acquired thrombophilic state. *J Breast Cancer* 2012;15:148–56.

27. Elit, LM, Lee AY, Swystun LL, et al. Dalteraprin low molecular weight heparin (LMWH) in ovarian cancer: A phase II randomized study. *Thromb Res* 2012; 130:894–900.

28. Scotte F, Rey JB, Launay-Vacher V. Thrombosis, cancer and renal insufficiency: low molecular weight heparin at the crossroads. *Support Care Cancer* 2012;20: 3033–42.

29. Agnelli G, George D, Kakkar A, et al. Semuloparin for thromboprophylaxis in patients receiving chemotherapy for cancer. *N Engl J Med* 2012;366:601–9.

30. Monagle P, Ignjatovic V, Savoia H. Hemostasis in neonates and children: pitfalls and dilemmas. *Blood Rev* 2010;24:63–8.

31. Monagle P, Chan AK, Goldenberg NA, et al. Antithrombotic therapy in neonates and children. *Chest* 2012;141:737S–801S.

32. O'Brien S, Kilma J, Gaines B, Betz S, Zenati M. Utilization of low-molecular-weight heparin prophylaxis in pediatric and adolescent trauma patients. *J Trauma Nurs* 2012;19:117–21.

33. Askegard-Giesmann J, O'Brien S, Wang W, Kenney B. Increased use of enoxaparin in pediatric trauma patients. *J Pediatr Surg* 2012;47:980–3.

34. Saltiel M. Dosing low molecular weight heparins in kidney disease. *J Pharm Pract* 2010;3:205–9.

35. Yildirim T, Kocak T, Buyukasik Y, et al. Are low-molecular-weight heparins appropriately dosed in patients with CKD stage 3 to 5? *Blood Coagul Fibrinolysis* 2012; 23:700–4.

36. Villa C, Camma C, Marietta M, et al. Enoxaparin prevents portal vein thrombosis and liver decompensation in patients with advanced liver cirrhosis. *Gastroenterology* 2012;143:1253–60.

37. Samama MM. Use of low-molecular-weight heparins and new anticoagulants in elderly patients with renal impairment. *Drugs Aging* 2011;28:177–93.

38. Chande N, MacDonald JK, Wang JJ, McDonald JW. Unfractionated or low molecular weight heparin for induction of remission in ulcerative colitis: a Cochrane inflammatory bowel disease and functional bowel disorders systemic review of randomized trials. *Inflamm Bowel Dis* 2011;17:1979–86.

39. Chande N, McDonald JW,Macdonald JK, Wang JJ. Unfractionated or low molecular weight heparin for induction of remission in ulcerative colitis. *Evid Based Med* 2011;16:71–2.

40. Olson JD, Arkin CF, Brandt JT. College of American Pathologist Conference XXXI on laboratory monitoring of anticoagulant therapy. Laboratory monitoring of unfractionated heparin therapy. *Arch Pathol Lab Med* 1998;122:782–98.

41. Laposata M, Green D, Van Cott EM, et al. College of American Pathologists Conference XXXI on laboratory monitoring of anticoagulant therapy. The clinical use of laboratory monitoring of low-molecular-weight heparin, danaparoid, hirudin and related compounds, and argatroban. *Arch Pathol Lab Med* 1998;122:799–807.

42. Walenga J, Fareed J, Messmore HL. Newer avenues in the monitoring of antithrombotic therapy: the role of automation. *Semin Thromb Hemost* 1983;9:346–54.

43. Marmur JD, Anand SC, Bagga RS. The activated clotting time can be used to monitor the low molecular weight heparin dalteparin after intravenous administration. *J Am Coll Cardiol* 2003;4:394–402.

44. Eikelboom JW, Weitz JI. Update on antithrombotic therapy. *Circulation* 2010; 121:1523–32.

45. Fareed J. Thethi I, Hoppensteadt D. Old versus new oral anticoagulants: focus on pharmacology. *Annu Rev Pharmacol Toxicol* 2012;52:79–99.

46. Walenga JM, Prechel M, Jeske WP, et al. Rivaroxaban – an oral, direct factor Xa inhibitor – has potential for the management of patients with heparin-induced thrombocytopenia. *Br J Haematol* 2008;143:92–9.

47. Fareed J, Leong W, Hoppensteadt DA, Jeske WP, Walenga J, Bick RL. Development of generic low molecular weight heparins: a perspective. *Hematol Oncol Clin North Am* 2005;19:53–68.

Index

Hemostasis and Thrombosis: Practical Guidelines in Clinical Management, First Edition.
Hussain I. Saba and Harold R. Roberts.
© 2014 John Wiley & Sons, Ltd. Published 2014 by John Wiley & Sons, Ltd.